Basic Dysrhythmias Interpretation and Management

Robert. J. Huszar, M.D.

Medical Director
Emergency Medical Services Program
New York State Department of Health

*with **91** Illustrations*

The C. V. Mosby Company
ST. LOUIS • WASHINGTON • TORONTO   1988

Editor: Richard A. Weimer
Assistant editor: Adrianne H. Cochran
Book design: Marta J. Huszar, Jo Ann Jakiela
Illustrator: Robert J. Huszar, M.D.
Cover design: Dan Beisel

Library of Congress Cataloging-in-Publication Data

```
Huszar, Robert J.
    Basic dysrhythmias.

    Includes index.
    1. Arrhythmia.  I. Title.  [DNLM: 1. Arrhythmia--
diagnosis.  2. Arrhythmia--therapy.  3. Electrocardi-
ography.  WG 330 H972b]
RC685.A65H89  1988          616.1'28          85-62612
ISBN 0-8016-2410-X
```

Printed in the United States of America

The C.V. Mosby Company
11830 Westline Industrial Drive, St. Louis, Missouri 63146

Library of Congress Cataloging in Publication Data

Basic Dysrhythmias: Interpretation and Management

ISBN 0-8016-2410-X

9   8   7   6

*This book is dedicated
to my wife, Jean*

Preface

Basic Dysrhythmias: Interpretation and Management is designed to help medical, nursing and paramedical personnel (physicians, nurses, residents, interns, medical students, paramedics, emergency medical technicians, cardiology technicians, and other allied health personnel) acquire the skills to analyze and identify common arrhythmias (or dysrhythmias). The term "arrhythmia," meaning an absence of rhythm, is used in this book by the author's preference instead of the more accurate term "dysrhythmia," meaning abnormality in rhythm. This choice was dictated by the fact that most medical editors prefer the term "arrhythmia."

The text is simply written, profusely illustrated with descriptive diagrams, and interspersed with numerous ECG drawings and tracings. Although the student who is being introduced to the interpretation of ECGs for the first time was continuously kept in mind during the preparation of the manuscript, the book should be of value as a reference to those already acquainted with the principles of electrocardiography.

The anatomy and electrophysiology of the heart is presented in Chapter 1 in a simplified manner yet, with sufficient detail to provide a sound basis for arrhythmia identification. In Chapter 2, the electrical basis of the electrocardiogram is discussed, and the ECG paper, leads, and artifacts are described. In the unique and detailed description of the components of the ECG in Chapter 3, numerous examples of the normal and abnormal waves, complexes, segments, and intervals are included to help prepare the reader to recognize the numerous variations of these components found in clinical electrocardiography. In Chapter 4, a detailed step-by-step method for identifying an arrhythmia is presented. In the description of individual arrhythmias in Chapter 5, numerous examples of each arrhythmia are included so that the reader can appreciate the various appearances that an arrhythmia may have. Chapter 6 includes the treatment of common arrhythmias presented in a protocol format, based on the current American Heart Association/American Red Cross standards. The reader is given an opportunity for self-evaluation in Chapter 7, which includes all the ECGs presented in the previous chapters plus new ones.

I wish to gratefully acknowledge the assistance of Timothy Frank, Kevin Kraus, and Andrew Stern, who reviewed the manuscript, and the following who supplied many of the original ECG tracings: Ann Charlebois, R.N., M.S., Cardiac Resuscitation Corporation (Wilsonville, Oregon), Ronald Baker, EMT-Paramedic and Paramedic Instructor, Troy Fire Department (Troy, New York), Earl Evans, Regional Emergency Medical Organization (Albany, New York), Anne Ficarelli, EMT-Paramedic and Paramedic Trainer, Mary Immaculate Hospital (New York City, New York), Joan C. Hillgardner, EMT-Paramedic, New York City Emergency Medical Services, Health and Hospitals Corporation (New York City, New York), John Spoor, M.D., Imogene Bassett Hospital (Cooperstown, New York), and the staff of the Cardiology Departments of Leonard Hospital (Troy, New York) and Saint Peter's Hospital (Albany, New York).

Special acknowledgment is given Marta Huszar for her expertise in providing the original graphic design of the book, Jo Ann Jakiela for her invaluable assistance in preparing the manuscript, and Eric Boehm for his typesetting skills. The illustrations and graphics were prepared by the author.

Contents

Contents

Basic Dysrhythmias Interpretation and Management

Chapter 1

Anatomy and Physiology of the Heart

Anatomy and Physiology of the Heart

The **heart,** whose sole purpose is to circulate blood through the **circulatory system** (the blood vessels of the body), consists of four hollow chambers. Two of the chambers are thin-walled, the **right** and **left atria,** and two are thick-walled and muscular, the **right** and **left ventricles.** The walls of the ventricles are composed of three layers of tissue: the innermost thin layer is called the **endocardium;** the middle thick, muscular layer, the **myocardium;** and the outermost thin layer, the **epicardium.** The walls of the left ventricle are more muscular and about three times thicker than those of the right ventricle. The atrial walls are also composed of three layers of tissue like those of the ventricles, but the middle muscular layer is much thinner. The two atria form the **base of the heart;** the ventricles form the **apex of the heart.**

Normally, the **interatrial septum** (a thin membranous wall) separates the two atria, and a thicker, more muscular wall, the **interventricular septum,** separates the two ventricles. The two septa, in effect, divide the heart into two pumping systems, the **right** and **left heart,** each one consisting of an atrium and a ventricle.

The right heart pumps blood into the **pulmonary circulation** (the blood vessels in the lungs and those carrying blood to and from the lungs), and the left heart pumps blood into the **systemic circulation** (the blood vessels in the rest of the body and those carrying blood to and from the body).

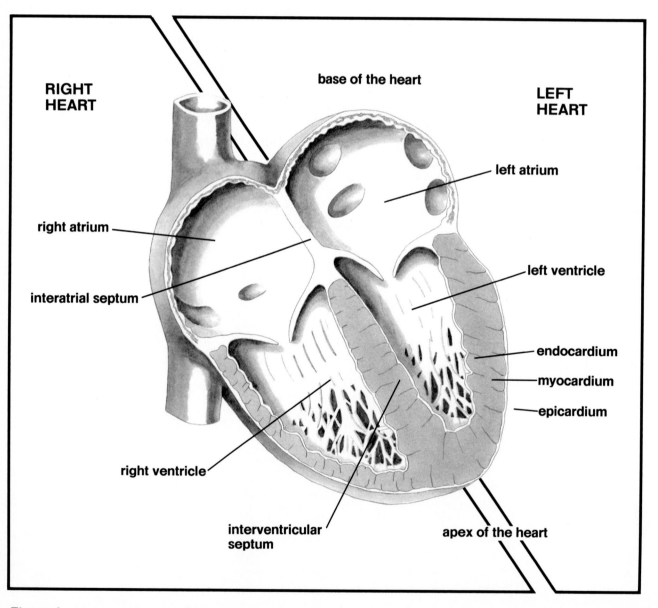

Figure 1. Anatomy of the Heart.

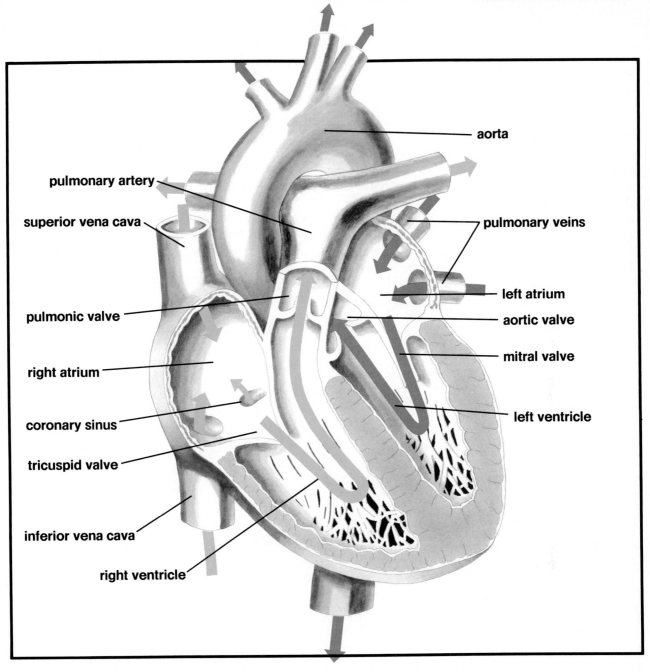

Figure 2. Circulation through the Heart.

The right atrium receives unoxygenated blood from the body via two of the body's largest veins (the **superior vena cava** and **inferior vena cava**) and from the heart itself by way of the **coronary sinus.** The blood is delivered to the right ventricle through the **tricuspid valve.** The right ventricle then pumps the unoxygenated blood through the **pulmonic valve** and into the lungs via the **pulmonary artery.** In the lungs, the blood picks up oxygen and releases excess carbon dioxide.

The left atrium receives the newly oxygenated blood from the lungs via the **pulmonary veins** and delivers it to the left ventricle through the **mitral valve.** The left ventricle then pumps the oxygenated blood out through the **aortic valve** and into the **aorta,** the largest artery in the body. From the aorta, the blood is distributed throughout the body where the blood releases oxygen and collects carbon dioxide.

The heart performs its pumping action over and over in a rhythmic sequence. First, the atria relax **(atrial diastole),** allowing the blood to pour in from the body and lungs. As the atria fill with blood, the atrial pressure rises and forces the tricuspid and mitral valves to open, allowing the blood to empty rapidly into the relaxed ventricles. Then, the atria contract **(atrial systole),** filling the ventricles to capacity. The period of dilatation and filling of the ventricles with blood is called **ventricular diastole.**

Following the contraction of the atria, the pressures in the atria and ventricles equalize and the tricuspid and mitral valves begin to close. Then, the ventricles contract vigorously, causing the ventricular pressure to rise sharply. The tricuspid and mitral valves close completely and the aortic and pulmonic valves snap open, allowing the blood to be ejected forcefully into the pulmonary and systemic circulation. Meanwhile, the atria are again relaxing and filling with blood. As soon as the ventricles empty of blood and begin to relax, the ventricular pressure falls, the aortic and pulmonic valves shut tightly, and the rhythmic cardiac sequence begins anew. The period during which the ventricles contract and empty of blood is called **ventricular systole.**

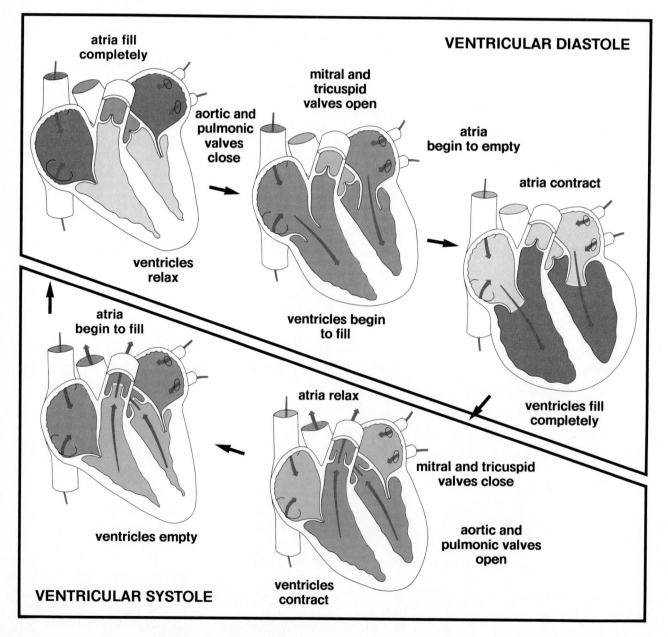

Figure 3. Ventricular Diastole and Systole.

Cardiac Cells

The heart is composed of **cylindrical cells** which partially divide into two or more branches at their ends; these connect with the branches of adjacent cells and form a branching and anastomosing network of cells. At the junctions where the branches join together are specialized cellular membranes called **intercalated disks;** these membranes are not found in any other cells. These structures contain **"gap junctions"** that permit very rapid conduction of electrical impulses from one cell to another. The ability of cardiac cells to conduct electrical impulses is called the **property of conductivity.**

Cardiac cells are covered by a semipermeable membrane which allows certain charged chemical particles (**ions**), such as sodium, potassium, and calcium ions, to flow in and out of the cells during the pumping action of the heart.

There are two basic kinds of cardiac cells in the heart—the **myocardial cells** and the **specialized cells of the electrical conduction system** of the heart described in the next section.

The myocardial cells contain **contractile filaments** that contract when the cells are electrically stimulated. This gives the myocardial cells the **property of contractility**—the ability to shorten and return to their original length. The myocardial cells form the thin muscular layer of the atrial wall and the much thicker muscular layer of the ventricular wall (the myocardium).

The force of myocardial contractility increases in response to certain drugs (e.g., sympathomimetics, digitalis, bretylium) and to certain physiologic conditions (e.g., increased venous return to the heart, exercise, emotion, hypovolemia, anemia). On the other hand, other drugs (e.g., quinidine, procainamide, beta-blockers, excess potassium) and physiologic conditions (e.g., shock, hypocalcemia, hypothyroidism) decrease the force of myocardial contractility.

The cells of the electrical conduction system do not contain contractile filaments and, therefore, cannot contract. Because these cells contain more gap junctions than do myocardial cells, they conduct electrical impulses extremely rapidly (at least six times faster than do myocardial cells).

Certain of the cells of the electrical conduction system are also capable of generating electrical impulses spontaneously. This capability, the **property of automaticity,** will be discussed in greater detail later in this chapter. Such cells are called **pacemaker cells.**

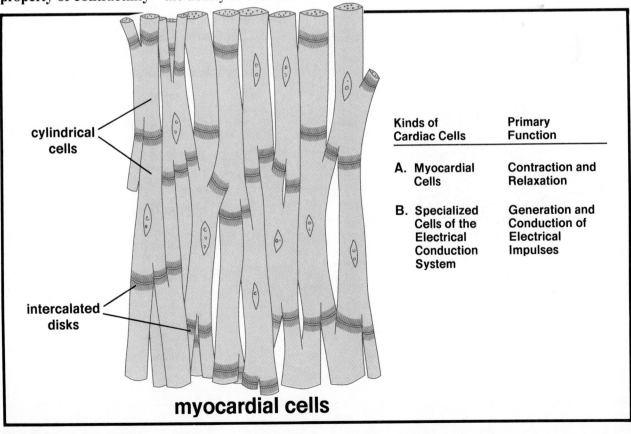

Kinds of Cardiac Cells	Primary Function
A. Myocardial Cells	Contraction and Relaxation
B. Specialized Cells of the Electrical Conduction System	Generation and Conduction of Electrical Impulses

cylindrical cells

intercalated disks

myocardial cells

Figure 4. Cardiac Cells.

Electrical Conduction System of the Heart

The **electrical conduction system** of the heart is composed of the **sinoatrial (SA) node, internodal atrial conduction tracts, interatrial conduction tract, atrioventricular (AV) node, bundle of His, right** and **left bundle branches,** and **Purkinje network.** The AV node and the bundle of His form the **atrioventricular (AV) junction.** The bundle of His, the right and left bundle branches, and the Purkinje network are also known as the **His-Purkinje system of the ventricles.** As its sole function, the electrical conduction system of the heart transmits minute **electrical impulses** from the SA node (where they are normally generated) to the atria and ventricles, causing them to contract.

The **SA node** lies in the wall of the right atrium near the inlet of the superior vena cava and consists of pacemaker cells that generate electrical impulses automatically and regularly.

The three **internodal atrial conduction tracts,** running through the walls of the right atrium between the SA node and the AV node, conduct the electrical impulses rapidly (approximately 0.03 second) from the SA node to the AV node. The **interatrial conduction tract (Bachmann's bundle),** a branch of one of the internodal atrial conduction tracts, extends across the atria, conducting the electrical impulses from the SA node to the left atrium.

The **AV node** lies partly in the right side of the interatrial septum in front of the opening of the coronary sinus and in the upper part of the interventricular septum above the base of the tricuspid valve. The primary function of the AV node is to relay the electrical impulses from the atria into the ventricles in an orderly and timely way. A ring of fibrous tissue insulates the remainder of the atria from the ventricles, preventing electrical impulses from entering the ventricles haphazardly.

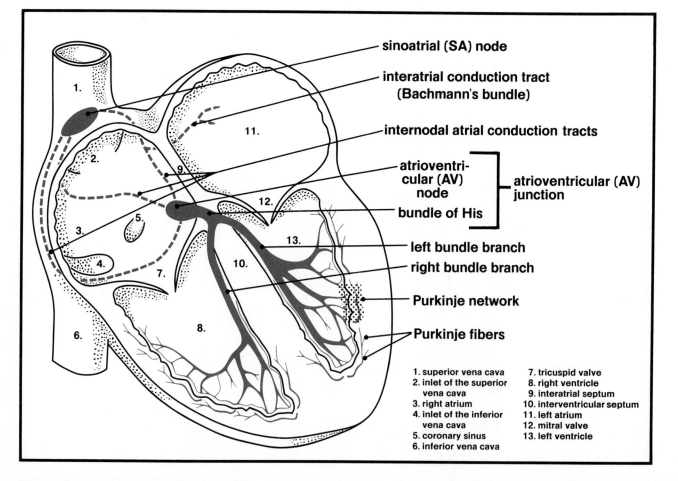

1. superior vena cava
2. inlet of the superior vena cava
3. right atrium
4. inlet of the inferior vena cava
5. coronary sinus
6. inferior vena cava
7. tricuspid valve
8. right ventricle
9. interatrial septum
10. interventricular septum
11. left atrium
12. mitral valve
13. left ventricle

Figure 5. Electrical Conduction System.

The electrical impulses travel at a relatively slow rate (0.06 to 0.12 second) through the AV node to reach the bundle of His. The delay is such that the atria can contract and empty and the ventricles fill before the ventricles contract. In addition, the delay protects the ventricles from being bombarded by an excessive number of electrical impulses from the atria.

The **bundle of His** lies in the upper part of the interventricular septum, connecting the AV node with the two bundle branches. Once the electrical impulses enter the bundle of His, they travel more rapidly (0.03 to 0.05 second) to the bundle branches.

The **right** and **left bundle branches** arise from the bundle of His, straddle the interventricular septum, and run down either side of the septum. These branches subdivide into smaller and smaller

branches, finally connecting with the **Purkinje network,** an intricate web of **Purkinje fibers** spread diffusely throughout the myocardium, whose ends terminate at the muscle fibers. The electrical impulses travel through the two bundle branches from the bundle of His to the Purkinje network in less then 0.01 second.

Electrophysiology of the Heart

Cardiac cells are capable of generating and conducting electrical impulses that are responsible for the contraction and relaxation of myocardial cells. These electrical impulses are the result of brief but rapid flow of positively charged ions (primarily those of sodium and potassium and, to a lesser extent, those of calcium) back and forth across

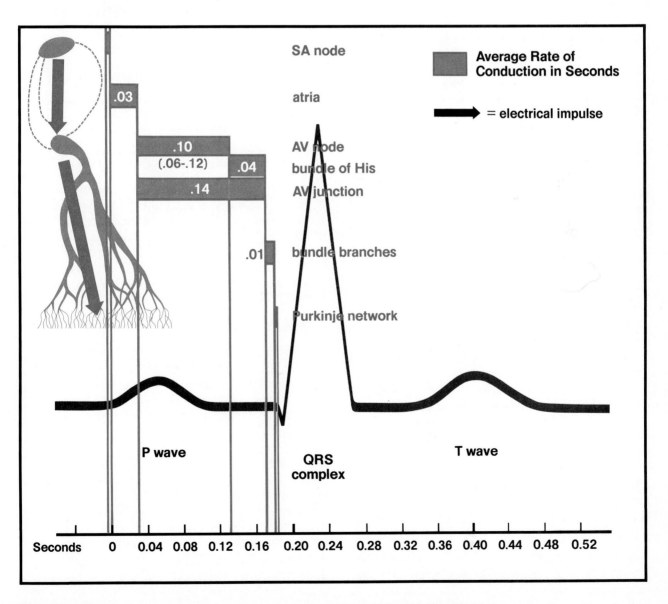

Figure 6. Relationship of the Electrical Impulse to the Electrical Conduction System.

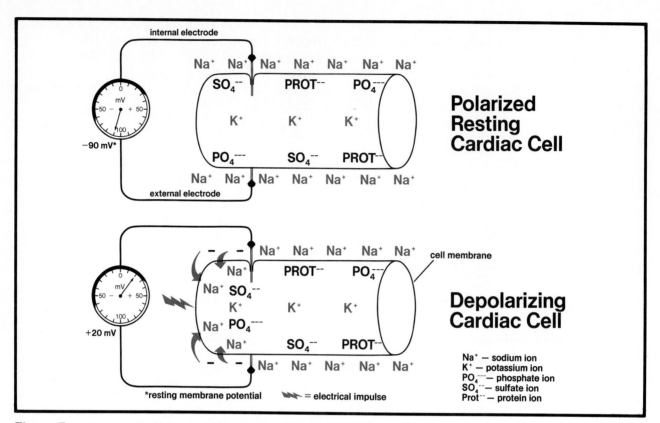

Figure 7. Membrane Potentials of Polarized and Depolarized Cardiac Cells.

the cardiac **cell membrane.** The difference in the concentration of such ions across the cell membrane at any given instant is called the **electrical potential (or voltage)** and is measured in **millivolts (mV).**

Resting State of the Cardiac Cell

When the cardiac cell (for example, a myocardial cell) is in the **resting state,** a high concentration of positively charged sodium ions (Na+) **(cations)** is present *outside* the cell. At the same time, a high concentration of both positively charged potassium ions (K+) and negatively charged ions (especially organic phosphate ions, organic sulfate ions, and protein ions) **(anions)** is present *inside* the cell. Under these conditions, where the interior of the cell is electrically negative with reference to its positive exterior, a **negative electrical potential** exists across the cell membrane. This is made possible by the cell membrane being impermeable to (1) positively charged sodium ions during the resting state and (2) negatively charged phosphate, sulfate, and protein ions at all times. When a cell membrane is impermeable to an ion, it does not permit the free flow of that ion across it.

The resting myocardial cell can be depicted as having a layer of positive ions surrounding the cell membrane and an equal number of negative ions lining the inside of the cell membrane directly

opposite each positive ion. When the ions are so aligned, the resting cell is called **"polarized."**

The electrical potential across the membrane of a resting cardiac cell is called the **resting membrane potential.** The resting membrane potential in atrial and ventricular myocardial cells and the cells of the electrical conduction system (except those of the SA and AV nodes) is normally -90 mV. It is somewhat less in the SA and AV nodal cells, -70 mV.

Depolarization and Repolarization

Upon stimulation by an electrical impulse, the membrane of a polarized myocardial cell, for example, becomes permeable to positively charged sodium ions, allowing sodium to flow into the cell. This causes the interior of the cell to become less negative. When the resting membrane potential drops from -90 mV to about -60 mV, large pores in the membrane (the so-called **fast sodium channels**) momentarily open. These channels facilitate the rapid, free flow of sodium across the cell membrane, resulting in a sudden large influx of positively charged sodium ions into the cell. This causes the exterior of the cell to become rapidly negative with respect to the now positive interior. The process by which the cell's resting, polarized state is reversed is called **depolarization.**

The fast sodium channels are typically found in the myocardial cells and the cells of the electrical conduction system other than those of the SA and AV nodes. The cells of the SA and AV nodes have, instead of fast sodium channels, **slow calcium-sodium channels** which open when the membrane potential drops to about -50 mV. They permit the entry of positively charged calcium and sodium ions into the cells during depolarization at a slow and gradual rate. The result is a slower rate of depolarization as compared to the depolarization of cardiac cells with fast sodium channels.

As soon as a cardiac cell depolarizes, positively charged potassium ions flow out of the cell, initiating a process by which the cell returns to its resting, polarized state. This process, called **repolarization,** involves a complex exchange of sodium, calcium, and potassium ions across the cell membrane.

Depolarization of one cardiac cell acts as an electrical impulse on adjacent cells and causes them to depolarize. The propagation of the electrical impulse from cell to cell produces an electric current, which flows in the direction of depolarization. As the cells repolarize, another electric current is produced. The direction of flow and magnitude of the currents generated by depolarization and repolarization of myocardial cells of the atria and ventricles can be detected by surface electrodes and recorded as the **electrocardiogram, (ECG).**

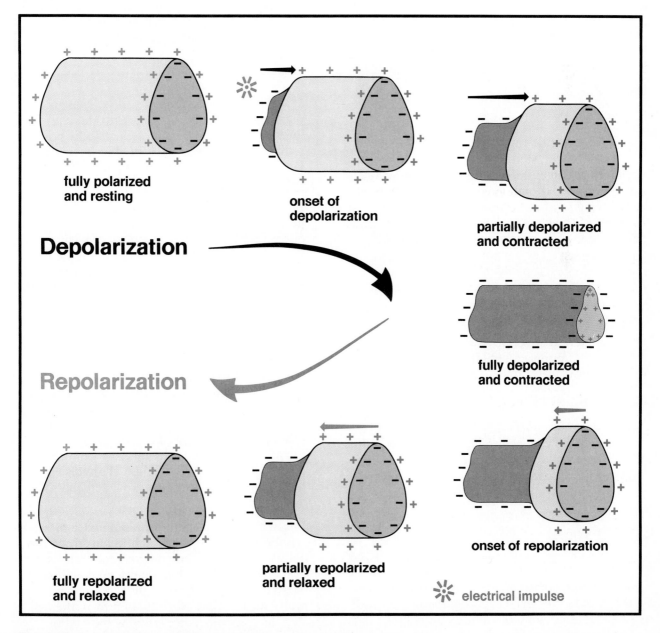

Figure 8. Depolarization and Repolarization of a Muscle Fiber.

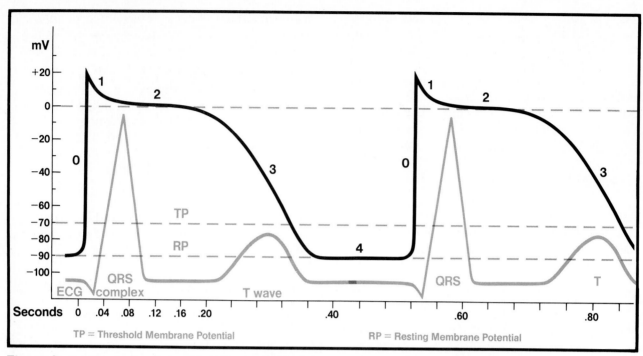

Figure 9. Cardiac Action Potential of Myocardial Cells

Threshold Potential

A cell need not be repolarized completely to its resting, polarized state before it can be stimulated to depolarize again. The cells of the SA and AV nodes can be depolarized when they have been repolarized to about -30 to -40 mV; the rest of the cells of the electrical conduction system of the heart and the myocardial cells can be depolarized when they have been repolarized to about -60 to -70 mV. The level to which a cell must be repolarized before it can be depolarized again is called the **threshold potential.**

It is important to note that a cardiac cell cannot be stimulated to generate or conduct an electrical impulse or to contract until it has been repolarized to a threshold potential.

Cardiac Action Potential

A **cardiac action potential** is a schematic representation of the changes in the membrane potential of a cardiac cell during depolarization and repolarization. The cardiac action potential is divided into five phases—phase 0 to phase 4.

The following is a description of the cardiac action potential of a typical myocardial cell.

Phase 0: Phase 0 (**depolarization phase**) is the sharp, tall upstroke of the action potential during which the cell membrane reaches the threshold potential, triggering the fast sodium channels to open momentarily and permit the rapid entry of sodium into the cell. As the

positively charged ions flow into the cell, the interior of the cell becomes electrically positive to about +20 mV with respect to its exterior. During the upstroke, the cell depolarizes and begins to contract.

Phase 1: During this phase (**early rapid repolarization phase**), the fast sodium channels close, terminating the rapid flow of sodium into the cell, followed by the loss of potassium from the cell. The net result is a decrease in the number of positive electrical charges within the cell and a drop in the membrane potential to about 0 mV.

Phase 2: This is the prolonged phase of slow repolarization (**plateau phase**) of the action potential of the myocardial cell, allowing it to finish contracting and begin relaxing. During phase 2, the membrane potential remains about 0 mV because of a very slow rate of repolarization. In a complicated exchange of ions across the cell membrane, calcium slowly enters the cell through the slow calcium channels as potassium continues to leave the cell and sodium to enter it.

Phase 3: Phase 3 is the **terminal phase of rapid repolarization,** during which the inside of the cell becomes markedly negative and the membrane potential once again returns to about -90 mV, its resting level. This is caused primarily by the flow of potassium from the cell. Repolarization is completed by the end of phase 3.

Phase 4: At the onset of phase 4 **(the period between action potentials),** the membrane has returned to its resting potential and the inside of the cell is once again negative (-90 mV) with respect to the outside. But there is still an excess of sodium in the cell and an excess of potassium outside. At this point, a mechanism known as the **"sodium-potassium pump"** is activated, transporting the excess sodium out of the cell and potassium back in. Because of this mechanism and the impermeability of the cell membrane to sodium during phase 4, the myocardial cell normally maintains a stable membrane potential between action potentials.

Refractory and Supernormal Periods

The time between the onset of depolarization and the end of repolarization is customarily divided into periods during which the cardiac cells can or cannot be stimulated to depolarize. These are the **refractory periods** (absolute and relative) and the **supernormal period.**

The refractory period of cardiac cells (for example, those of the ventricles) extends from phase 0 of the cardiac action potential to the end of phase 3 (beginning with the onset of the QRS complex

and ending with the end of the T wave) and is divided into the absolute and relative refractory periods. During the **absolute refractory period (ARP),** which ends midway through phase 3 (corresponding to about the peak of the T wave), cardiac cells have not repolarized to their threshold potential and, therefore, cannot be stimulated to depolarize. In other words, myocardial cells cannot contract and the cells of the electrical conduction system cannot conduct an electrical impulse during the absolute refractory period.

During the **relative refractory period (RRP),** which extends through the second half of phase 3 (corresponding to the downslope of the T wave), cardiac cells, having repolarized to their threshold potential, can be stimulated to depolarize if the stimulus is strong enough. This period is also called the **vulnerable period of repolarization.**

During a short portion of phase 3, just before the cells return to their resting potential, a stimulus weaker than is normally required can depolarize cardiac cells. This portion of repolarization is called the **supernormal period.**

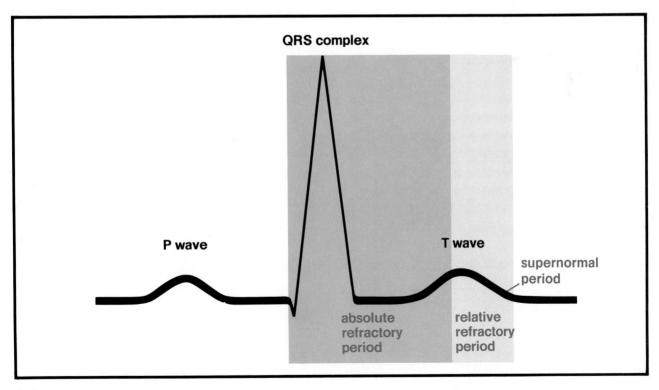

Figure 10. Refractory Periods.

Excitability and Automaticity

The capability of a resting, polarized cardiac cell to depolarize in response to an electrical stimulus is called the **property of excitability.** All cardiac cells have this property.

The capability of a cardiac cell to depolarize spontaneously during phase 4—to reach threshold potential and to depolarize completely without being externally stimulated—is called the **property of automaticity.** (This could also be called the **property of self-excitation.**)

Spontaneous depolarization depends on the ability of the cell membrane to become permeable to sodium during phase 4, thus allowing a steady leakage of sodium ions into the cell. This causes the resting membrane potential to become progressively less negative. As soon as the threshold potential is reached, rapid depolarization of the cell (phase 0) occurs. The rate of spontaneous depolarization is dependent on the **slope of phase 4 depolarization.** The steeper the slope of phase 4 depolarization, the faster is the rate of spontaneous depolarization and the **rate of impulse formation (the firing rate).** The flatter the slope, the slower the firing rate.

Automaticity is normally common to the pacemaker cells located in the SA node, some parts of the internodal atrial conduction tracts and AV node, and all parts of the bundle of His, bundle branches, and Purkinje network. The pacemaker cells other than those in the SA node hold this property in reserve should the SA node fail to function properly. For this reason, they are called **latent (or subsidiary) pacemaker cells.** Myocardial cells, which do not normally have the capability to depolarize spontaneously during phase 4, are called **nonpacemaker cells.**

Increase in **sympathetic activity** and administration of **catecholamines** increase the slope of phase 4 depolarization, resulting in an increase in the automaticity of the pacemaker cells and their firing rate. On the other hand, an increase in **parasympathetic activity** and administration of such drugs as lidocaine, procainamide, and quinidine decrease the slope of phase 4 depolarization, causing a decrease in the automaticity and firing rate of the pacemaker cells.

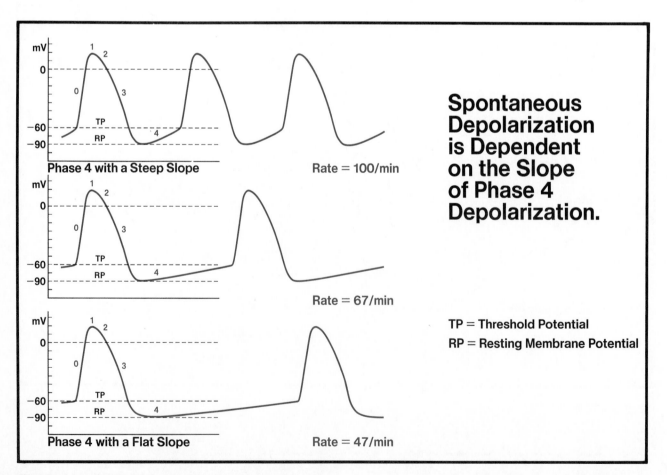

Phase 4 with a Steep Slope   Rate = 100/min

Rate = 67/min

Phase 4 with a Flat Slope   Rate = 47/min

Spontaneous Depolarization is Dependent on the Slope of Phase 4 Depolarization.

TP = Threshold Potential

RP = Resting Membrane Potential

Figure 11. Cardiac Action Potential of Pacemaker Cells.

Dominant and Escape Pacemakers of the Heart

Normally, the pacemaker cells with the fastest firing rate control the heart rate at any given time. Each time these pacemaker cells generate an electrical impulse the slower firing pacemaker cells are depolarized before they can do so spontaneously. This phenomenon is called **overdrive suppression.**

The **SA node** is normally the **dominant** and **primary pacemaker of the heart** because it possesses the highest level of automaticity, that is, its rate of automatic firing (60 to 100 times a minute) is normally greater than that of the latent pacemaker cells. If the SA node fails to generate electrical impulses at its normal rate or stops functioning entirely, latent pacemaker cells in the **AV junction** will usually assume the role of pacemaker of the heart but at a slower rate (40 to 60 times a minute). Such a pacemaker is called an **escape pacemaker.** If the AV junction is unable to do so because of disease, an escape pacemaker in the electrical conduction system below the AV junction (i.e., the **bundle branches** and **Purkinje network**) may take over at a still slower rate (less than 40 times a minute). In general, the farther the escape pacemaker is from the SA node, the slower it generates electrical impulses.

The rate at which the SA node or an escape pacemaker normally generates electrical impulses is called the pacemaker's **inherent firing rate.** A beat or a series of beats arising from an escape pacemaker is called an **escape beat** or **rhythm** and is identified according to its site of origin, e.g., junctional, ventricular.

Mechanisms of Abnormal Electrical Impulse Formation

There are three basic mechanisms by which abnormal electrical impulses can be generated in the heart: **enhanced automaticity, reentry,** and **triggered activity.** These may occur under certain circumstances in any part of the heart and cause abnormal **ectopic beats** and **rhythms** called

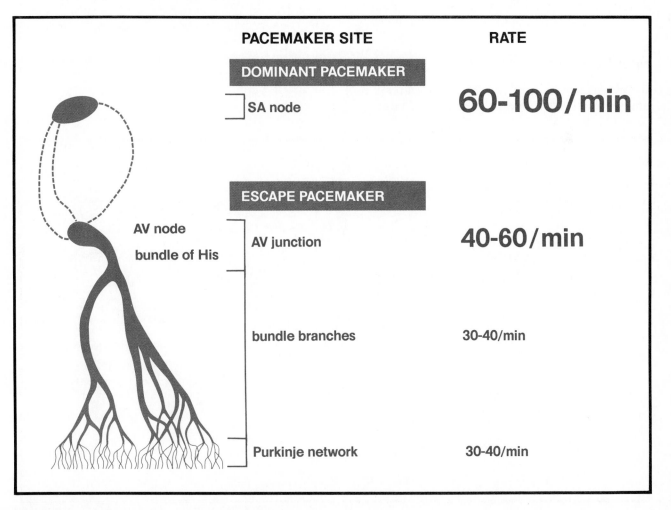

PACEMAKER SITE	RATE
DOMINANT PACEMAKER	
SA node	**60-100/min**
ESCAPE PACEMAKER	
AV junction	**40-60/min**
bundle branches	30-40/min
Purkinje network	30-40/min

AV node
bundle of His

Figure 12. Dominant and Escape Pacemakers.

premature contractions, rhythms, tachycardias, flutters, and **fibrillations.** Such **arrhythmias*** are identified according to their site of origin, e.g., sinus, atrial, junctional, ventricular.

Enhanced Automaticity

Enhanced automaticity is an abnormal condition of latent pacemaker cells in which their firing rate is increased beyond their inherent rate. This occurs when the cell membrane becomes abnormally permeable to sodium during phase 4. The result is an abnormally high leakage of sodium ions into the cells and, consequently, a sharp rise in the phase 4 slope of spontaneous depolarization. Even myocardial cells which do not ordinarily possess automaticity (nonpacemaker cells) may acquire this property under certain conditions and depolarize spontaneously. Enhanced automaticity can cause atrial, junctional, and ventricular ectopic beats and rhythms.

Common causes of enhanced automaticity are an increase in catecholamines, digitalis toxicity, hypoxia, hypercapnia, myocardial ischemia or infarction, stretching of the heart, hypokalemia, hypocalcemia, heating or cooling of the heart, and atropine.

Reentry

Reentry is a condition in which the progression of an electrical impulse is delayed or blocked (or both) in one or more segments of the electrical conduction system while the electrical impulse is conducted normally through the rest of the conduction system. This results in the delayed electrical impulse entering cardiac cells which have just been depolarized by the normally conducted impulse and, if they have repolarized sufficiently, depolarizing them prematurely and producing ectopic beats and rhythms.

The reentry mechanism can result in the abnormal generation of single or repetitive electrical impulses in the SA node, atria, AV junction, bundle branches, and Purkinje network. This produces sinus, atrial, junctional or ventricular ectopic beats and rhythms. If the delay in the conduction of the electrical impulse is constant for each beat, the abnormal beat will always follow the normal one at exactly the same interval of time. This is called **fixed coupling** and **bigeminal rhythm,** or simply **bigeminy.** In addition, a **reentry tachycardia,** for example, typically starts and stops abruptly.

Myocardial ischemia and hyperkalemia are the two most common causes of delay or block in the conduction of an electrical impulse through the electrical conduction system responsible for the reentry mechanism. Both can cause a decrease in the rate of rise of the action potential of cardiac cells during phase 0, resulting in a delay or block in impulse conduction.

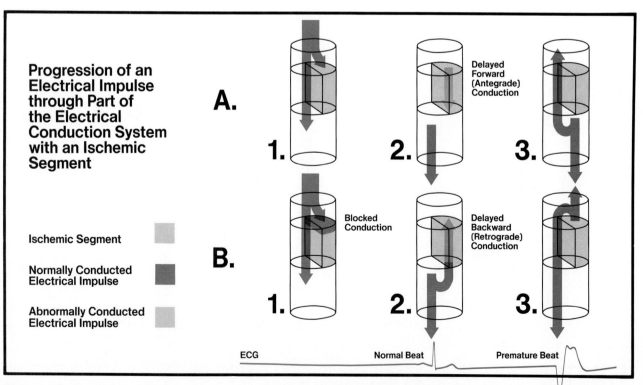

Figure 13. Examples of Reentry Mechanism. A. Delayed Conduction. B. Blocked and Delayed Conduction.

Triggered Activity

Triggered activity is an abnormal condition of latent pacemaker and myocardial cells (nonpacemaker cells) in which the cells may depolarize more than once following stimulation by a single electrical impulse. The level of phase 4 membrane action potential spontaneously and rhythmically increases after the first depolarization until it reaches threshold potential, causing the cells to depolarize. This phenomenon, called **afterdepolarization,** can occur immediately following depolarization (**early afterdepolarization**) or late in phase 4 (**delayed afterdepolarization**).

Triggered activity can result in atrial or ventricular ectopic beats occurring singly, in groups of two (**paired** or **coupled beats**), or in bursts of three or more beats (**paroxysms of beats** or **tachycardia**).

Common causes of triggered activity, like enhanced automaticity, are an increase in catecholamines, digitalis toxicity, hypoxia, myocardial ischemia or injury, and stretching or cooling of the heart.

*The term "arrhythmia," meaning an absence of rhythm, is used in this book by preference instead of the more accurate term "dysrhythmias," meaning abnormality in rhythm. This choice was dictated by the fact that most medical editors prefer the term "arrhythmia."

Chapter 2

The Electrocardiogram

**Electrical Basis
of the Electrocardiogram**

Components of the Electrocardiogram

ECG Paper

ECG Leads

Artifacts

Electrical Basis of the Electrocardiogram

The **electrocardiogram (ECG)** is a graphic record of the direction and magnitude of the **electrical activity** (also referred to as **electric current**) that is generated by the **depolarization** and **repolarization** of the atria and ventricles. This electrical activity is readily detected by electrodes attached to the skin. But neither the electrical activity that results from the generation and transmission of **electrical impulses** (which are too feeble to be detected electrically) nor the mechanical contractions and relaxations of the atria and ventricles (which do not generate electrical activity) appear in the electrocardiogram.

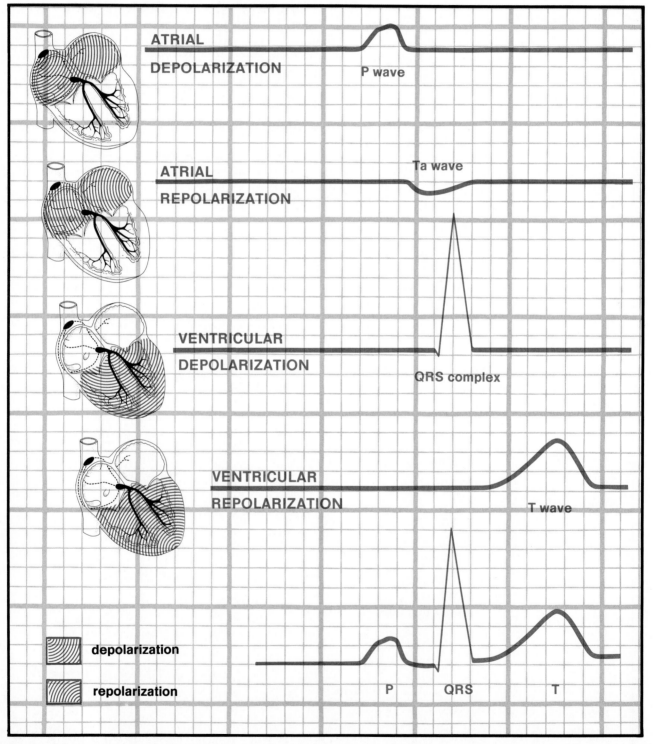

Figure 14. Electrical Basis of the ECG.

Components of the Electrocardiogram

After the electrical activity generated by depolarization and repolarization of the atria and ventricles is detected by electrodes, it is amplified, displayed on an oscilloscope, and recorded on ECG paper as waves and complexes. The electrical activity generated by atrial depolarization is recorded as the **P wave,** and that generated by ventricular depolarization, the **Q, R,** and **S waves**—the **QRS complex.** Atrial repolarization is recorded as the **atrial T wave (Ta),** and ventricular repolarization is recorded as the **ventricular T wave,** or simply, the **T wave.** Because atrial repolarization normally occurs during ventricular depolarization, the atrial T wave is buried or hidden in the QRS complex.

In a normal cardiac cycle, the P wave occurs first, followed by the QRS complex and the T wave.

The sections of the ECG between the waves and complexes are called **segments** and **intervals:** the **P-R segment,** the **S-T segment,** the **T-P segment,** the **P-R interval,** and the **R-R interval** (see Chapter 3). Intervals include waves and complexes, whereas, segments do not.

When electrical activity is not being detected, the ECG is a straight, flat line—the **isoelectric line** or **baseline.**

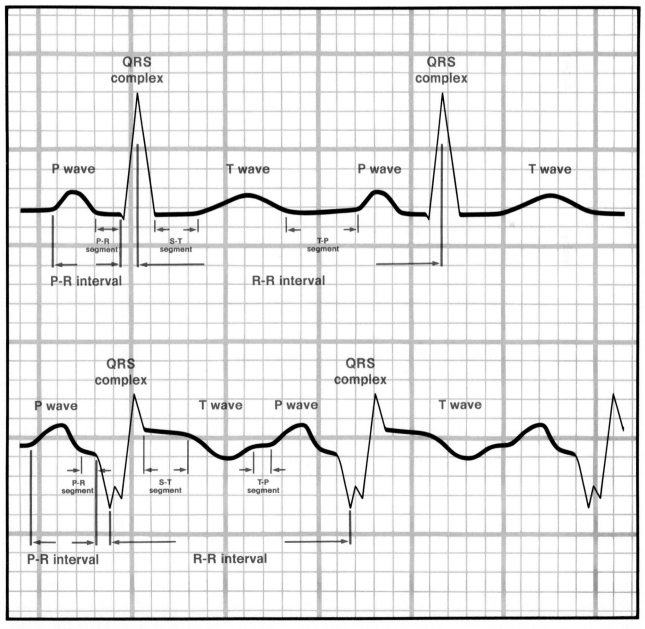

Figure 15. Components of the ECG.

The paper used in recording electrocardiograms has a **grid** to permit the measurement of time, in seconds (sec), along the horizontal lines and voltage (amplitude), in millimeters (mm), along the vertical lines.

The grid consists of intersecting dark and light vertical and horizontal lines that form large and small squares. When the ECG is recorded at the standard paper speed of 25 mm/sec, the **dark vertical lines** are **0.20 second (5 mm)** apart, and the **light vertical lines** are **0.04 second (1 mm)** apart. The **dark horizontal lines** are **5 mm** apart,

and the **light horizontal lines** are **1 mm** apart. One **large square** is **5 x 5 mm,** and one **small square** is **1 x 1 mm.** Conventionally, the sensitivity of the ECG machine is adjusted (**standardized**) so that a **1-millivolt (mV)** electrical signal produces a **10-mm** deflection (two large squares) on the ECG.

Printed along one edge of the ECG paper, usually the upper one, are regularly spaced short, vertical lines denoting intervals of time. When the ECG is recorded at the **standard paper speed,** the distance between two consecutive short vertical lines is **75 mm (3 sec),** and that between every third short vertical line is **150 mm (6 sec).**

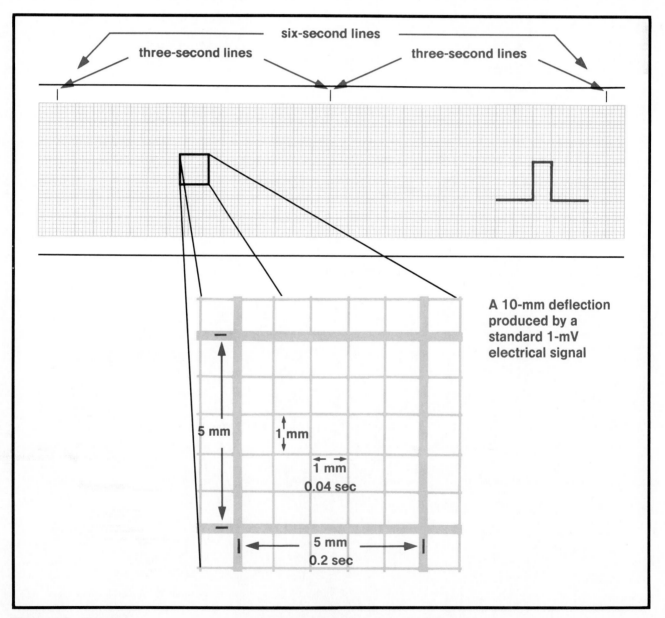

Figure 16. ECG Paper.

ECG Leads

An ECG lead consists of two surface electrodes of opposite polarity (one positive and the other negative) or one positive surface electrode and a reference point. A lead composed of two electrodes of opposite polarity is called a **bipolar lead;** a lead composed of a single positive electrode and a reference point is a **unipolar lead.**

For a routine analysis of the heart's electrical activity, an ECG recorded from twelve separate leads is used. A **12-lead ECG** consists of **three bipolar limb leads (I, II,** and **III), three unipolar limb leads (AVR, AVL,** and **AVF),** and **six unipolar chest leads,** also called **precordial** or **V leads,** (**V₁, V₂, V₃, V₄, V₅,** and **V₆).**

When monitoring the heart solely for arrhythmias, **Lead II** is commonly used, especially in the pre-hospital phase of emergency care. Lead II is obtained by attaching the negative electrode to the right arm and the positive electrode to the left leg. (Lead II may also be obtained by attaching the negative electrode to the right shoulder or upper right anterior chest wall and the positive electrode to the left thigh or lower left anterior chest wall at the intersection of the fourth intercostal space and the midclavicular line.) To eliminate or reduce electrical interference (**"noise"**) in the electrocardiogram when using Lead II for monitoring, a third, electrically neutral electrode (**ground electrode),** is attached to an extremity, usually the left arm or right leg, or to the chest.

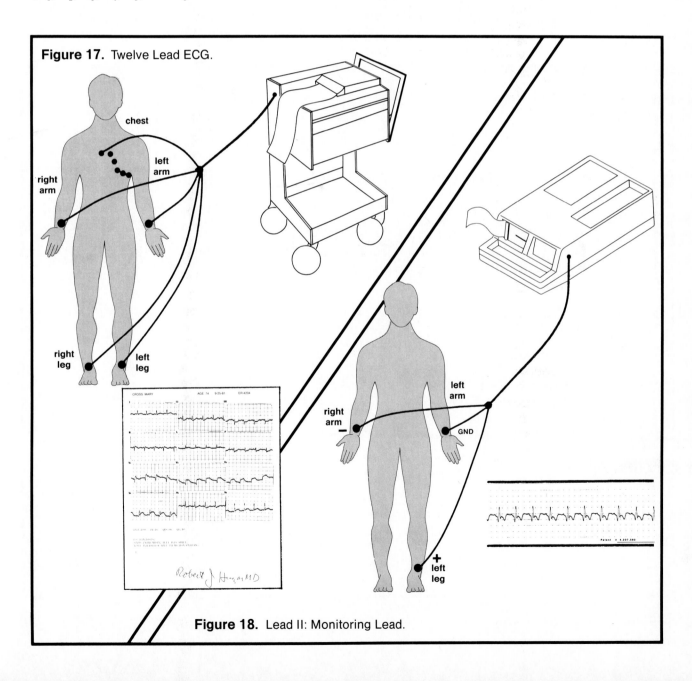

Figure 17. Twelve Lead ECG.

Figure 18. Lead II: Monitoring Lead.

When an electric current flows toward the positive electrode of a lead, a positive (upright) deflection is recorded on the electrocardiogram. Conversely, a negative (downward) deflection is recorded when an electric current flows away from the positive electrode. If the positive ECG electrode is attached to the left leg, all electric currents generated in the heart that flow toward the left leg will be recorded as positive (upright) deflections; those that flow away from the left leg will be recorded as negative (downward) deflections.

It should be noted here that since normal depolarization of the atria and ventricles generally progresses from the right upper chest downward toward the left leg, the electric currents generated during normal depolarization of the heart will, for the most part, flow toward the left leg and be recorded as two positive (upright) deflections—a positive (upright) **P wave** and the **R wave**—in Lead II.

Since normal depolarization of the ventricles initially may progress away from the left leg for a short period of time, a small negative (inverted) deflection may occur before the R wave—the **Q wave**—in Lead II. In addition, depending on the position of the heart in the chest, normal ventricular depolarization may also progress away from the left leg during the last phase of ventricular depolarization, producing a negative (inverted) deflection after the R wave—the **S wave.**

Note: The ECG components and strips shown in this book are depicted as they would appear in Lead II.

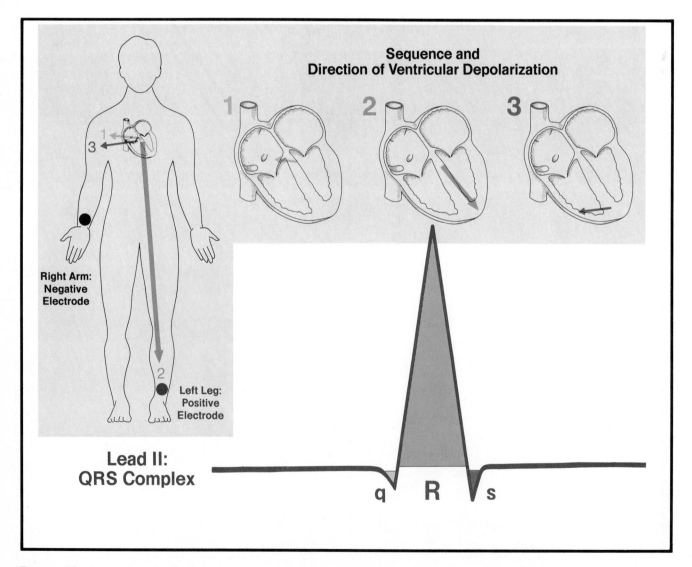

Figure 19. Sequence and Direction of Normal Ventricular Depolarization and the QRS Complex.

Artifacts

Abnormal waves and spikes in an ECG that result from sources other than the electrical activity of the heart and interfere with or distort the components of the ECG are called **artifacts.** The causes of artifacts are muscle tremor, alternating current (AC) interference, loose electrodes, biotelemetry-related interference, and external chest compression.

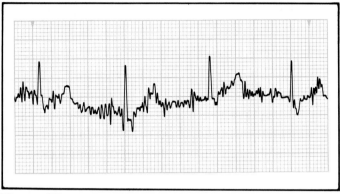

Figure 20. Muscle Tremor.

Muscle tremor can occur in tense or nervous patients or those shivering from cold and give the ECG a finely or coarsely jagged appearance.

AC interference can occur when a poorly grounded, AC-operated ECG machine is used or when an ECG is obtained near high tension wires or transformers. This results in a thick baseline composed of 60-cycle waves.

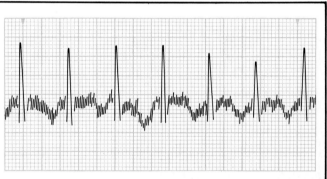

Figure 21. AC Interference.

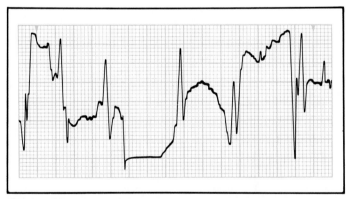

Figure 22. Loose Electrodes.

Loose electrodes or electrodes that are in poor electrical contact with the skin because of insufficient or dried electrode paste or jelly can cause multiple, sharp spikes and waves in the ECG.

Biotelemetry-related interference that occurs when ECG signals are poorly received over a biotelemetry system can result in sharp spikes and waves and a jagged appearance of the ECG. Such interference can occur when the ECG transmitter's power is low because of weak batteries or when the ECG transmitter is used in the outer fringes of the reception area of the base station receiver.

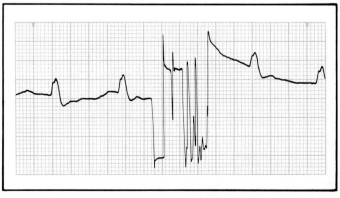

Figure 23. Biotelemetry.

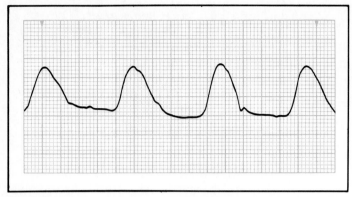

External chest compressions during cardio-pulmonary resuscitation cause regularly spaced, wide, upright waves, synchronous with the downward compressions of the chest.

Figure 24. External Chest Compression.

Chapter 3

Components of the Electrocardiogram

Normal Components

    P Wave
    Normal Sinus P Wave

    QRS Complex
    Normal QRS Complex

    T Wave
    Normal T Wave

    U Wave

    P-R Interval
    Normal P-R Interval

    R-R Interval

    S-T Segment
    Normal S-T Segment

    P-R Segment

    T-P Segment

Abnormal Components

    Abnormal Sinus P Wave

    Ectopic P Wave

    Abnormal QRS Complex

    Abnormal T Wave

    Abnormal P-R Interval

    Abnormal S-T Segment

Normal Components of the Electrocardiogram

P Wave

Definition

A **P wave** represents **depolarization of the right and left atria.**

Normal Sinus P Wave

Characteristics

1. Pacemaker Site: The pacemaker site is the SA node.

2. Relationship to Cardiac Anatomy and Physiology: A **normal sinus P wave** represents **normal depolarization of the atria.** Depolarization of the atria begins near the SA node and progresses across the atria from right to left and downward. The first part of the normal sinus P wave represents depolarization of the right atrium; the second part represents depolarization of the left atrium. During the P wave, the electrical impulse progresses from the SA node through the internodal atrial conduction tracts and most of the AV node. The P wave normally occurs during ventricular diastole.

Description

1. Onset and End: The onset of the P wave is identified as the first abrupt or gradual deviation from the baseline. The point where the wave returns to the baseline marks the end of the P wave.

2. Direction: The direction is positive (upright) in Lead II.

3. Duration: The duration is 0.10 second or less.

4. Amplitude: The amplitude is 0.5 to 2.5 mm in Lead II. The normal P wave is rarely over 2 mm high.

5. Shape: The shape is smooth and rounded.

6. P Wave-QRS Complex Relationship: A QRS complex normally follows each sinus P wave, but in certain arrhythmias, such as AV blocks (see Chapter 5), a QRS complex may not follow each sinus P wave.

7. P-R Interval: The P-R interval may be normal (0.12 to 0.20 second) or abnormal (greater than 0.20 second).

Significance

A normal sinus P wave indicates that the electrical impulse responsible for the P wave originated in the SA node and that normal depolarization of the right and left atria has occurred.

Notes

NORMAL SINUS P WAVE

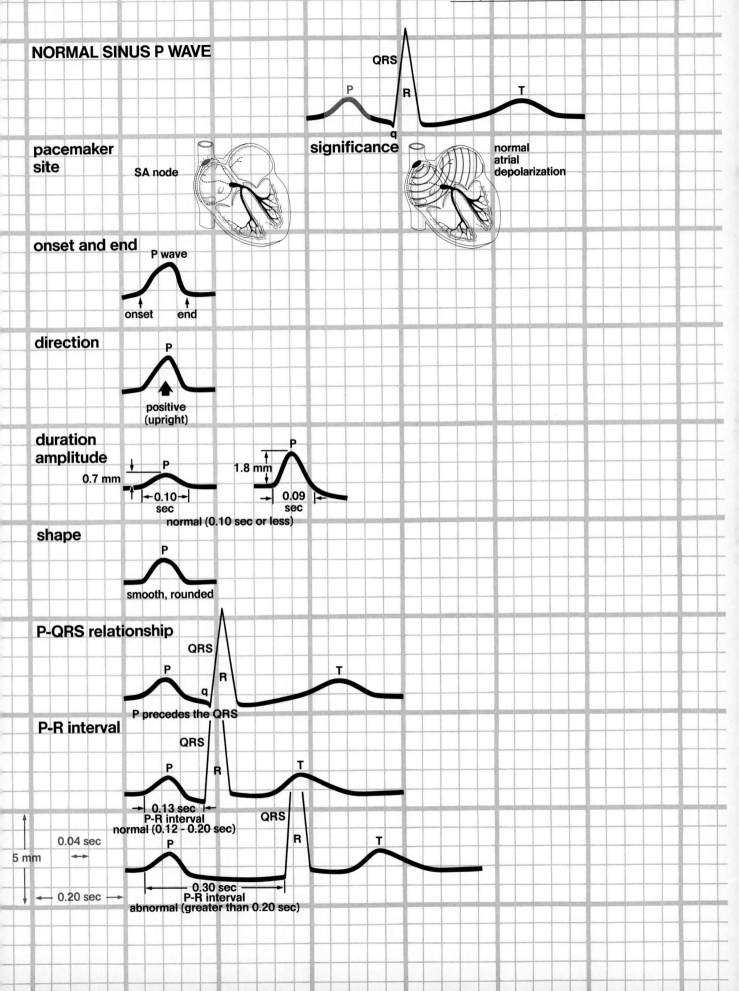

QRS

P   R   T

q

pacemaker site   SA node

significance   normal atrial depolarization

onset and end   P wave   onset   end

direction   P   positive (upright)

duration amplitude   0.7 mm   P |←0.10→| sec   1.8 mm   P   0.09 sec   normal (0.10 sec or less)

shape   P   smooth, rounded

P-QRS relationship   QRS   P   R   q   T   P precedes the QRS

P-R interval   QRS   P   R   T |→ 0.13 sec |←   P-R interval   normal (0.12 - 0.20 sec)

QRS   P   R   T |← 0.30 sec →| P-R interval   abnormal (greater than 0.20 sec)

5 mm   0.04 sec |→ 0.20 sec →|

QRS Complex

Definition

A **QRS complex** represents **depolarization of the right and left ventricles.**

Normal QRS Complex

Characteristics

1. Pacemaker Site: The pacemaker site of a normal QRS complex is the SA node or an ectopic pacemaker in the atria or AV junction.

2. Relationship to Cardiac Anatomy and Physiology: A **normal QRS complex** represents **normal depolarization of the ventricles.** Depolarization begins in the left side of the interventricular septum near the AV junction and progresses across the interventricular septum from left to right. Then, beginning at the endocardial surface of the ventricles, depolarization progresses through the ventricular walls to the epicardial surface. The first short part of the QRS complex, usually the Q wave, represents depolarization of the interventricular septum; the rest of the QRS complex represents the simultaneous depolarization of the right and left ventricles. Because the left ventricle is larger than the right ventricle and has more muscle mass, the QRS complex represents, for the most part, depolarization of the left ventricle.

The electrical impulse that causes normal ventricular depolarization originates above the ventricles in the SA node or an ectopic pacemaker in the atria or AV junction and has normal conduction down the right and left bundle branches to the Purkinje network. The QRS complex occurs before ventricular systole.

Description

1. Onset and End: The onset of the QRS complex is identified as the point where the first wave of the complex just begins to deviate, abruptly or gradually, from the baseline. The end of the QRS complex is the point where the last wave of the complex begins to flatten out (sharply or gradually)

at, above, or below the baseline. This point, the junction between the QRS complex and the S-T segment, is called the **"junction" or "J" point.**

2. Components: The QRS complex consists of one or more of the following: positive (upright) deflections called R waves and negative (inverted) deflections called Q, S, and QS waves.

> **a. R wave:** The R wave is the first positive deflection in the QRS complex. Subsequent positive deflections that extend above the baseline are called **R prime (R′), R double prime (R′′)**, and so forth.
>
> **b. Q wave:** The Q wave is the first negative deflection in the QRS complex not preceded by an R wave.
>
> **c. S wave:** The S wave is the first negative deflection that extends below the baseline in the QRS complex following an R wave. Subsequent negative deflections are called **S prime (S′), S double prime (S′′)**, and so forth.
>
> **d. QS wave:** A QS wave is a QRS complex that consists entirely of a single, large negative deflection.
>
> *Note: Although there may be only one Q wave, there can be more than one R wave and one S wave in the QRS complex.*
>
> **e. Notch:** A notch in the R wave is a negative deflection that does not extend below the baseline; a notch in the S wave is a positive deflection that does not extend above the baseline.

The waves comprising the QRS complex are usually identified by upper or lower case letters depending on the relative size of the waves. **Large waves** that form the major deflections are identified by **upper case letters** (QS, R, S); **small waves** that are less than one-half the amplitude of the major deflections are identified by **lower case letters** (q, r, s). Thus, the ventricular depolarization complex can be described more accurately by using upper and lower case letters assigned to the waves, for example, qR, Rs, qRs.

NORMAL QRS COMPLEX

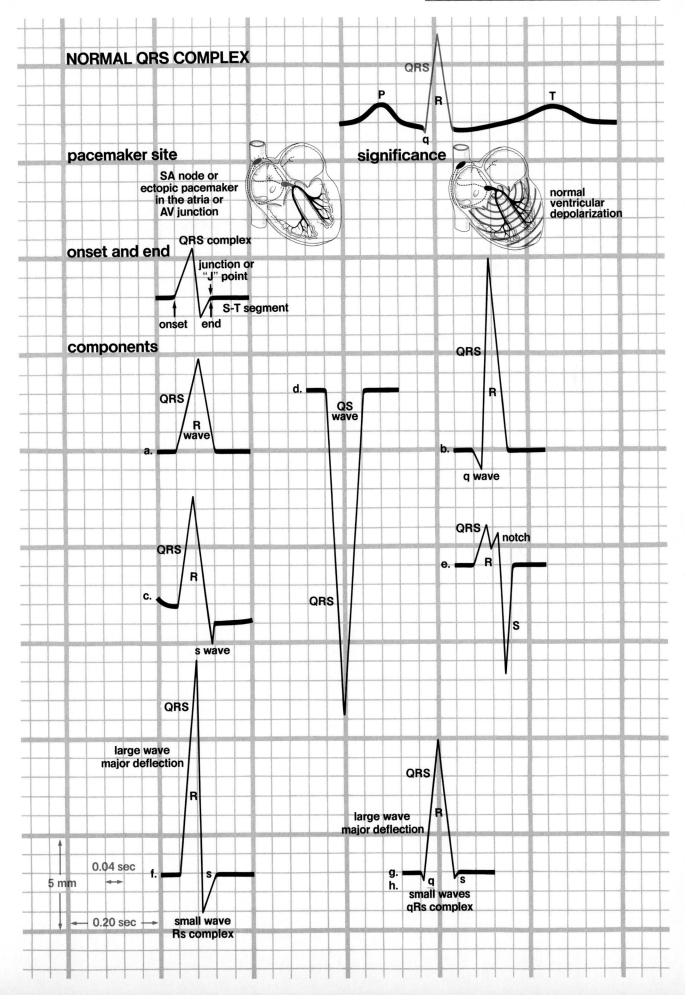

QRS

P   R   T

q

pacemaker site

SA node or
ectopic pacemaker
in the atria or
AV junction

significance

normal
ventricular
depolarization

onset and end

QRS complex

junction or
"J" point

S-T segment

onset   end

components

QRS

R
wave

a.

d.

QS
wave

QRS

R

b.

q wave

QRS

R

c.

s wave

QRS

QRS   notch

e.   R

S

QRS

large wave
major deflection

R

f.   s

QRS

large wave
major deflection

R

g.
h.   q   s
small waves
qRs complex

5 mm

0.04 sec

0.20 sec

small wave
Rs complex

Normal QRS Complex—Cont.

3. Direction: The direction of the QRS complex may be predominantly positive (upright), predominantly negative (inverted), or biphasic (partly positive, partly negative). A predominantly positive QRS complex, for example, has more area encompassed by the R wave, the major deflection, than is encompassed by the Q and S waves.

4. Duration: The duration of the QRS complex is 0.10 second or less (0.06 to 0.10 second) in adults and 0.08 second or less in children. The QRS complex is measured from the onset of the Q or R wave to the end of the last wave of the complex or the J point. The duration of the Q wave does not normally exceed 0.04 second.

5. Amplitude: The amplitude of the R or S wave in the QRS complex in Lead II may vary from 1 to 2 mm to 15 mm or more. The normal Q wave is less than 25% of the amplitude of the R wave.

6. Shape: The waves in the QRS complex are generally narrow and sharply pointed.

Significance

A normal QRS complex indicates that the electrical impulse has progressed normally from the bundle of His to the Purkinje network through the right and left bundle branches and that normal depolarization of the right and left ventricles has occurred.

Notes

NORMAL QRS COMPLEX—CONT.

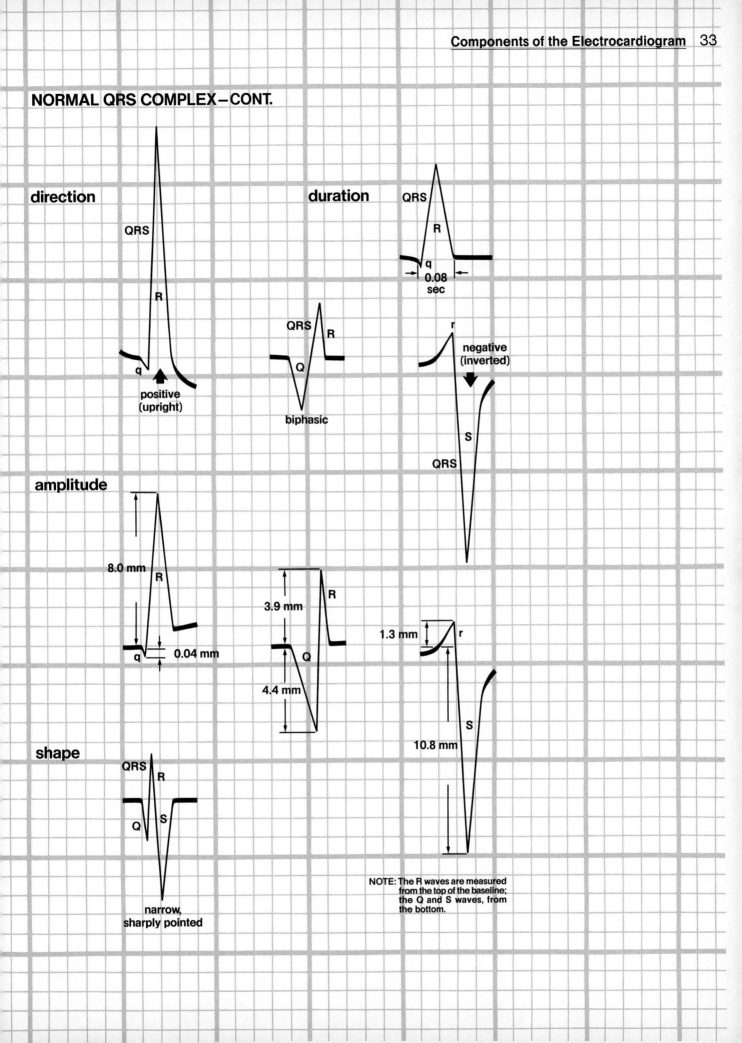

direction

QRS
R
q
positive
(upright)

QRS   R
Q
biphasic

duration

QRS
R
q
0.08
sec

r
negative
(inverted)
S
QRS

amplitude

8.0 mm
R
q   0.04 mm

3.9 mm
R
Q
4.4 mm

1.3 mm   r
S
10.8 mm

shape

QRS   R
Q   S
narrow,
sharply pointed

NOTE: The R waves are measured
from the top of the baseline;
the Q and S waves, from
the bottom.

T Wave

Definition

A **T wave** represents **ventricular repolarization.**

Normal T Wave

Characteristics

1. Relationship to Cardiac Anatomy and Physiology: A **normal T wave** represents **normal repolarization of the ventricles.** Repolarization begins at the epicardial surface of the ventricles and progresses inwardly through the ventricular walls to the endocardial surface. The T wave occurs during the last part of ventricular systole.

Description

1. Onset and End: The onset of the T wave is identified as the first abrupt or gradual deviation from the S-T segment (or the point where the slope of the S-T segment appears to become abruptly or gradually steeper). If the S-T segment is absent, the T wave begins at the end of the QRS complex (or the **J point**). The point where the T wave returns to the baseline marks the end of the T wave. In the absence of an S-T segment, the T wave is sometimes called the **S-T, T wave.** Often the onset and end of the T wave are difficult to determine with certainty.

2. Direction: The direction of the normal T wave is positive (upright) in Lead II.

3. Duration: The duration is 0.10 to 0.25 second or greater.

4. Amplitude: The amplitude is less than 5 mm.

5. Shape: The normal T wave is sharply or bluntly rounded and slightly asymmetrical. Ordinarily, the first, upward part of the T wave is longer than the second, downward part.

6. T Wave-QRS Complex Relationship: The T wave always follows the QRS complex.

Significance

A normal T wave preceded by a normal S-T segment indicates that normal repolarization of the right and left ventricles has occurred.

Notes

NORMAL T WAVE

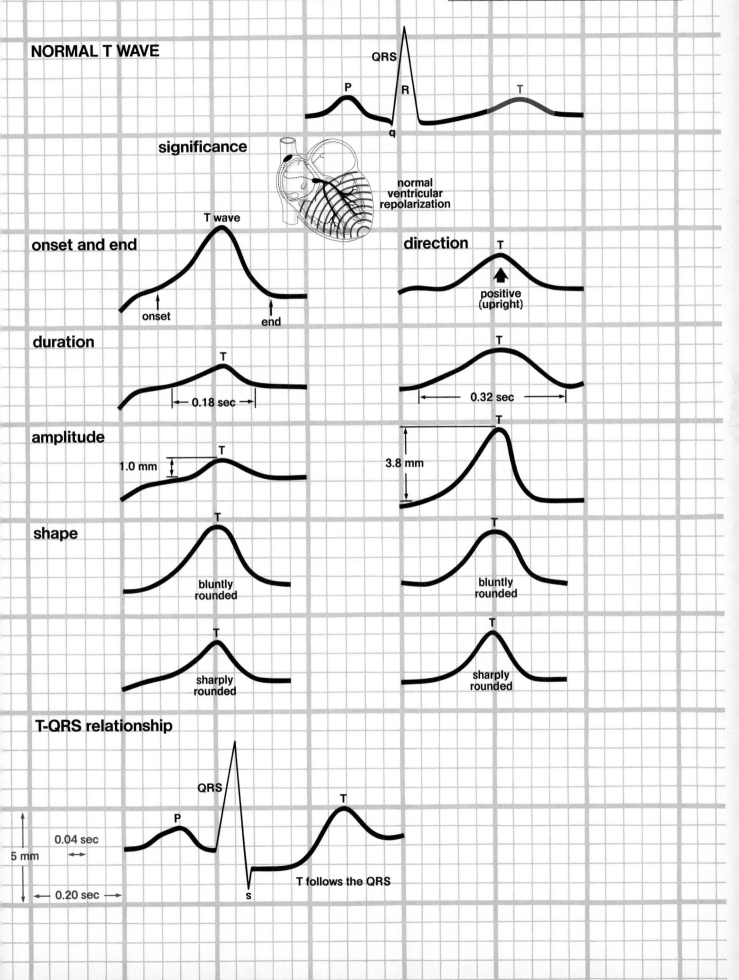

QRS

P

R

T

q

significance

normal
ventricular
repolarization

onset and end

T wave

onset

end

direction

T

positive
(upright)

duration

T

|← 0.18 sec →|

T

|← 0.32 sec →|

amplitude

1.0 mm

T

3.8 mm

T

shape

T

bluntly
rounded

T

bluntly
rounded

T

sharply
rounded

T

sharply
rounded

T-QRS relationship

QRS

P

T

0.04 sec

5 mm

|← 0.20 sec →|

s

T follows the QRS

U Wave

Definition

A **U wave** probably represents the **final stage of repolarization of the ventricles.**

Characteristics

1. Relationship to Cardiac Anatomy and Physiology: A U wave probably represents repolarization of a small segment of the ventricles (such as the papillary muscles or ventricular septum) after most of the right and left ventricles have been repolarized. Although uncommon and not easily identified, the U wave can best be seen when the heart rate is slow.

Description

1. Onset and End: The onset of the U wave is identified as the first abrupt or gradual deviation from the baseline or the downward slope of the T wave. The point where the U wave returns to the baseline or downward slope of the T wave marks the end of the U wave.

2. Direction: The direction of a normal U wave is positive (upright), the same as that of the preceding normal T wave in Lead II. An abnormal U wave may be flat or negative (inverted).

3. Duration: The duration is not determined routinely.

4. Amplitude: The amplitude of a normal U wave is usually less than 2 mm and always smaller than that of the preceding T wave in Lead II. A U wave taller than 2 mm is considered to be abnormal.

5. Shape: The U wave is rounded and symmetrical.

6. U Wave-T Wave-P Wave Relationship: The U wave always follows the peak of the T wave and occurs before the next P wave.

Significance

A U wave indicates that repolarization of the ventricles has occurred. An abnormally tall U wave may be present in hypokalemia, cardiomyopathy, left ventricular hypertrophy, and diabetes and may follow administration of digitalis and quinidine.

Notes

U WAVE

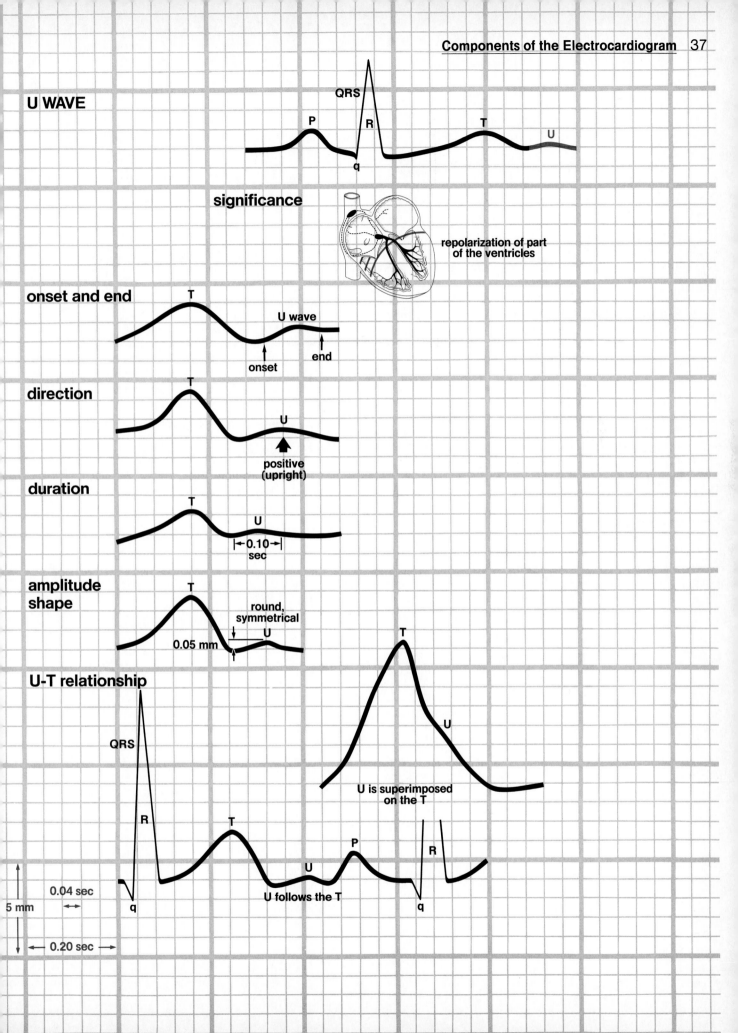

QRS

P R T U

q

significance

repolarization of part
of the ventricles

onset and end

T

U wave

onset end

direction

T

U

positive
(upright)

duration

T

U

|←0.10→|
sec

amplitude
shape

T

round,
symmetrical

U

0.05 mm

U-T relationship

QRS

R

T

P

U

R

q

U follows the T

q

T

U

U is superimposed
on the T

0.04 sec

5 mm

0.20 sec

P-R Interval

Definition

A **P-R interval** represents the time of progression of the electrical impulse from the SA node through the entire electrical conduction system of the heart to the ventricular myocardium and includes the depolarization of the atria.

Normal P-R Interval

Characteristics

1. Relationship to Cardiac Anatomy and Physiology: A **normal P-R interval** represents the time from the onset of atrial depolarization to the onset of ventricular depolarization during which the electrical impulse progresses normally from the SA node through the internodal atrial conduction tracts, AV junction, bundle branches, and Purkinje network to the ventricular myocardium. The P-R interval includes a P wave and the following short, usually flat (isoelectric) segment—the P-R segment.

Description

1. Onset and End: The P-R interval begins with the onset of the P wave and ends with the onset of the QRS complex.

2. Duration: The duration of the normal P-R interval is 0.12 to 0.20 second and is dependent on the heart rate. When the heart rate is fast, the P-R interval is normally shorter than when the heart rate is slow (Example: heart rate 120, P-R interval 0.16 second; heart rate 60, P-R interval 0.20 second).

Significance

A normal P-R interval indicates that the electrical impulse originated in the SA node or an ectopic pacemaker in the adjacent atria and has progressed normally through the electrical conduction system of the heart to the ventricular myocardium. The major significance of a normal P-R interval is that the electrical impulse has been conducted through the AV node and bundle of His normally and without delay.

Notes

NORMAL P-R INTERVAL

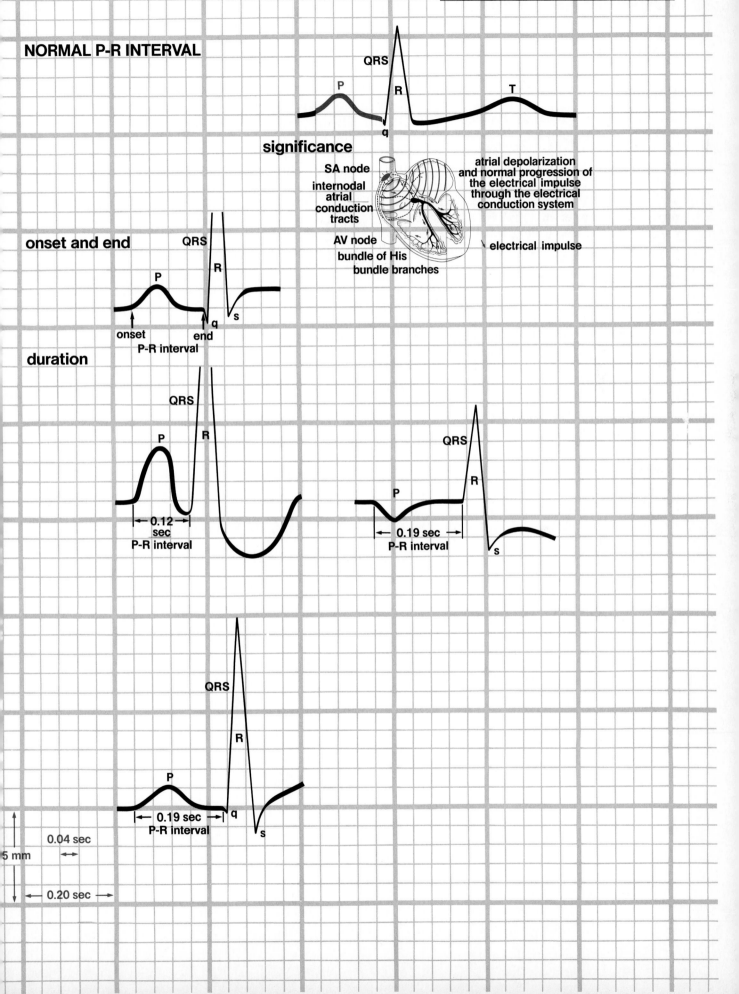

significance

SA node
internodal
atrial
conduction
tracts

AV node
bundle of His
bundle branches

atrial depolarization
and normal progression of
the electrical impulse
through the electrical
conduction system

electrical impulse

onset and end

QRS
R
P
q
s
onset   end
P-R interval

duration

QRS
P   R
|← 0.12 →|
sec
P-R interval

QRS
P   R
|← 0.19 sec →|
P-R interval
s

QRS
R
P
|← 0.19 sec →| q
P-R interval
s

0.04 sec
5 mm
|← 0.20 sec →|

R-R Interval

Definition

An **R-R interval** represents the time between two successive ventricular depolarizations.

Characteristics

1. Relationship to Cardiac Anatomy and Physiology: An R-R interval normally represents **one cardiac cycle** during which the ventricles contract and relax once.

Description

1. Onset and End: The onset of the R-R interval is generally considered to be the peak of one R wave; the end, the peak of the succeeding R wave.

2. Duration: The duration is dependent on the heart rate. When the heart rate is fast, the R-R interval is shorter than when the heart rate is slow (Example: heart rate 120, R-R interval 0.50 second; heart rate 60, R-R interval 1.0 second). The R-R intervals may be equal or unequal in duration depending on the underlying rhythm.

Significance

An R-R interval represents the time between two successive ventricular depolarizations.

Notes

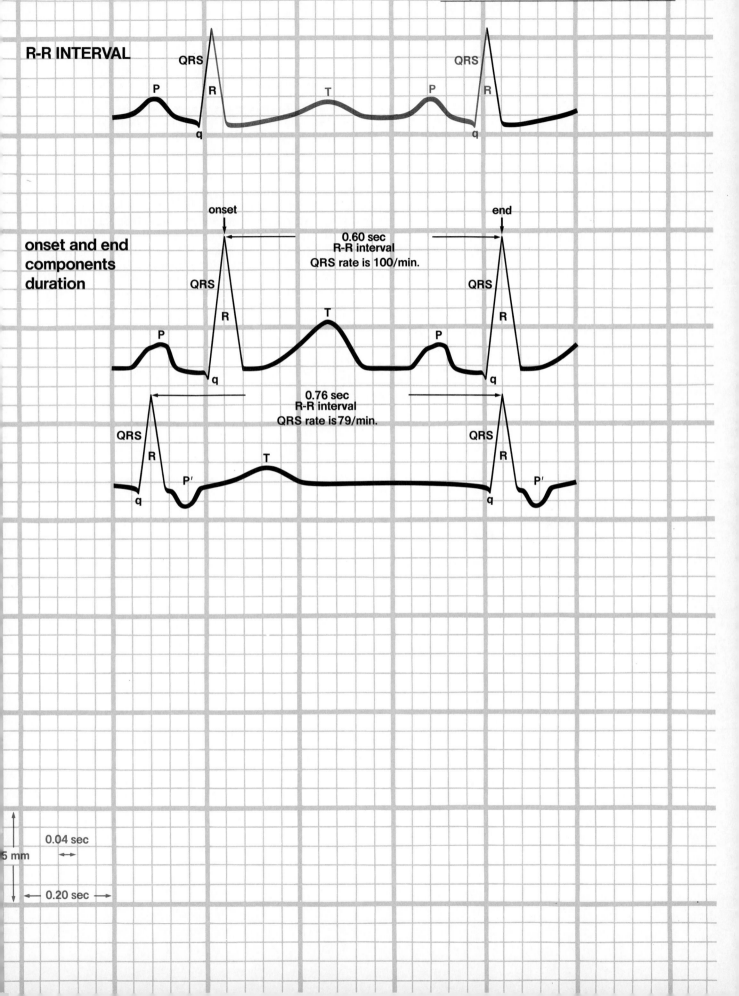

R-R INTERVAL

QRS
P
R
T
P
QRS
R
q
q

onset and end components duration

onset
end
0.60 sec
R-R interval
QRS rate is 100/min.

QRS
QRS
R
T
R
P
P
q
q

0.76 sec
R-R interval
QRS rate is 79/min.

QRS
R
P'
T
QRS
R
P'
q
q

0.04 sec
5 mm
0.20 sec

S-T Segment

Definition

An **S-T segment** represents the **early part of repolarization of the right and left ventricles.**

Normal S-T Segment

Characteristics

1. Relationship to Cardiac Anatomy and Physiology: The S-T segment represents the early part of ventricular repolarization.

Description

1. Onset and End: The S-T segment begins with the end of the QRS complex and ends with the onset of the T wave. The junction between the QRS complex and the S-T segment is called the **"junction" or "J" point.**

2. Duration: The duration is about 0.20 second or less and is dependent on the heart rate. When the heart rate is fast, the S-T segment is shorter than when the heart rate is slow.

3. Amplitude: Normally, the S-T segment is flat (isoelectric). However, it may be slightly elevated (by less than 0.25 mm at its onset) or slightly depressed (by less than 1.0 mm at its onset or 0.08 second after the **J point**) and still be normal. The T-P segment is normally used as a baseline reference for the determination of the amplitude of the S-T segment. However, if the T-P segment is absent because of a very rapid heart rate, the P-R segment is used instead.

4. Appearance: If slightly elevated, the S-T segment may be flat, concave, or arched. If slightly depressed, the S-T segment may be flat, sagging, or downsloping.

Significance

A normal S-T segment followed by a normal T wave indicates that normal repolarization of the right and left ventricles has occurred.

Notes

NORMAL S-T SEGMENT

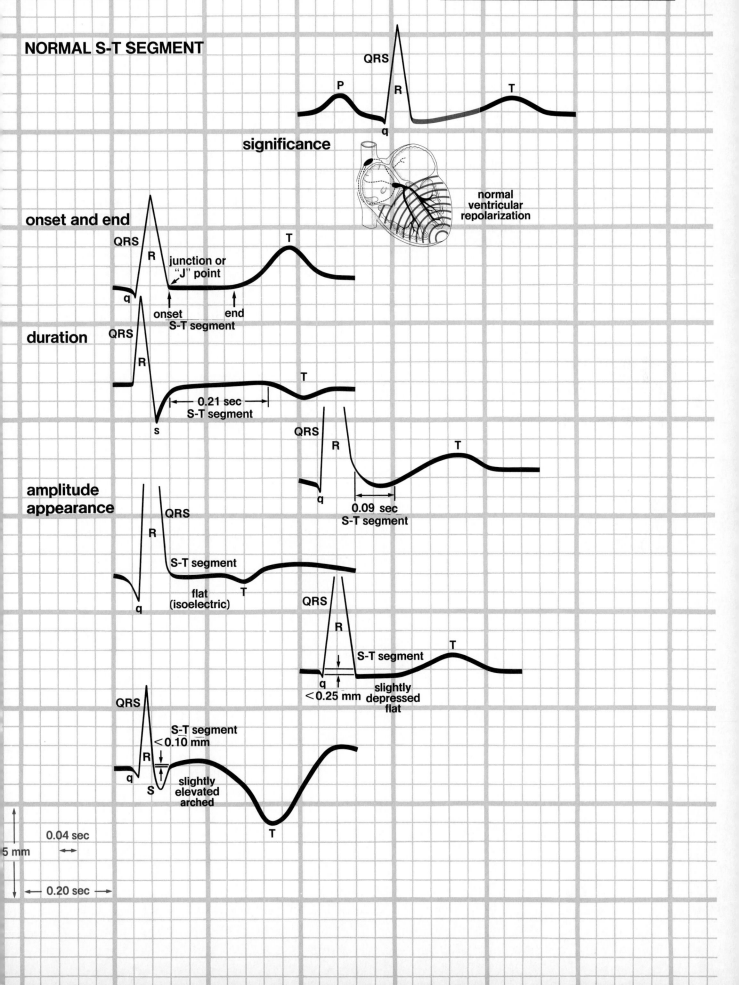

significance

normal
ventricular
repolarization

onset and end

QRS
R
junction or
"J" point
q
onset
end
S-T segment
T

duration

QRS
R
0.21 sec
S-T segment
T
s

QRS
R
0.09 sec
S-T segment
T
q

**amplitude
appearance**

QRS
R
S-T segment
flat
(isoelectric)
T
q

QRS
R
S-T segment
<0.25 mm
slightly
depressed
flat
T
q

QRS
R
S-T segment
<0.10 mm
slightly
elevated
arched
q
S
T

0.04 sec

5 mm

0.20 sec

P-R Segment

Definition

A **P-R segment** represents the time of progression of the electrical impulse from the AV node through the bundle of His, bundle branches, and Purkinje network to the ventricular myocardium.

Characteristics

1. Relationship to Cardiac Anatomy and Physiology: The P-R segment represents the time from the end of atrial depolarization to the onset of ventricular depolarization during which the electrical impulse progresses from the AV node through the bundle of His, bundle branches, and Purkinje network to the ventricular myocardium.

Description

1. Onset and End: The onset of the P-R segment begins with the end of the P wave and ends with the onset of the QRS complex.

2. Duration: The duration normally varies from about 0.02 to 0.10 second. It may be greater than 0.10 second if there is a delay in the progression of the electrical impulse through the AV node or bundle of His.

3. Amplitude: Normally, the P-R segment is flat (isoelectric).

Significance

A P-R segment of 0.10-second duration or less indicates that the electrical impulse has been conducted through the AV junction normally and without delay. A P-R segment exceeding 0.10 second in duration indicates a delay in the conduction of the electrical impulse through the AV junction.

Notes

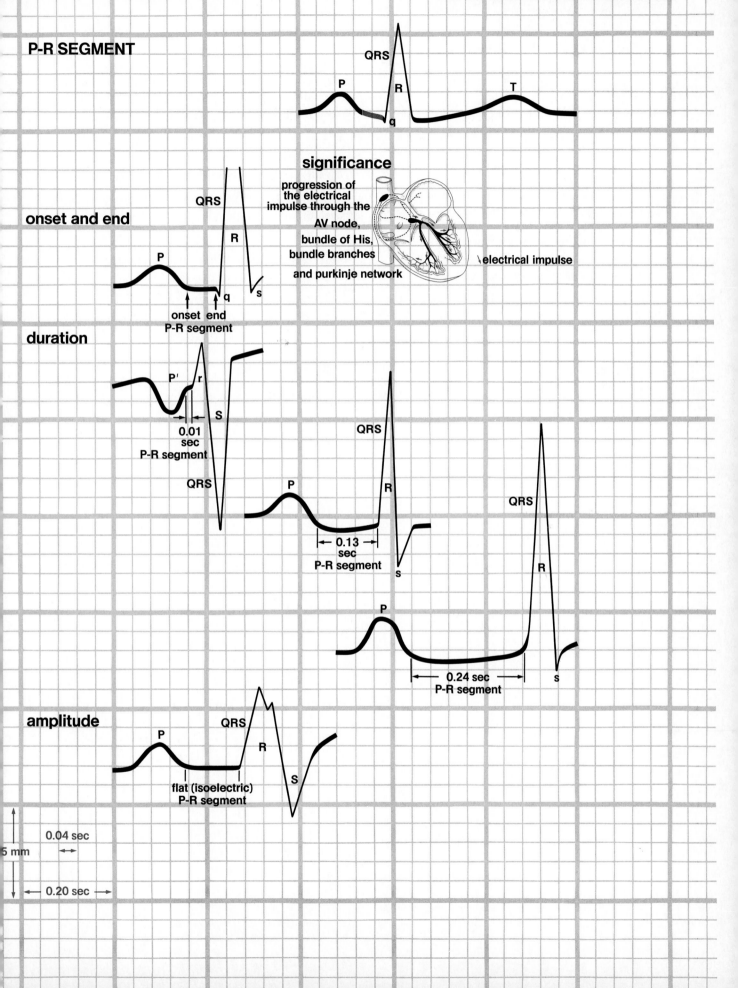

P-R SEGMENT

QRS

P

R

T

q

onset and end

QRS

R

P

q

s

significance

progression of
the electrical
impulse through the

AV node,
bundle of His,
bundle branches

and purkinje network

electrical impulse

onset end
P-R segment

duration

P' r

S

0.01
sec
P-R segment

QRS

QRS

P

R

0.13
sec
P-R segment

s

QRS

R

P

0.24 sec
P-R segment

s

amplitude

P

QRS

R

S

flat (isoelectric)
P-R segment

0.04 sec

5 mm

0.20 sec

T-P Segment

Definition

A **T-P segment** is the interval between two successive P-QRS-T complexes during which electrical activity of the heart is absent.

Characteristics

1. Relationship to Cardiac Anatomy and Physiology: A T-P segment represents the time from the end of ventricular repolarization to the onset of atrial depolarization during which electrical activity of the heart is absent.

Description

1. Onset and End: The T-P segment begins with the end of the T wave and ends with the onset of the P wave.

2. Duration: The duration is 0.0 to 0.40 second or greater and is dependent on the heart rate. When the heart rate is fast, the T-P segment is shorter than when the heart rate is slow (Example: heart rate about 120 or greater, T-P segment 0 second; heart rate about 60 or less, T-P segment 0.40 second or greater).

3. Amplitude: Usually, the T-P segment is flat (isoelectric).

Significance

A T-P segment indicates the absence of any electrical activity of the heart. The T-P segment is used as the baseline reference for the determination of S-T segment elevation or depression.

Notes

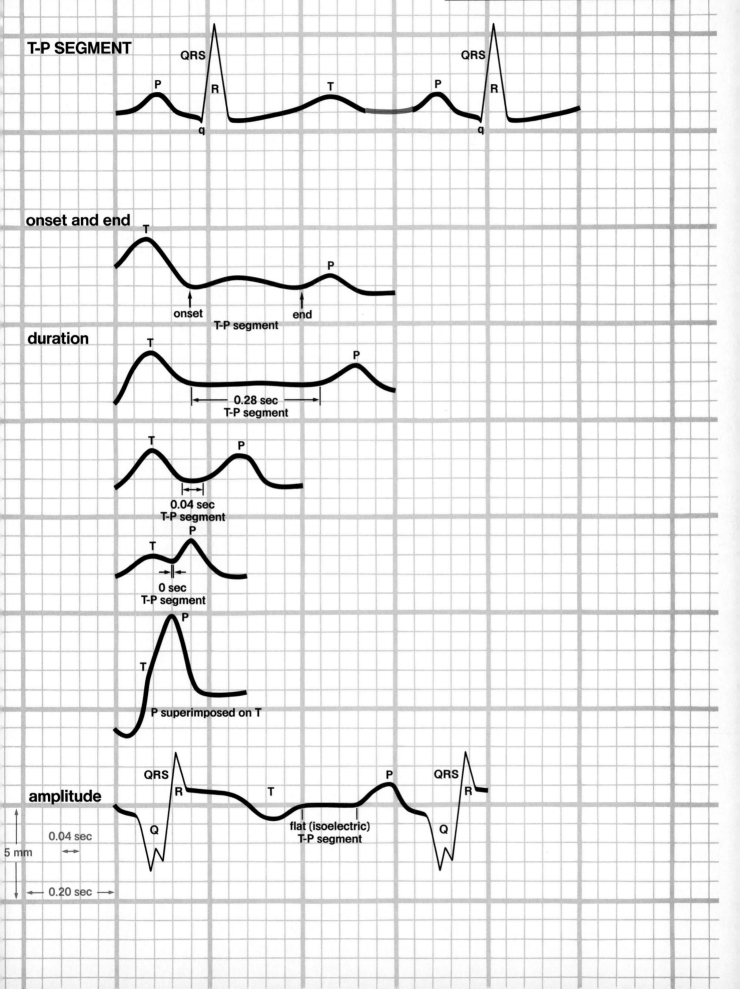

T-P SEGMENT

QRS

P

R

q

T

P

QRS

R

q

onset and end

T

P

onset

end

T-P segment

duration

T

P

0.28 sec
T-P segment

T

P

0.04 sec
T-P segment

T

P

0 sec
T-P segment

P

T

P superimposed on T

amplitude

QRS

R

Q

T

flat (isoelectric)
T-P segment

P

QRS

R

Q

0.04 sec

5 mm

0.20 sec

Abnormal Components
of the Electrocardiogram

Abnormal Sinus P Wave

Characteristics

1. Pacemaker Site: The pacemaker site is the SA node.

2. Relationship to Cardiac Anatomy and Physiology: An **abnormal sinus P wave** represents **depolarization of altered, damaged, or abnormal atria.**

Increased right atrial pressure and right atrial dilatation and hypertrophy (right atrial overload) — as found in chronic obstructive pulmonary disease, status asthmaticus, acute pulmonary embolism, and acute pulmonary edema — may result in tall and symmetrically peaked P waves (**P pulmonale**). Abnormally tall P waves may also occur in sinus tachycardia (see Chapter 5).

Increased left atrial pressure and left atrial dilatation and hypertrophy (left atrial overload) — as found in hypertension, mitral and aortic valvular disease, acute myocardial infarction, and pulmonary edema secondary to left heart failure — may cause wide, notched P waves (**P mitrale**). Such P waves may also result from a delay or block of the progression of electrical impulses through the interatrial conduction tract between the right and left atria:

Description

1. Onset and End: The onset of the abnormal sinus P wave is identified as the first abrupt or gradual deviation from the baseline. The point where the wave flattens out to join with the P-R segment marks the end of the abnormal sinus P wave.

2. Direction: The direction is positive (upright) in Lead II.

3. Duration: The duration may be normal (0.10 second or less) or greater than 0.10 second.

4. Amplitude: The amplitude may be normal (0.5 to 2.5 mm) or greater than 2.5 mm in Lead II. By definition, a P pulmonale is 2.5 mm or greater in amplitude.

5. Shape: The abnormal sinus P wave may be tall and symmetrically peaked or may be wide and notched.

6. P Wave-QRS Complex Relationship: The P wave-QRS complex relationship is the same as that of a normal sinus P wave.

7. P-R Interval: The P-R interval may be normal (0.12 to 0.20 second) or abnormal (greater than 0.20 second).

Significance

An abnormal sinus P wave indicates that the electrical impulse responsible for the P wave originated in the SA node and that depolarization of altered, damaged, or abnormal atria has occurred.

Notes

ABNORMAL SINUS P WAVE

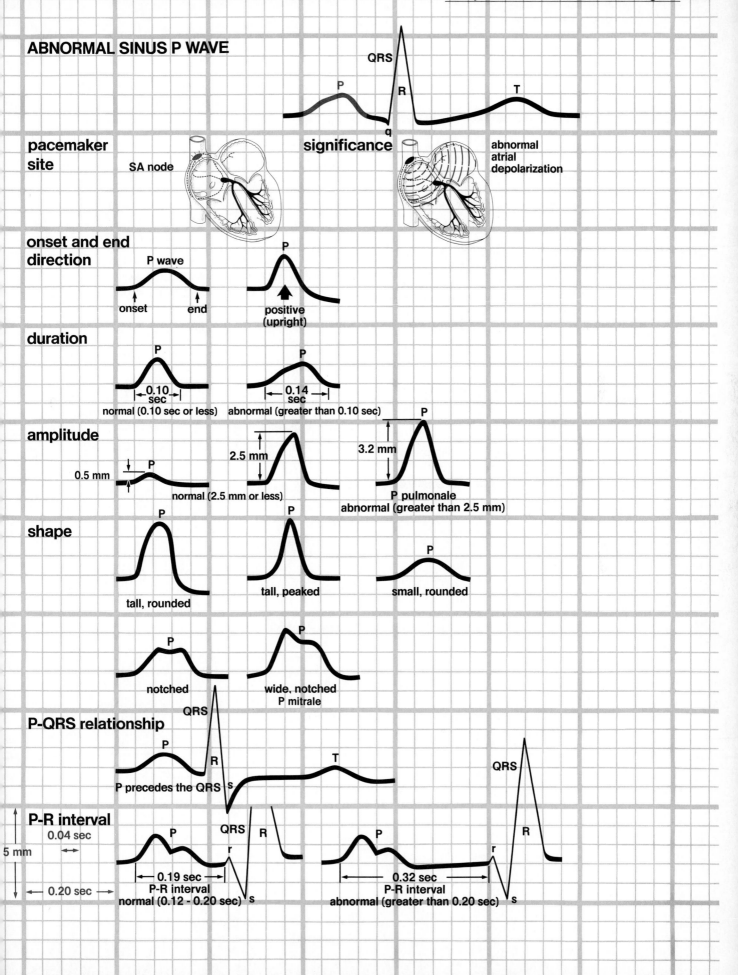

pacemaker site

SA node

significance

abnormal atrial depolarization

onset and end direction

P wave

onset   end

positive (upright)

duration

P

0.10 sec

normal (0.10 sec or less)

P

0.14 sec

abnormal (greater than 0.10 sec)

amplitude

0.5 mm   P

2.5 mm

normal (2.5 mm or less)

3.2 mm   P

P pulmonale abnormal (greater than 2.5 mm)

shape

P

tall, rounded

P

tall, peaked

P

small, rounded

P

notched

P

wide, notched P mitrale

P-QRS relationship

QRS

P   R   T

P precedes the QRS   s

QRS

P-R interval

0.04 sec

5 mm

0.20 sec

P   QRS   R

r

0.19 sec P-R interval normal (0.12 - 0.20 sec)   s

P   QRS   R

r

0.32 sec P-R interval abnormal (greater than 0.20 sec)   s

Ectopic P Wave (P Prime or P′)

Characteristics

1. Pacemaker Site: The pacemaker site is an ectopic pacemaker in the atria outside of the SA node or in the AV junction or ventricles.

2. Relationship to Cardiac Anatomy and Physiology: An **ectopic P wave (P′)** represents **atrial depolarization occurring in an abnormal direction or sequence or both.** If the ectopic pacemaker is in the atria, depolarization of the atria may occur in a normal direction (right to left and downward) or in a retrograde direction (left to right and upward), depending on the ectopic pacemaker's location. If the ectopic pacemaker is in the AV junction or ventricles, the electrical impulse travels upward through the AV junction into the atria **(retrograde conduction),** causing retrograde atrial depolarization.

Ectopic P waves occur in various atrial, junctional, and ventricular arrhythmias, including wandering atrial pacemaker, premature atrial contractions, nonparoxysmal atrial tachycardia, paroxysmal atrial tachycardia, premature junctional contractions, junctional escape rhythm, nonparoxysmal junctional tachycardia, paroxysmal junctional tachycardia, and, occasionally, premature ventricular contractions (see Chapter 5 for details).

Description

1. Onset and End: The onset of the abnormal ectopic P wave is identified as the first abrupt or gradual deviation from the baseline. The point where the wave flattens out to join with the P-R segment marks the end of the abnormal ectopic P wave.

2. Direction: The ectopic P wave may be either positive (upright) or negative (inverted) in Lead II if the ectopic pacemaker is in the atria; it is negative (inverted) if the ectopic pacemaker is in the AV junction or ventricles.

Generally, if the ectopic pacemaker is in the left atrium or in the lower right atrium near the AV node, the ectopic P wave is negative (inverted). If the ectopic pacemaker is in any other part of the right atrium, the ectopic P wave is positive (upright) and may resemble a normal sinus P wave.

3. Duration: The duration is 0.10 second or less.

4. Amplitude: The amplitude is usually less than 2.5 mm in Lead II, but it may be greater.

5. Shape: The ectopic P wave may be smooth and rounded, peaked, or dimple-shaped.

6. P′ Wave-QRS Complex Relationship: The ectopic P wave may precede, be buried in, or follow the QRS complex with which it is associated. If the ectopic P wave is buried in the QRS complex, it is not seen and is said to be hidden or invisible. The ectopic P wave may also be superimposed on the preceding T wave resulting in a T wave that differs in amplitude and shape from the other T waves not so affected.

7. P′-R Interval: Generally, the **P′-R interval** is normal (0.12 to 0.20 second) if the ectopic pacemaker is in the upper or middle part of the atria and slightly less than 0.12 second if it is in the lower part of the atria, close to the AV node. If the ectopic pacemaker is in the upper part of the AV junction, the ectopic P wave usually precedes the QRS complex, and the P′-R interval is less than 0.12 second. If the ectopic pacemaker is in the lower part of the AV junction or in the ventricles, the ectopic P wave usually follows the QRS complex, and an R-P′ interval is present; it is usually less than 0.21 second.

Significance

An ectopic P wave indicates that the electrical impulse responsible for the ectopic P wave originated in part of the atria outside the SA node or in the AV junction or ventricles and that depolarization of the right and left atria has occurred in an abnormal direction or sequence or both.

Notes

ECTOPIC P WAVE (P PRIME OR P')

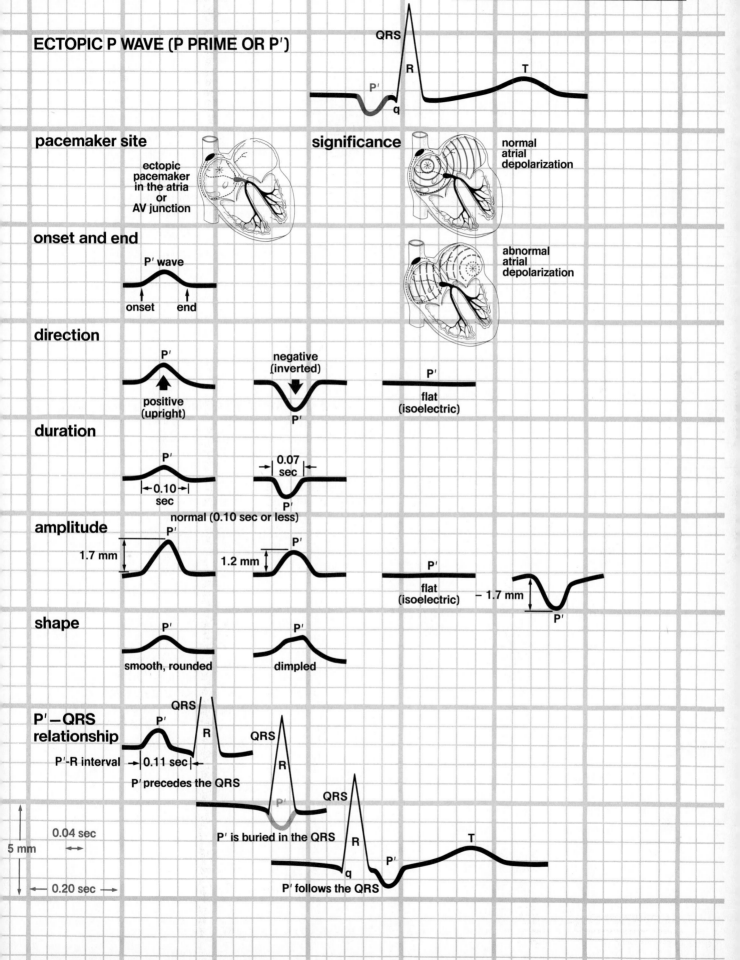

pacemaker site

ectopic
pacemaker
in the atria
or
AV junction

significance

normal
atrial
depolarization

abnormal
atrial
depolarization

onset and end

P' wave

onset   end

direction

P'

positive
(upright)

negative
(inverted)

P'

P'

flat
(isoelectric)

duration

P'

|← 0.10 →|
sec

0.07
sec

P'

normal (0.10 sec or less)

amplitude

P'

1.7 mm

P'

1.2 mm

P'

flat
(isoelectric)

− 1.7 mm

P'

shape

P'

smooth, rounded

P'

dimpled

P'−QRS relationship

QRS

P'   R

P'-R interval →|0.11 sec|←

P' precedes the QRS

QRS

R

P'   QRS

P' is buried in the QRS

QRS

R

q   P'   T

P' follows the QRS

0.04 sec

5 mm

|← 0.20 sec →|

Abnormal QRS Complex

Characteristics

1. Pacemaker Site: The pacemaker site is the SA node or an ectopic pacemaker in the atria, AV junction, bundle branches, Purkinje network, or ventricular myocardium.

2. Relationship to Cardiac Anatomy and Physiology: An **abnormal QRS complex** represents **abnormal depolarization of the ventricles** because of (a) a partial or complete block in the conduction of electrical impulses through a bundle branch (**bundle branch block** and **aberrant ventricular conduction**), (b) abnormal conduction of electrical impulses from the atria to the ventricles through abnormal anatomical pathways bypassing the AV node and bundle of His (**anomalous AV conduction** or **preexcitation syndrome**), or (c) an electrical impulse originating in a **ventricular ectopic pacemaker.**

(a) **Bundle branch block** results from partial or complete block in conduction of the electrical impulse from the bundle of His to the Purkinje network through the right or left bundle branch while conduction continues uninterrupted through the unaffected bundle branch. A block in one bundle branch causes the ventricle on that side to be depolarized later than the other.

For example, in **complete left bundle branch block,** because of a block in conduction through the left bundle branch, depolarization of the left ventricle is delayed, resulting in an abnormal QRS complex—one that is greater than 0.12 second in duration and appears bizarre, that is, abnormal in size and shape. On the other hand, in **complete right bundle branch block,** the block is in the right bundle branch and, thus, depolarization of the right ventricle is delayed.

In **partial** or **incomplete bundle branch block,** conduction of the electrical impulse is only partially blocked, resulting in less of a delay in depolarization of the ventricle on the side of the block than in complete bundle branch block. Consequently, the QRS complex is greater than 0.10 second but less than 0.12 second in duration and often appears normal.

Complete and incomplete bundle branch block may be present in normal sinus rhythm and in any **supraventricular arrhythmia,** that is, any arrhythmia arising in the SA node, atria, or AV junction. Certain of these supraventricular arrhythmias with bundle branch block may mimic ventricular arrhythmias (see Chapter 5).

Aberrant ventricular conduction is a transient inability of the right or left bundle branch to conduct an electrical impulse normally when that impulse arrives at the bundle branch while it is still refractory after conducting a previous electrical impulse. This results in an abnormal QRS complex often resembling an incomplete or complete bundle branch block.

Aberrant ventricular conduction usually occurs in supraventricular arrhythmias such as premature atrial and junctional contractions, nonparoxysmal atrial tachycardia, paroxysmal atrial tachycardia, atrial flutter, atrial fibrillation, nonparoxysmal junctional tachycardia, and paroxysmal junctional tachycardia. These supraventricular arrhythmias with aberrant ventricular conduction may mimic ventricular arrhythmias (see Chapter 5).

(b) **Anomalous AV conduction** or **preexcitation syndrome** is a clinical condition associated with abnormal conduction pathways between the atria and ventricles that bypass the AV node and bundle of His and allow the electrical impulses to initiate depolarization of the ventricles earlier than usual. This results in a P-R interval of less than 0.12 second, a QRS complex greater than 0.10 second, and an abnormal slurring of the onset of the QRS complex (**delta wave**).

Supraventricular tachycardia and atrial flutter and fibrillation with anomalous AV conduction may resemble ventricular tachycardia (see Chapter 5).

(c) An electrical impulse originating in an ectopic pacemaker in the bundle branches, Purkinje network, or myocardium of one of the ventricles depolarizes that ventricle earlier than the other and produces an abnormal QRS complex that is greater than 0.12 second in duration and appears bizarre. Such QRS complexes typically occur in ventricular arrhythmias such as accelerated idioventricular rhythm, ventricular escape rhythm, ventricular tachycardia, and premature ventricular contractions (see Chapter 5).

Description

1. Onset and End: The onset and end of the abnormal QRS complex are the same as those of a normal QRS complex.

ABNORMAL QRS COMPLEX

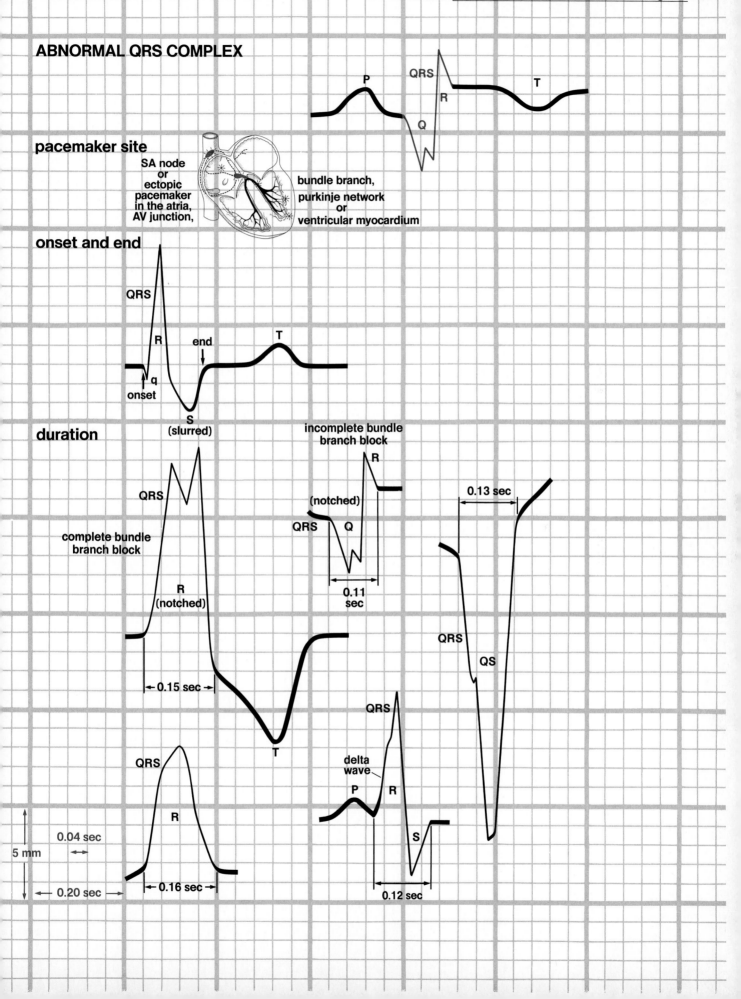

pacemaker site

SA node
or
ectopic
pacemaker
in the atria,
AV junction,

bundle branch,
purkinje network
or
ventricular myocardium

onset and end

QRS

R

q
onset

end

T

S
(slurred)

duration

QRS

complete bundle
branch block

R
(notched)

← 0.15 sec →

T

QRS

R

0.04 sec

5 mm

← 0.20 sec →

← 0.16 sec →

incomplete bundle
branch block

R

(notched)

QRS   Q

0.11
sec

0.13 sec

QRS

QS

delta
wave

P   R

QRS

S

0.12 sec

Abnormal QRS Complex—Cont.

2. Duration: The duration of the abnormal QRS complex is greater than 0.10 second. If a bundle branch block is present and the duration of the QRS complex is between 0.10 and 0.12 seconds, the bundle branch block is called **"incomplete."** If the duration of the QRS complex is greater than 0.12 second, the bundle branch block is called **"complete."**

The duration of a QRS complex caused by an electrical impulse originating in an ectopic pacemaker in the Purkinje network or ventricular myocardium is always greater than 0.12 second; typically, it is 0.16 second or greater. However, if the electrical impulse originates in a bundle branch, the duration of the QRS complex may be only slightly greater than 0.10 second.

3. Direction: The direction of the abnormal QRS complex may be predominantly positive (upright), predominantly negative (inverted), or biphasic (partly positive, partly negative).

ABNORMAL QRS COMPLEX – CONT.

direction

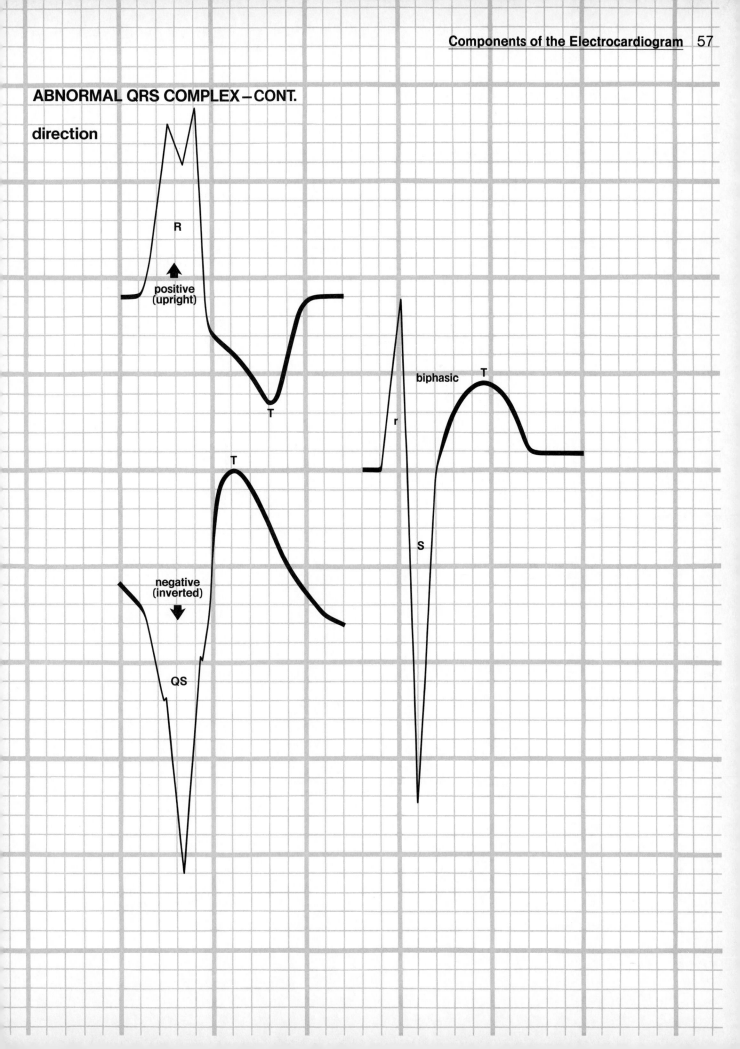

R

positive
(upright)

T

biphasic   T

r

negative
(inverted)

T

S

QS

Abnormal QRS Complex—Cont.

4. Amplitude: The amplitude of the waves in the abnormal QRS complex varies from 1 to 2 mm to 20 mm or more.

5. Shape: An abnormal QRS complex varies widely in shape, from one that appears quite normal—narrow and sharply pointed (as in incomplete bundle branch block)—to one that is wide and bizarre, slurred and notched (as in complete bundle branch block and ventricular arrhythmias).

Significance

An abnormal QRS complex indicates that abnormal depolarization of the ventricles has occurred because of (1) a block in the progression of the electrical impulse from the bundle of His to the Purkinje network through the right or left bundle branch (bundle branch block, aberrant ventricular conduction), (2) the progression of the electrical impulse from the atria to the ventricles through an abnormal conduction pathway (anomalous AV conduction or preexcitation syndrome), or (3) the origination of the electrical impulse responsible for the ventricular depolarization in a ventricular ectopic pacemaker.

Notes

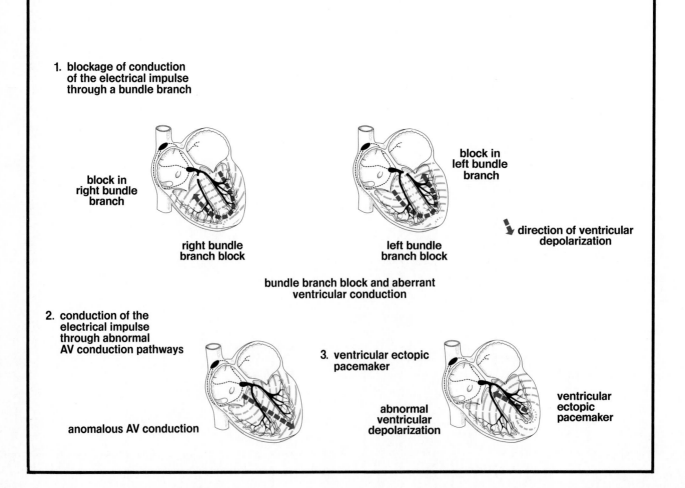

1. blockage of conduction of the electrical impulse through a bundle branch

block in right bundle branch

right bundle branch block

block in left bundle branch

direction of ventricular depolarization

left bundle branch block

bundle branch block and aberrant ventricular conduction

2. conduction of the electrical impulse through abnormal AV conduction pathways

anomalous AV conduction

3. ventricular ectopic pacemaker

abnormal ventricular depolarization

ventricular ectopic pacemaker

ABNORMAL QRS COMPLEX – CONT.

amplitude

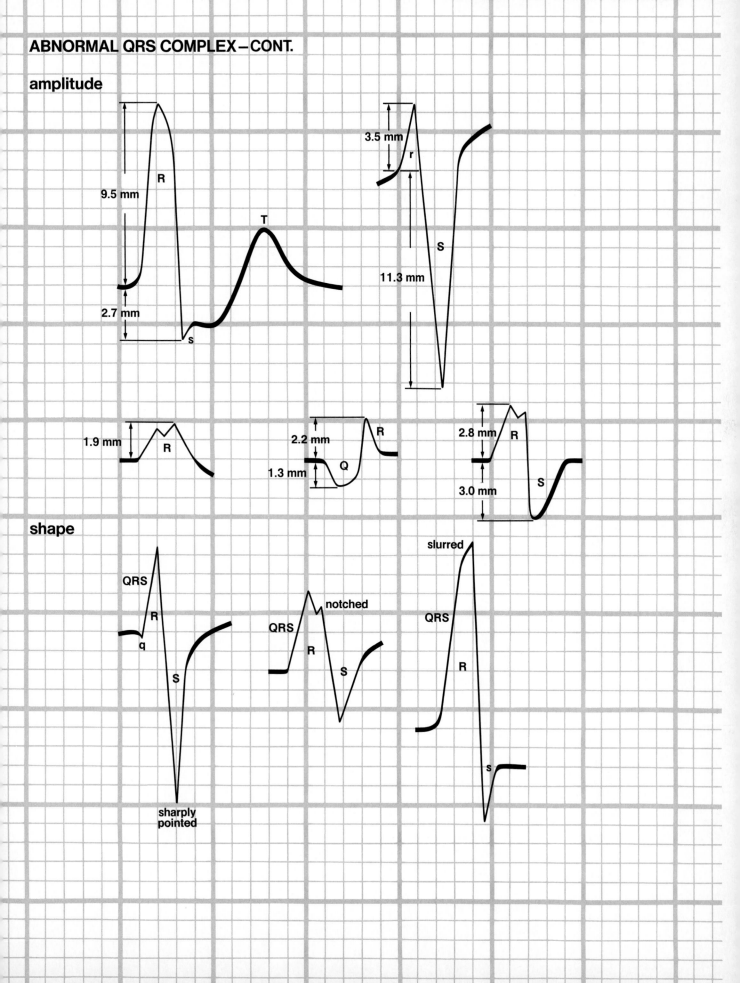

shape

Abnormal T Wave

Characteristics

1. Relationship to Cardiac Anatomy and Physiology: An **abnormal T wave** represents **abnormal ventricular repolarization.** Repolarization may begin at the epicardial surface of the ventricles and progress inwardly through the ventricular walls to the endocardial surface, as it normally does, or it may begin at the endocardial surface of the ventricles and progress through the ventricular walls to the epicardial surface. Abnormal ventricular repolarization may result from myocardial ischemia, acute myocardial infarction, myocarditis, pericarditis, ventricular enlargement (hypertrophy), electrolyte imbalance (e.g., excess serum potassium), administration of certain cardiac drugs (e.g., quinidine, procainamide); it also commonly occurs where there is abnormal depolarization of the ventricles (as in bundle branch block and ectopic ventricular arrhythmias). Abnormal ventricular repolarization may also occur in athletes and persons who are hyperventilating.

Description

1. Onset and End: The onset and end of an abnormal T wave are the same as those of a normal T wave.

2. Direction: The abnormal T wave may be positive (upright) and abnormally tall or low, negative (inverted), or biphasic (partially positive and partially negative) in Lead II. The abnormal T wave may or may not be in the same direction as that of the QRS complex. The T wave following an abnormal QRS complex is almost always opposite in direction to it and abnormally wide and tall or deeply inverted.

3. Amplitude: The amplitude varies.

ABNORMAL T WAVE

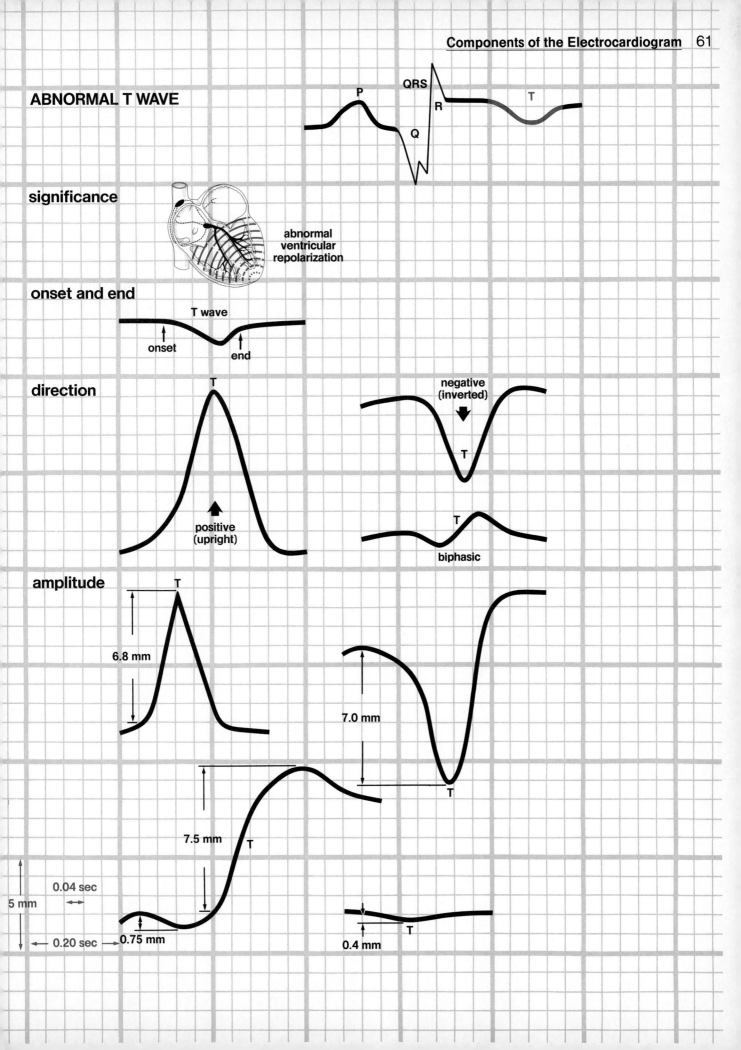

significance

abnormal
ventricular
repolarization

onset and end

T wave

onset

end

direction

T

positive
(upright)

negative
(inverted)

T

T

biphasic

amplitude

T

6.8 mm

7.0 mm

T

7.5 mm

T

0.04 sec

5 mm

0.20 sec

0.75 mm

0.4 mm

T

4. Duration: The duration is 0.10 to 0.25 second or greater.

5. Shape: The abnormal T wave may be rounded, blunt, sharply peaked, wide, or notched.

6. T Wave-QRS Complex Relationship: The abnormal T wave always follows the QRS complex.

Significance

An abnormal T wave indicates that abnormal repolarization of the ventricles has occurred.

Notes

ABNORMAL T WAVE—CONT.

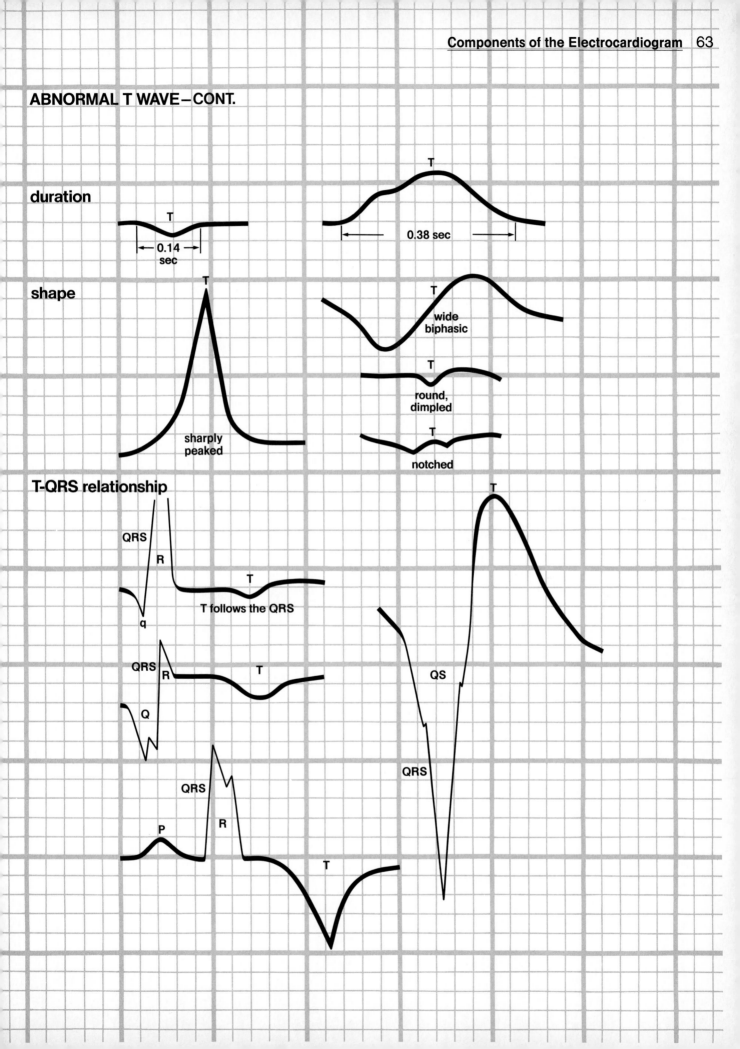

duration

T

0.14 sec

0.38 sec

shape

T

sharply peaked

T
wide biphasic

T
round, dimpled

T
notched

T-QRS relationship

QRS

R

q

T

T follows the QRS

QRS R

Q

T

T

QS

QRS

QRS

R

P

T

Abnormal P-R Interval

Characteristics

1. Relationship to Cardiac Anatomy and Physiology: A P-R interval greater than 0.20 second represents delayed progression of the electrical impulse through the AV node or bundle of His. The P wave associated with a prolonged P-R interval may be normal or abnormal.

A P-R interval less than 0.12 second is commonly present when the electrical impulse originates in an ectopic pacemaker in the atria close to the AV node or in the AV junction. Negative (inverted) P waves in Lead II are commonly associated with abnormally short P-R intervals.

A P-R interval less than 0.12 second also occurs if the electrical impulse progresses from the atria to the ventricles through abnormal conduction pathways, which bypass the AV node and bundle of His, and depolarizes the ventricles earlier than usual. In this AV conduction abnormality—called the **anomalous AV conduction** or **preexcitation syndrome**—the short P-R interval is commonly followed by a wide, abnormally shaped QRS complex. The P waves in this condition may be positive (upright) or negative (inverted) in Lead II.

Description

1. Onset and End: The onset and end of the **abnormal P-R interval** are the same as those of a normal P-R interval.

2. Duration: The duration of the abnormal P-R interval may be greater than 0.20 second or less than 0.12 second.

Significance

An abnormally long P-R interval indicates that a delay of progression of the electrical impulse through the AV node or bundle of His is present. An abnormally short P-R interval indicates that the electrical impulse originated in an ectopic pacemaker in the atria near the AV node or in the AV junction or that the electrical impulse progressed from the atria to the ventricles through atrioventricular conduction pathways other than the AV node and bundle of His.

Notes

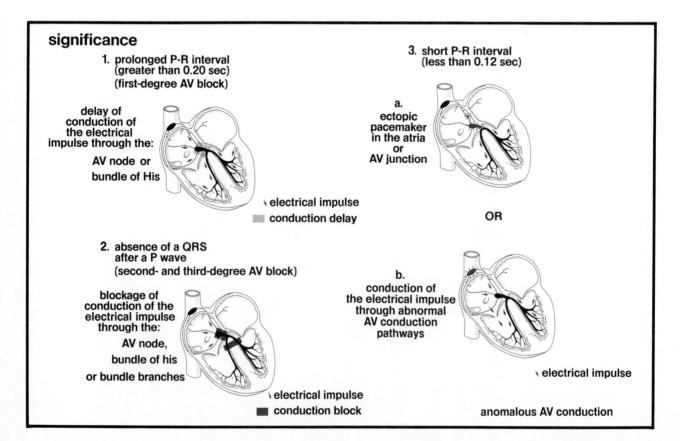

significance

1. prolonged P-R interval
   (greater than 0.20 sec)
   (first-degree AV block)

delay of conduction of the electrical impulse through the:

AV node or bundle of His

electrical impulse
conduction delay

2. absence of a QRS after a P wave
   (second- and third-degree AV block)

blockage of conduction of the electrical impulse through the:

AV node, bundle of his or bundle branches

electrical impulse
conduction block

3. short P-R interval
   (less than 0.12 sec)

a. ectopic pacemaker in the atria or AV junction

OR

b. conduction of the electrical impulse through abnormal AV conduction pathways

electrical impulse

anomalous AV conduction

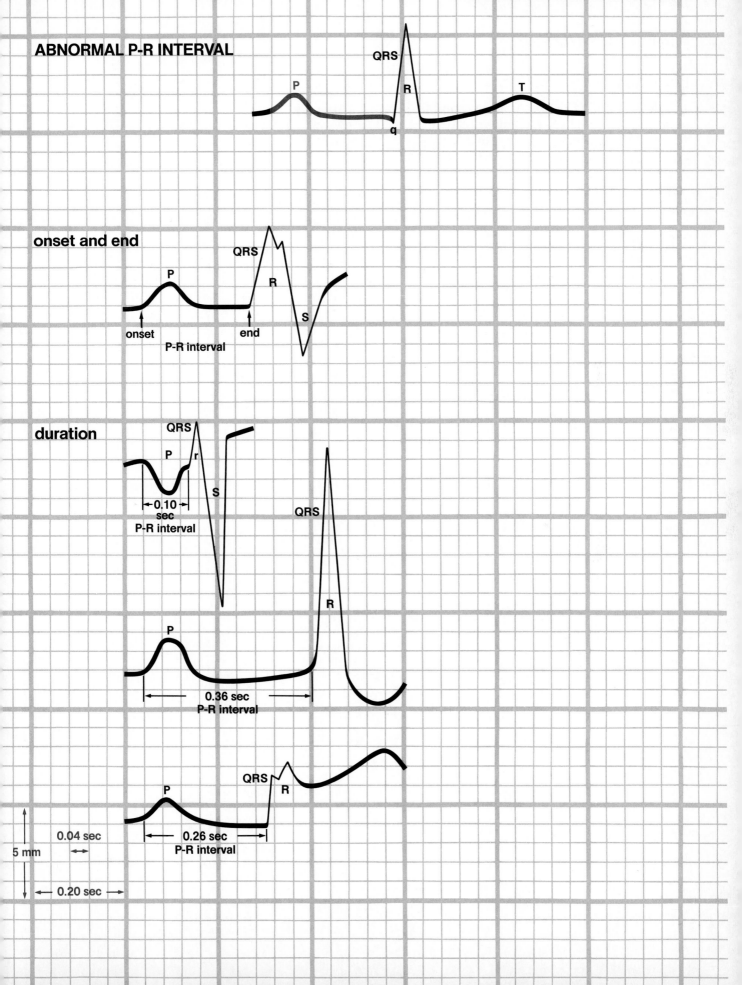

ABNORMAL P-R INTERVAL

QRS

P   R   T

q

onset and end

QRS

P   R

S

onset   end
P-R interval

duration

QRS

P   r

S

0.10
sec
P-R interval

QRS

R

P

0.36 sec
P-R interval

QRS

R

P

5 mm

0.04 sec

P

0.26 sec
P-R interval

0.20 sec

Abnormal S-T Segment

Characteristics

1. Relationship to Cardiac Anatomy and Physiology: An **abnormal S-T segment** represents **abnormal ventricular repolarization,** a result of myocardial ischemia, acute myocardial infarction, ventricular fibrosis or aneurysm, pericarditis, left ventricular enlargement (hypertrophy), or administration of digitalis.

Description

1. Onset and End: The onset and end of the abnormal S-T segment are the same as those of a normal S-T segment.

2. Duration: The duration is 0.20 second or less.

ABNORMAL S-T SEGMENT

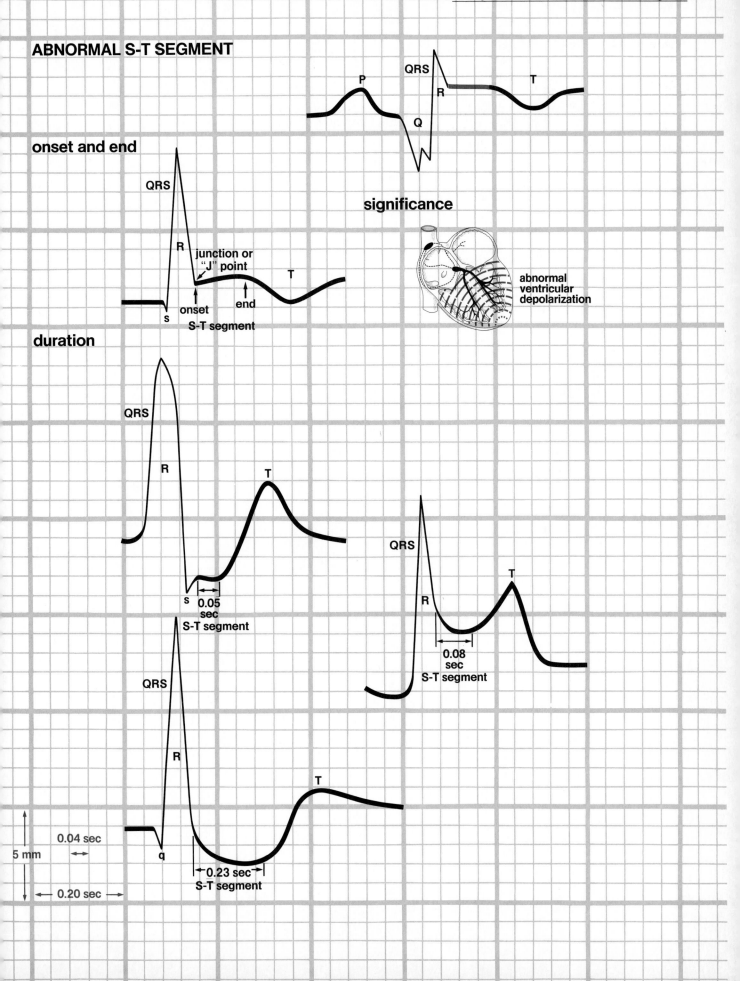

onset and end

QRS

R

junction or "J" point

onset

S-T segment

end

T

s

significance

abnormal ventricular depolarization

duration

QRS

R

T

s   0.05 sec

S-T segment

QRS

R

T

0.08 sec

S-T segment

QRS

R

T

q

0.23 sec

S-T segment

5 mm

0.04 sec

0.20 sec

3. Amplitude: The abnormal S-T segment is elevated by 0.25 mm or more at its onset or depressed by 1.0 mm or more at its onset or 0.08 second after the **J point.**

4. Appearance: If elevated, the S-T segment may be flat, concave, or arched. If depressed, the S-T segment may be flat, sagging, or downsloping.

Significance

An abnormal S-T segment indicates that abnormal ventricular repolarization has occurred. The most common causes of an abnormal S-T segment are coronary artery disease (coronary insufficiency, myocardial infarction), left ventricular hypertrophy, digitalis effect, and pericarditis.

Notes

ABNORMAL S-T SEGMENT – CONT.

amplitude

appearance

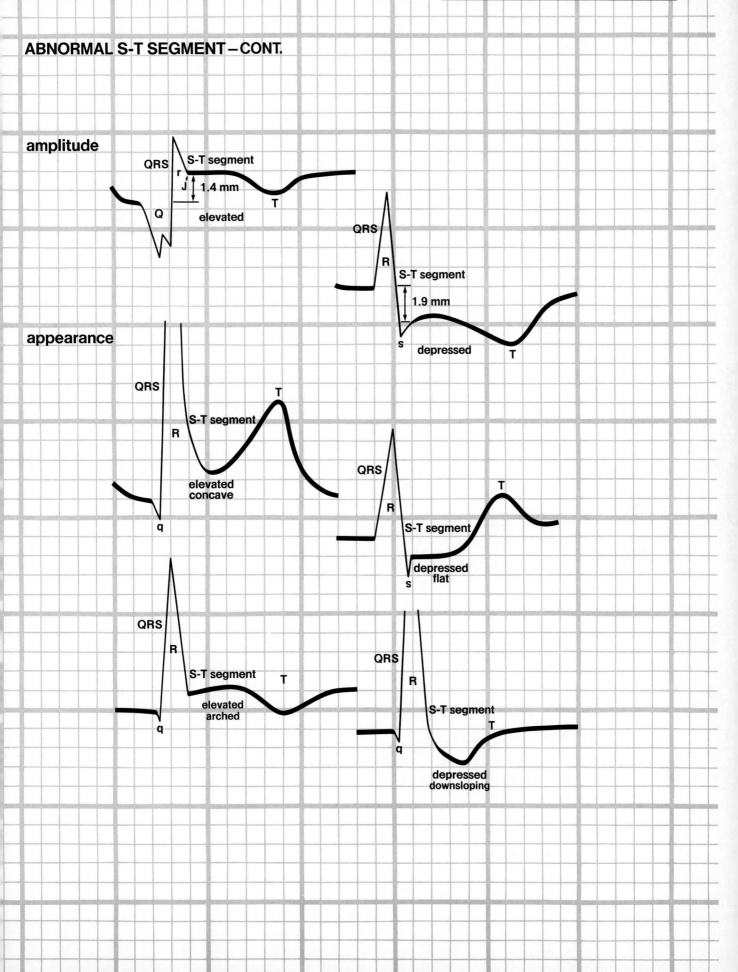

Chapter 4

Arrhythmia Determination

Step One
Identify the QRS Complex

Step Two
Determine the Heart Rate

Step Three
Determine the Ventricular Rhythm

Step Four
Identify the P Waves

Step Five
Determine the P-R Interval

Step Six
Determine the Pacemaker Site of the Arrhythmia

Step Seven
Identify the Arrhythmia

Arrhythmia Determination

The steps used to determine the identity of an arrhythmia are as follows:

- **Step one: Identify the QRS complex.**
- **Step two: Determine the heart rate.**
- **Step three: Determine the ventricular rhythm.**
- **Step four: Identify the P waves.**
- **Step five: Determine the P-R or R-P interval.**
- **Step six: Determine the pacemaker site.**
- **Step seven: Identify the arrhythmia.**

Step One
Identify the QRS Complex

The QRS complexes, consisting of one or more positive and negative deflections called Q, R, and S waves, are identified.

The duration and shape of the QRS complexes are noted. The QRS complexes may be normal (0.10 second or less wide) or abnormal (greater than 0.10 second wide and bizarre-appearing). The QRS complexes of **ventricular arrhythmias** are typically wide and bizarre. The QRS complexes may also be wide and bizarre in a **supraventricular arrhythmia**—one that originates in the SA node or an ectopic pacemaker in the atria or AV junction—if a **bundle branch block** or **aberrant ventricular conduction** is present. Less commonly, **anomalous AV conduction** is the cause of abnormal QRS complexes in arrhythmias originating in the SA node or atria.

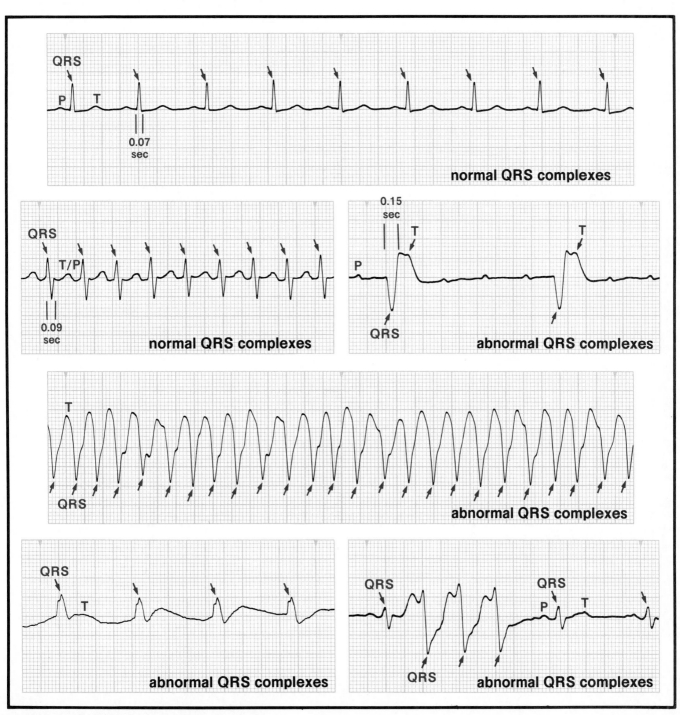

Figure 25. Identifying the QRS Complexes.

Step Two
Determine the Heart Rate

The heart rate, as calculated using the ECG, is the number of ventricular depolarizations (QRS complexes) or beats occurring in one minute.

The heart rate can be determined by using the six-second count method, a heart rate calculator ruler, the R-R interval method, or the triplicate method.

The Six-second Count Method

The **six-second count method** is the simplest way of determining the heart rate and is generally considered the fastest, with the exception of the heart rate calculator ruler method. The six-second count method, however, is the least accurate. This method can be used when the rhythm is either regular or irregular.

The short, vertical lines at the top of most ECG papers divide the ECG paper strip into **three-second intervals** when the paper is run at a standard speed of 25 mm per second. Two of these intervals are equal to a **six-second interval.**

The heart rate is calculated by determining the number of QRS complexes in a six-second interval and multiplying this number by ten. The result is the heart rate in beats per minute. The heart rate calculated by this method is almost always an approximation of the actual heart rate.

Example. If there are eight QRS complexes in a six-second interval, the heart rate is: 8 x 10 = 80 beats per minute.

To obtain a more accurate heart rate when the rate is extremely slow and/or the rhythm is grossly irregular, the number of QRS complexes should be determined in a longer interval, such as a **twelve-second interval,** and the multiplier should be adjusted accordingly.

Example. If there are six QRS complexes in a twelve-second interval, the heart rate is: 6 x 5 = 30 beats per minute.

A heart rate less than 60 beats per minute indicates **bradycardia;** a heart rate above 100 per minute indicates **tachycardia.**

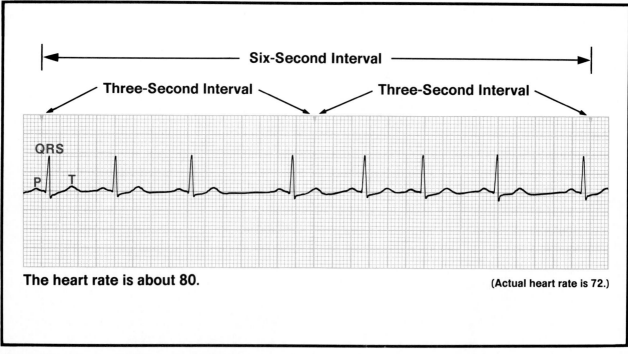

The heart rate is about 80.   (Actual heart rate is 72.)

Figure 26. Three- and Six-Second Intervals.

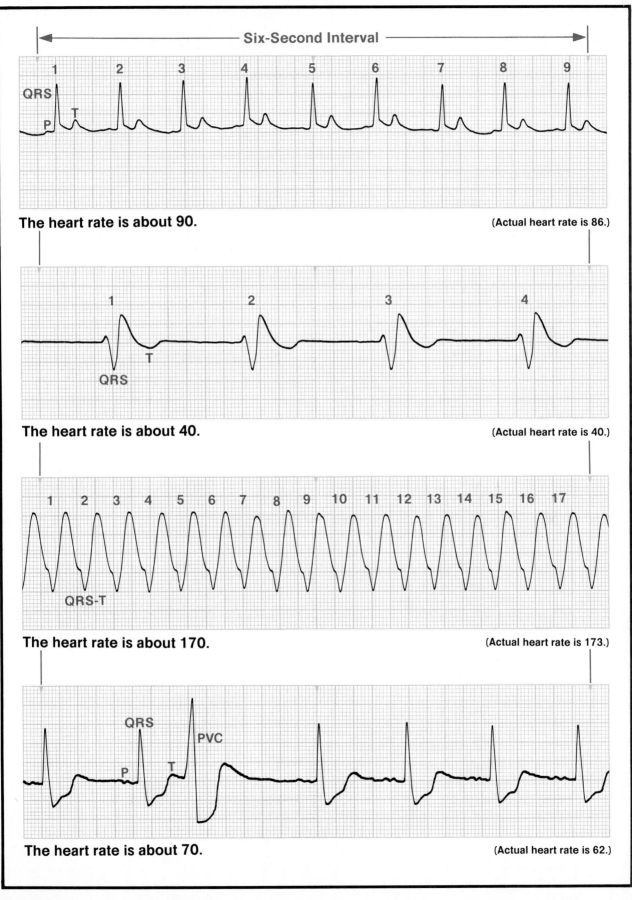

Six-Second Interval

The heart rate is about 90.   (Actual heart rate is 86.)

The heart rate is about 40.   (Actual heart rate is 40.)

The heart rate is about 170.   (Actual heart rate is 173.)

The heart rate is about 70.   (Actual heart rate is 62.)

Figure 27. Six-Second Count Method.

Heart Rate Calculator Ruler Method

A **heart rate calculator ruler** is a device that can be used to determine the heart rate rapidly and accurately. This method is most accurate if the rhythm is regular. Several different kinds of heart rate calculator rulers are available, and the directions supplied with the rulers should be followed.

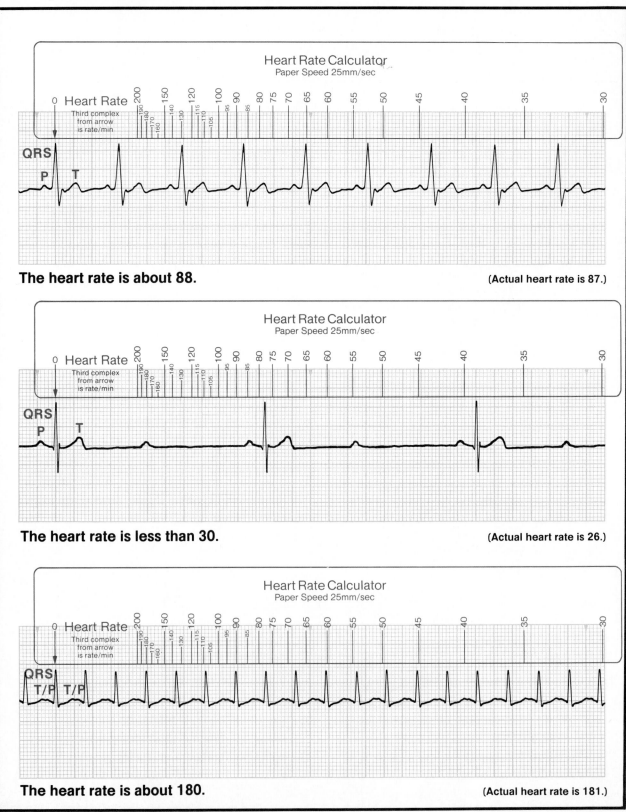

The heart rate is about 88.   (Actual heart rate is 87.)

The heart rate is less than 30.   (Actual heart rate is 26.)

The heart rate is about 180.   (Actual heart rate is 181.)

Figure 28. Heart Rate Calculator Ruler Method.

R-R Interval Method

The **R-R interval** may be used four different ways to determine the heart rate. The rhythm must be regular if the calculation of the heart rate is to be accurate. The four ways are as follows:

1. Measure the distance in seconds between the peaks of two consecutive R waves, and divide this number into sixty to obtain the heart rate.

Example. If the distance between the peaks of two consecutive R waves is 0.56 second, the heart rate is:
$$60/0.56 = 107 \text{ beats per minute.}$$

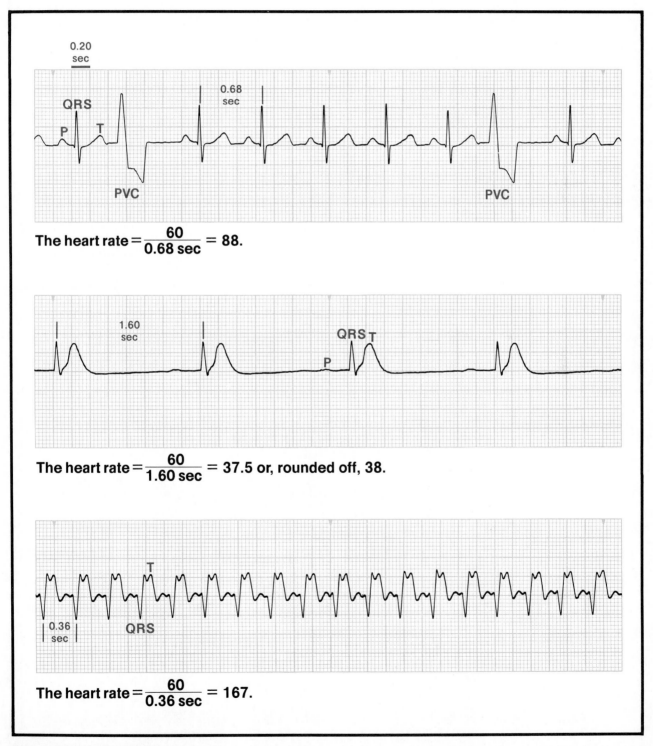

The heart rate $= \dfrac{60}{0.68 \text{ sec}} = 88.$

The heart rate $= \dfrac{60}{1.60 \text{ sec}} = 37.5$ or, rounded off, 38.

The heart rate $= \dfrac{60}{0.36 \text{ sec}} = 167.$

Figure 29. R-R Interval Method 1.

2. Count the large squares between the peaks of two consecutive R waves, and divide this number into 300 to obtain the heart rate.

Example. If there are 2.5 large squares between the peaks of two consecutive R waves, the heart rate is:
300/2.5 = 120 beats per minute.

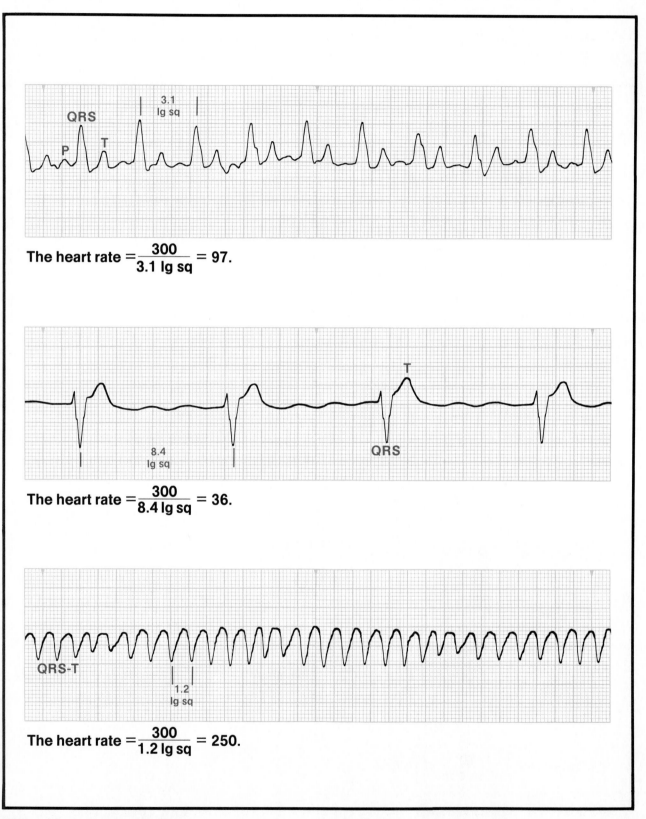

The heart rate $= \dfrac{300}{3.1 \text{ lg sq}} = 97.$

The heart rate $= \dfrac{300}{8.4 \text{ lg sq}} = 36.$

The heart rate $= \dfrac{300}{1.2 \text{ lg sq}} = 250.$

Figure 30. R-R Interval Method 2.

3. Count the small squares between the peaks of two consecutive R waves, and divide this number into 1,500 to obtain the heart rate.

Example. If there are nineteen small squares between the peaks of two consecutive R waves, the heart rate is: 1,500/19 = 78.9 or, rounded off, 80 beats per minute.

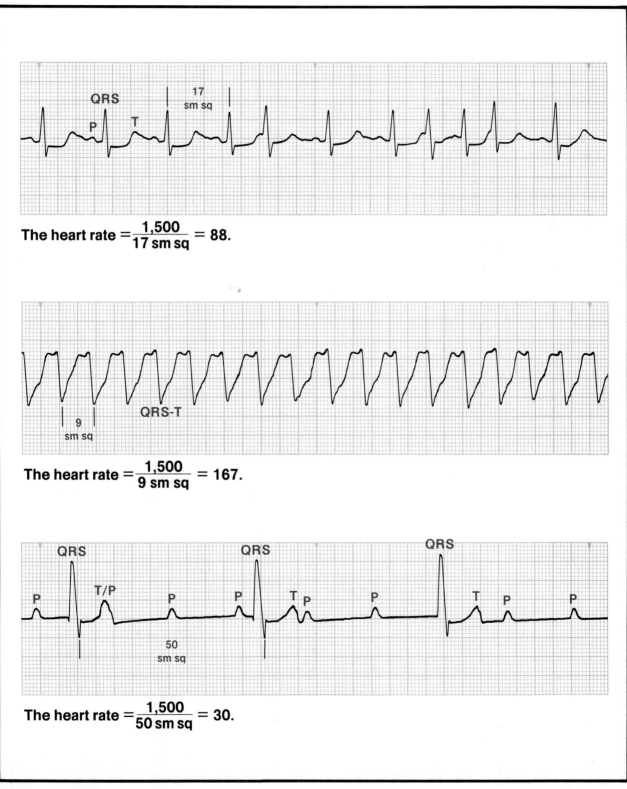

The heart rate $= \dfrac{1,500}{17 \text{ sm sq}} = 88.$

The heart rate $= \dfrac{1,500}{9 \text{ sm sq}} = 167.$

The heart rate $= \dfrac{1,500}{50 \text{ sm sq}} = 30.$

Figure 31. R-R Interval Method 3.

4. Count the small squares between the peaks of two consecutive R waves, and, using a **rate conversion table,** convert the number of small squares into the heart rate.

Example. If there are seventeen small squares between the peaks of two consecutive R waves, the heart rate is 88 beats per minute.

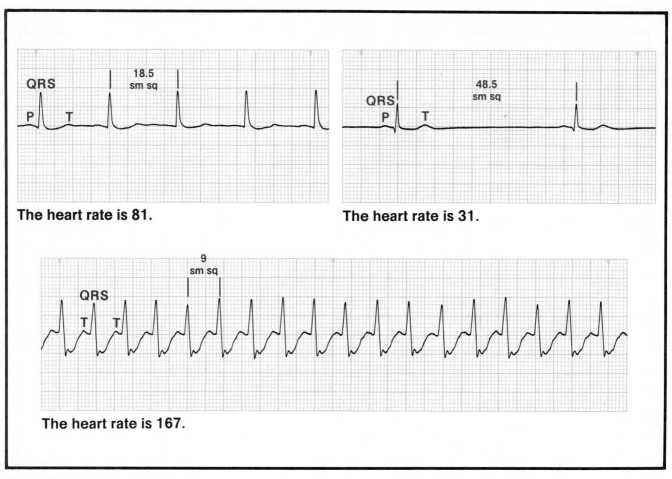

Figure 32. R-R Interval Method 4.

SMALL SQUARES	HEART RATE PER MINUTE	SMALL SQUARES	HEART RATE PER MINUTE	SMALL SQUARES	HEART RATE PER MINUTE
5	300	20	75	35	43
6	250	21	71	36	42
7	214	22	68	37	41
8	188	23	65	38	40
9	167	24	63	39	39
10	150	25	60	40	38
11	136	26	58	41	37
12	125	27	56	42	36
13	115	28	54	44	34
14	107	29	52	45	33
15	100	30	50	46	33
16	94	31	48	47	32
17	88	32	47	48	31
18	83	33	46	49	31
19	79	34	44	50	30

Figure 33. Rate Conversion Table.

Triplicate Method

The **triplicate method** of determining the heart rate will be accurate only if the rhythm is regular.

The heart rate per minute is determined as follows:

1. Select an R wave that lines up with a dark vertical line, and label it "**A.**"

2. Number the next six dark vertical lines consecutively from left to right: "**300,**" "**150,**" "**100,**" "**75,**" "**60,**" and "**50.**" These numbers represent heart rate in beats per minute.

3. Identify the first R wave to the right of the R wave labeled "A," and label this R wave "**B.**"

4. Identify the numbered dark vertical lines on either side of the R wave labeled "**B.**"

5. Estimate the distance of the R wave labeled "**B**" from the nearest of the two adjacent numbered dark vertical lines with respect to the total distance between them, for example, one-quarter, one-third, or one-half of the total distance.

6. Estimate the heart rate by equating the estimated distance of the R wave labeled "**B**" from the nearest adjacent numbered, dark vertical line to beats per minute.

Examples. If the R wave labeled "B" is half way between the "150" dark vertical line and the "100" dark vertical line, the heart rate is about 125 beats per minute.

If the R wave labeled "B" is a third of the way between the "75" dark vertical line and the "60" dark vertical line, the heart rate is about 70 beats per minute.

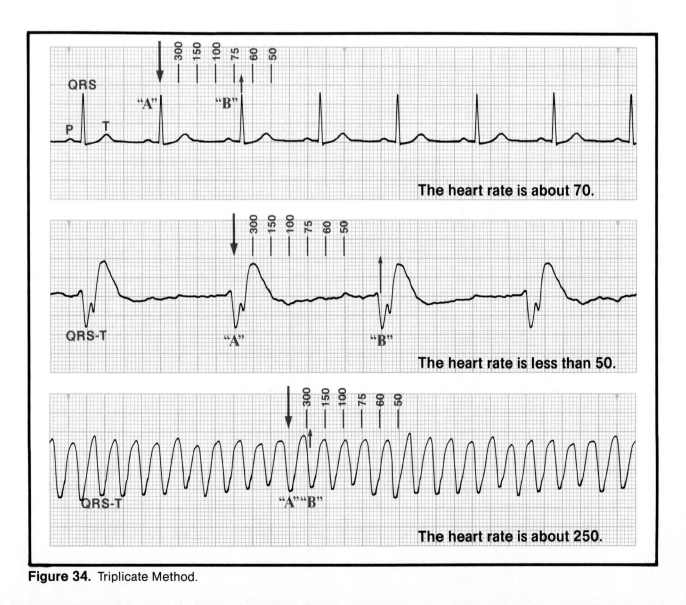

Figure 34. Triplicate Method.

Step Three
Determine the Ventricular Rhythm

The rhythm is determined by comparing the R-R intervals to each other using **ECG calipers** or, if calipers are not available, a **pencil and paper.** First, an R-R interval (preferably one located on the left side of the ECG strip for the sake of convenience) is measured. Second, the R-R intervals in the rest of the strip are compared to the one first measured in a systematic way from left to right.

If ECG calipers are used, one tip of the calipers

is placed on the peak of one R wave; the other is adjusted so that it rests on the peak of the adjacent R wave. Without changing the distance between the tips of the calipers, the other R-R intervals are compared to the R-R interval first measured. If a pencil and paper are used, the straight edge of the paper is placed near the peaks of the R waves and the distance between two consecutive R waves (the R-R interval) is marked off. This R-R interval is then compared to the other R-R intervals in the ECG strip.

If the shortest and longest R-R intervals vary by less than 0.16 seconds (four small squares) in a

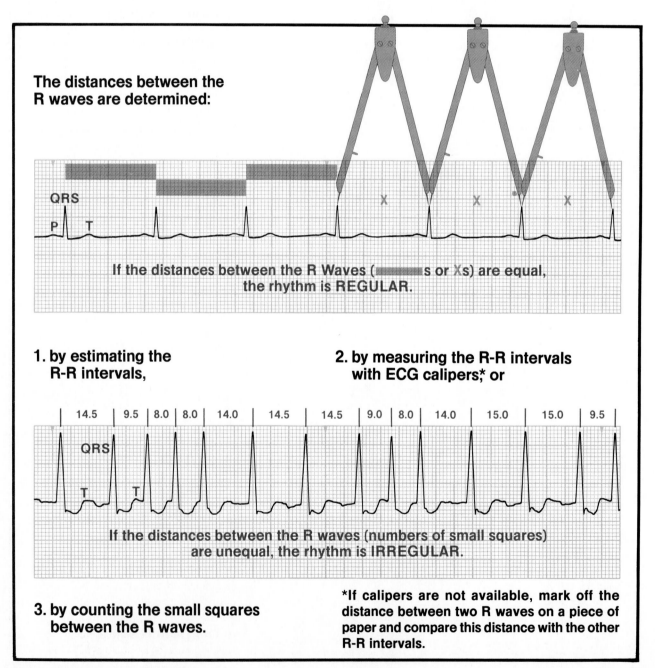

The distances between the R waves are determined:

If the distances between the R Waves (▬▬s or Xs) are equal, the rhythm is REGULAR.

1. by estimating the R-R intervals,

2. by measuring the R-R intervals with ECG calipers;* or

| 14.5 | 9.5 | 8.0 | 8.0 | 14.0 | 14.5 | 14.5 | 9.0 | 8.0 | 14.0 | 15.0 | 15.0 | 9.5 |

If the distances between the R waves (numbers of small squares) are unequal, the rhythm is IRREGULAR.

3. by counting the small squares between the R waves.

*If calipers are not available, mark off the distance between two R waves on a piece of paper and compare this distance with the other R-R intervals.

Figure 35. Determining the Rhythm.

given ECG strip, the rhythm is considered to be "**essentially regular.**" (Thus, the R-R intervals of an "essentially regular" rhythm may be precisely equal or slightly unequal.) If the shortest and longest R-R intervals vary by more than 0.16 seconds, the rhythm is considered to be **irregular.** The rhythm may be **slightly irregular, occasionally irregular, regularly irregular,** or **irregularly irregular.** Other terms to describe an irregularly irregular rhythm are **grossly** and **totally irregular.**

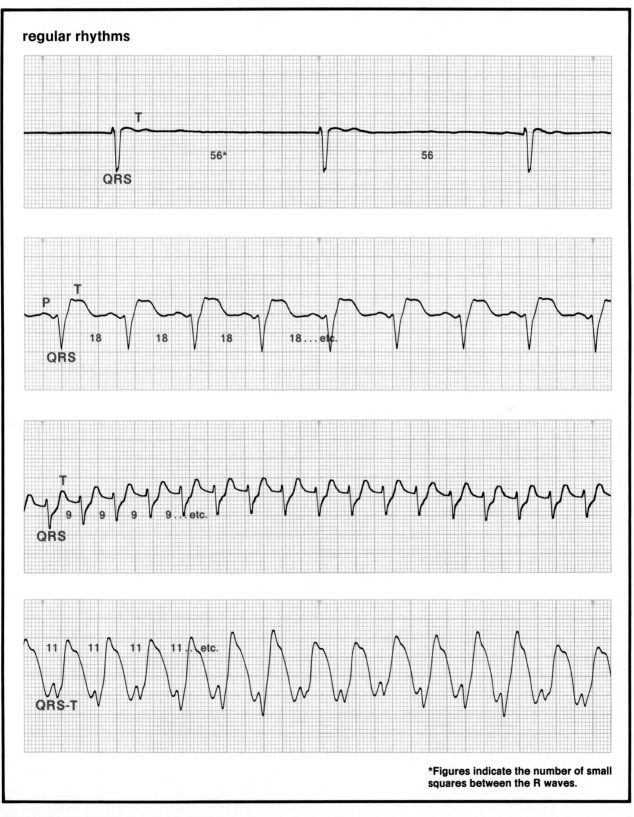

Figure 36. The Different Rhythms.

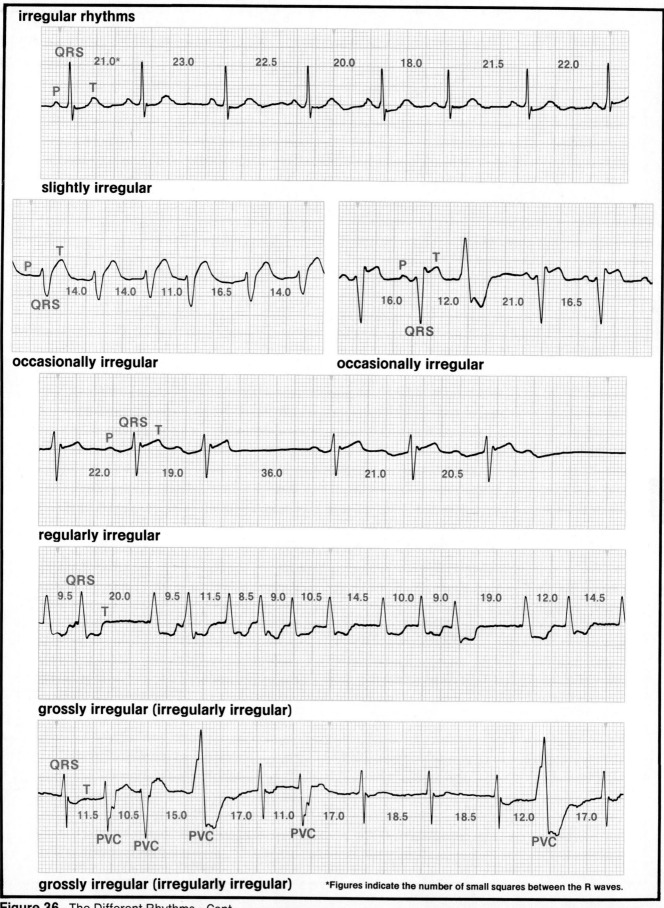

Figure 36. The Different Rhythms—Cont.

Step Four
Identify the P Waves

A normal P wave is a positive, smoothly rounded wave appearing before each QRS complex or singly without a QRS complex following it. It is 0.5 to 2.5 mm high and 0.10 second or less wide.

An abnormal P wave may be positive, negative, or flat (isoelectric); it may be smoothly rounded,

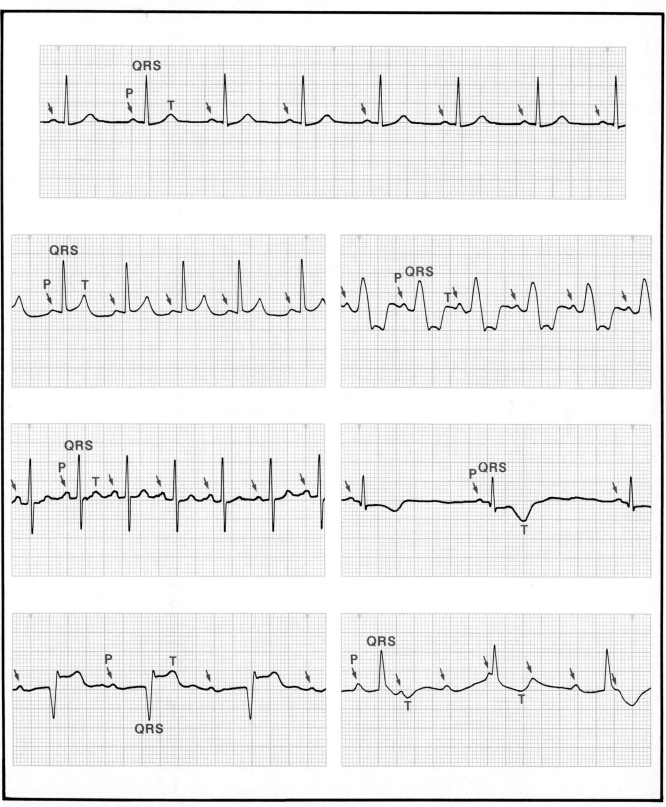

Figure 37. Normal P Waves.

peaked, or deformed and appear before, during, or after each QRS complex or singly without a QRS complex following it. Its height may be normal (0.5 to 2.5 mm) or abnormal (less than 0.5 mm or greater than 2.5 mm). Its duration may be normal (0.10 second or less) or abnormal (greater than 0.10 second).

Determine the atrial rate and rhythm and whether each QRS complex is regularly accompanied by a P wave.

If P waves are absent, determine if **atrial flutter** or **fibrillation waves** are present.

Atrial flutter or **F waves** are typically negative, V-shaped waves followed by positive, sharply pointed atrial T waves in Lead II. The rate of the

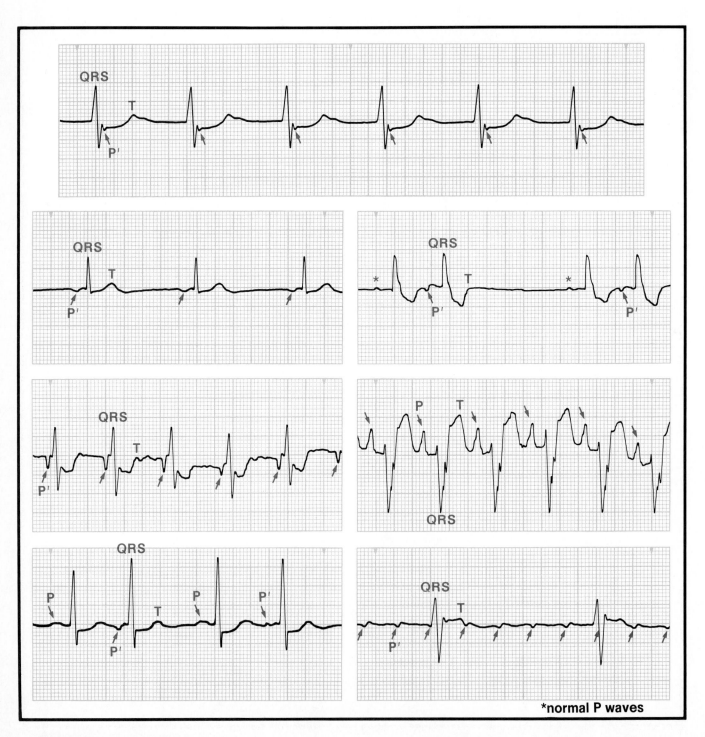

Figure 38. Abnormal P Waves.

F waves is usually between 240 to 350 per minute. QRS complexes commonly occur regularly after every other or every fourth F wave or irregularly at varying F wave-to-QRS complex ratios (**variable AV block**).

Atrial fibrillation or **f waves** are irregularly shaped, rounded, and dissimilar waves. If they are less than 1 mm high, the f waves are called "**fine**" **fibrillatory waves;** if they are greater than 1 mm

high, they are called "**coarse" fibrillatory waves.** If the f waves are extremely fine, they may not be identified as such, and the sections of the ECG between the T waves and QRS complexes may appear only slightly wavy or even flat (isoelectric). The f wave rate is usually between 350 to 600 (average 400) per minute. Typically, in atrial fibrillation, the QRS complexes occur irregularly with no set pattern.

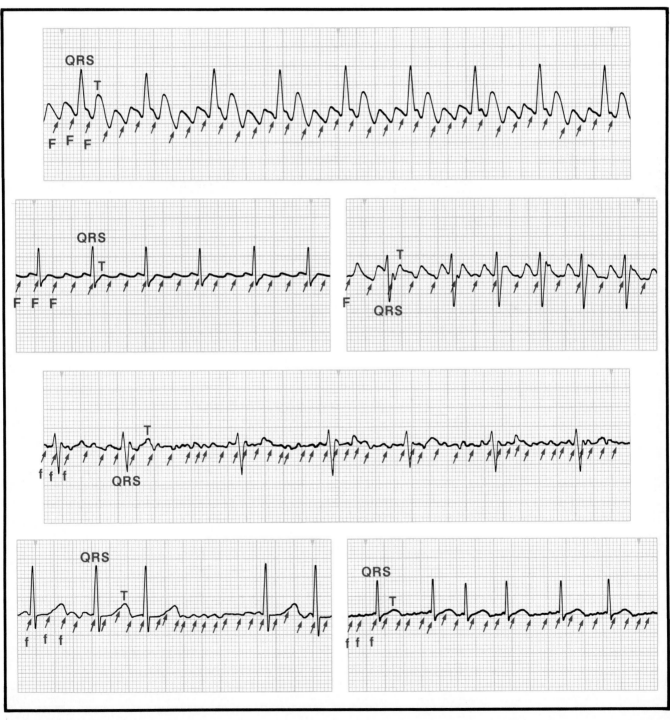

Figure 39. F and f waves.

Step Five
Determine the P-R Interval

The P-R interval is determined by measuring the distance in seconds between the onset of the P wave and the onset of the first wave of the QRS complex, be it a Q, R, or S wave.

A normal P-R interval is 0.12 to 0.20 second in duration and indicates that the electrical impulse causing the P wave originated in the SA node or in an ectopic pacemaker in the upper or middle part of the atria. When the heart rate is fast, the P-R interval is shorter than when the heart rate is slow.

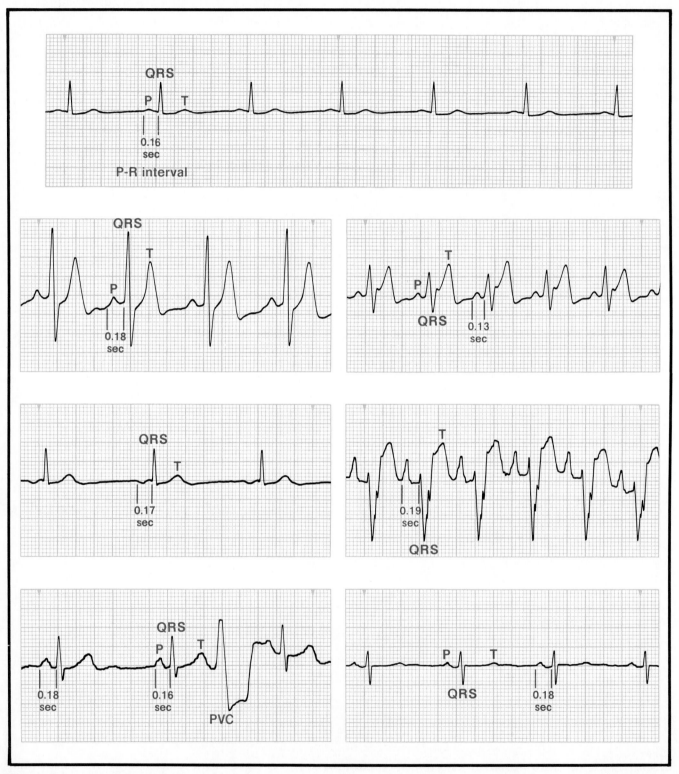

Figure 40. Normal P-R Intervals.

A P-R interval less than 0.12 second or greater than 0.20 second is abnormal. An abnormally prolonged P-R interval indicates a delay in the conduction of the electrical impulse through the AV node or bundle of His (**AV block**). A P-R interval less than 0.12 second indicates that the electrical impulse has originated in an ectopic pacemaker in the lower part of the atria or in the AV junction or that the electrical impulse progressed from the atria to the ventricles through atrioventricular (AV) conduction pathways other than the AV node and bundle of His (**anomalous AV conduction**).

If a P wave follows the QRS complex, an R-P′ interval is present, indicating that the electrical impulse responsible for the P′ wave and QRS complex has originated in an ectopic pacemaker in the AV junction or ventricles. An R-P′ interval is usually 0.20 second or less.

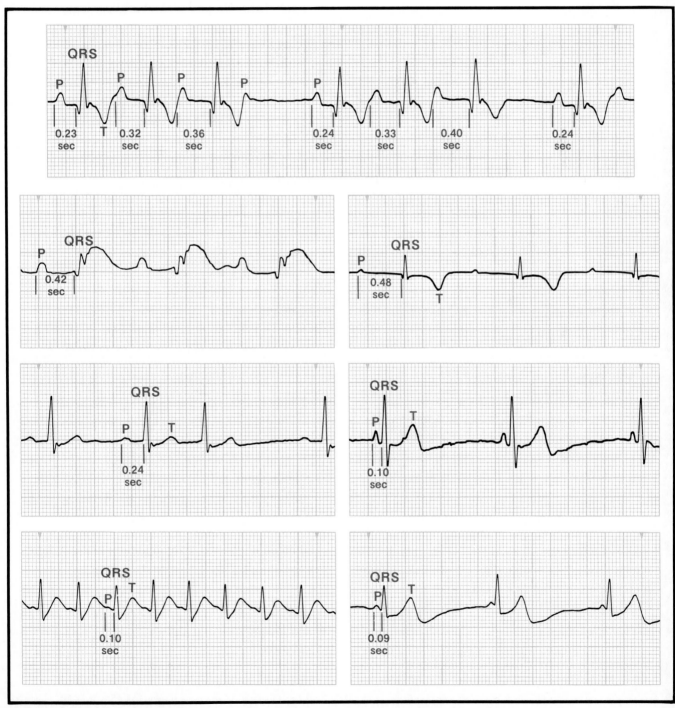

Figure 41. Abnormal P-R Intervals.

Step Six
Determine the Pacemaker Site of the Arrhythmia

If P waves are associated with the QRS complexes —that is, the P waves regularly precede or follow the QRS complexes—the pacemaker site of the arrhythmia is that of the P waves. The electrical impulses causing the P waves may have originated in the SA node or in an ectopic pacemaker in the atria, AV junction, or ventricles. The site of origin of the electrical impulses responsible for the P waves can usually be deduced by noting the direction of the P waves in Lead II, the relationship of the P waves to the QRS complexes, and the P-R interval.

- If the P waves are upright (positive) in Lead II and precede the QRS complexes and the P-R interval is 0.12 to 0.20 second or greater, the electrical impulses responsible for the P waves may have originated in the SA node or in an ectopic pacemaker in the atria. If an anomalous AV conduction is present, however, the P-R interval will be less than 0.12 second.

- If the P waves are negative (inverted) in Lead II and precede the QRS complexes and the P-R interval is less than 0.12 second, the electrical impulses responsible for the P waves may have originated in an ectopic pacemaker in the lower part of the atria near the AV junction or in the upper part of the AV junction.

- If the P waves are negative (inverted) in Lead II and follow the QRS complexes, the electrical impulses responsible for the P waves may have originated in an ectopic pacemaker in the lower part of the AV junction or in the ventricles.

- If the P waves have no set relationship to the QRS complexes, occurring at a rate different from that of the QRS complexes (a condition called **atrioventricular (AV) dissociation**), the electrical impulses responsible for the P waves may have originated in the SA node or in an ectopic pacemaker in the atria.

- If atrial flutter or fibrillation waves are present, the electrical impulses responsible for them have originated in the atria.

Table 4.1—Determination of the Pacemaker Site of Arrhythmias with P Waves Associated with the QRS Complexes

Pacemaker Site	Direction of the P wave in Lead II	P/QRS Relationship	P-R Interval
SA Node OR Atria	Positive (Upright)	P Precedes QRS Complex	0.12-0.20 Sec or Greater OR Less than 0.12 Sec*
Lower Atria OR Upper AV Junction	Negative (Inverted)	P Precedes QRS Complex	Less than 0.12 Sec
Lower AV Junction OR Ventricles	Negative (Inverted)	P Follows QRS Complex	None

*Associated with anomalous AV conduction

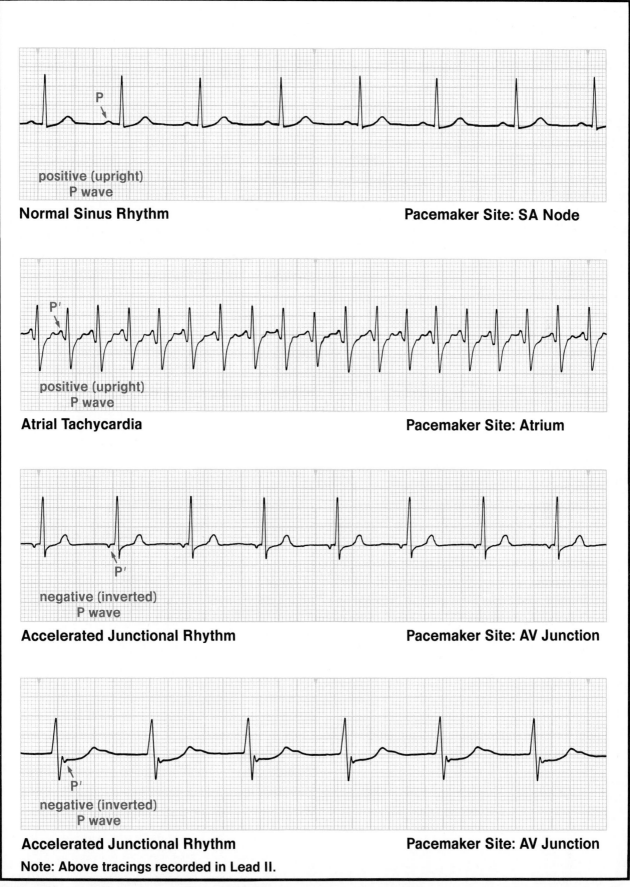

Figure 42. Examples of Arrhythmias with P waves associated with the QRS complexes and their pacemaker sites.

If the QRS complexes have no relationship to the P waves, occurring at a rate different from that of the P waves, or if P waves are absent, the electrical impulses causing the QRS complexes may have originated in the AV junction or ventricles (i.e., bundle branch, Purkinje network, or ventricular myocardium). The site of origin of the electrical impulses responsible for such QRS complexes can be deduced by noting the duration and shape of the QRS complex and whether or not a preexisting bundle branch block or aberrant ventricular conduction is present. Often, the pacemaker site of wide and bizarre QRS complexes, occurring independently of the P waves or in their absence, cannot be determined with accuracy based on an ECG obtained from a single monitoring lead.

- If the QRS complexes are 0.10 second or less in duration, the electrical impulses responsible for the QRS complexes most likely have origi-

nated in the AV junction.

- If the QRS complexes are between 0.10 and 0.12 second in duration, the electrical impulses responsible for the QRS complexes may have originated in the AV junction (in which case, a preexisting incomplete bundle branch block or an aberrant ventricular conduction is present) or in a bundle branch in the ventricles near the bundle of His.

- If the QRS complexes are greater than 0.12 second in duration and appear bizarre, the electrical impulses responsible for the QRS complexes may have originated in the AV junction (in which case, a preexisting complete bundle branch block or an aberrant ventricular conduction is present) or in the Purkinje network or ventricular myocardium.

Table 4.2.—Determination of the Pacemaker Site of QRS Complexes Not Associated with P Waves

Pacemaker Site	QRS Complex Duration	QRS Complex Appearance
AV Junction	0.10 Sec or Less	Normal
AV Junction* OR Bundle Branch	0.10-0.12 Sec	Normal
AV Junction† OR Purkinje Network, Ventricular Myocardium	Greater than 0.12 Sec	Bizarre

*In association with a preexisting incomplete bundle branch block or an aberrant ventricular conduction

†In association with a preexisting complete bundle branch block or an aberrant ventricular conduction

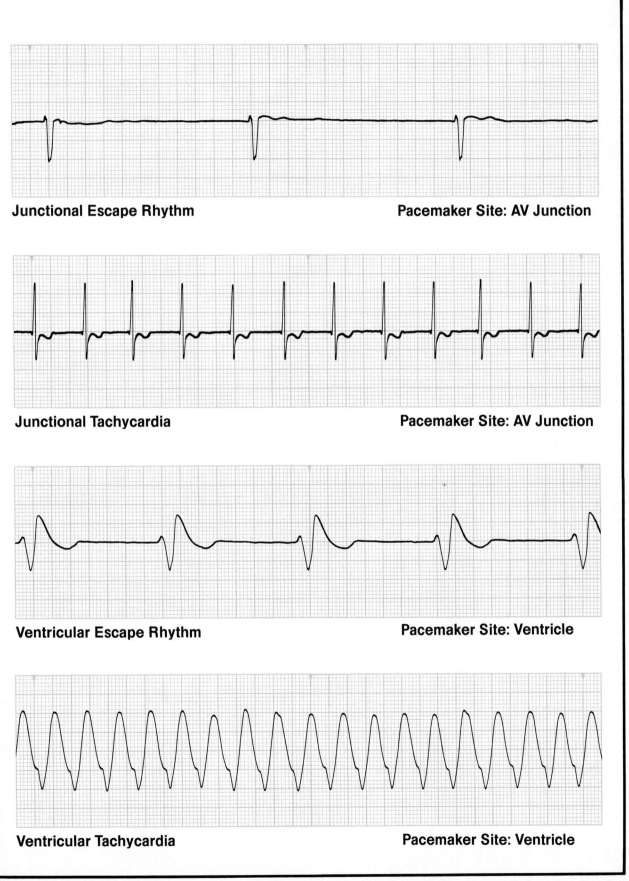

Junctional Escape Rhythm　　　　　　　**Pacemaker Site: AV Junction**

Junctional Tachycardia　　　　　　　**Pacemaker Site: AV Junction**

Ventricular Escape Rhythm　　　　　　　**Pacemaker Site: Ventricle**

Ventricular Tachycardia　　　　　　　**Pacemaker Site: Ventricle**

Figure 43. Examples of Arrhythmias with QRS complexes not associated with P waves and their pacemaker sites.

Step Seven
Identify the Arrhythmia

The identification of arrhythmias is presented in detail in the next chapter, Chapter 5.

Chapter 5

Arrhythmia Identification

Normal Sinus Rhythm (NSR)

Sinus Arrhythmia

Sinus Bradycardia

**Sinus Arrest and
Sinoatrial (SA) Exit Block**

Sinus Tachycardia

Wandering Atrial Pacemaker (WAP)

Premature Atrial Contractions (PACs)

**Atrial Tachycardia (AT)
(Nonparoxysmal Atrial Tachycardia,
Paroxysmal Atrial Tachycardia [PAT])**

Atrial Flutter (AF)

Atrial Fibrillation

Premature Junctional Contractions (PJCs)

Junctional Escape Rhythm

**Nonparoxysmal Junctional Tachycardia
(Accelerated Junctional Rhythm,
Junctional Tachycardia)**

Paroxysmal Junctional Tachycardia (PJT)

Premature Ventricular Contractions (PVCs)

Ventricular Tachycardia (VT)

Ventricular Fibrillation (VF)

Accelerated Idioventricular Rhythm (AIVR)

Ventricular Escape Rhythm

Ventricular Asystole

First-degree AV Block

**Second-degree AV Block
Type I AV Block (Wenckebach)**

**Second-degree AV Block
Type II AV Block**

**Second-degree AV Block
2:1 and High-degree (Advanced) AV Block**

Third-degree AV Block

Pacemaker Rhythm

Normal Sinus Rhythm (NSR)

Heart Rate: The heart rate is 60 to 100 beats per minute.

Rhythm: The atrial and ventricular rhythms are essentially regular.

Pacemaker Site: The pacemaker site is the SA node.

P Waves: The sinus P waves are identical and precede each QRS complex. They are positive (upright) in Lead II.

P-R Intervals: The P-R intervals are normal (0.12 to 0.20 second) and generally constant but may vary slightly with the heart rate.

R-R and P-P Intervals: The R-R intervals may be equal or vary slightly. The difference between the longest and shortest R-R (or P-P) interval is less than 0.16 second in normal sinus rhythm.

QRS Complexes: The QRS complexes are typically normal (0.10 second or less) unless a preexisting bundle branch block is present, in which case, the QRS complexes are abnormal (greater than 0.10 second). A QRS complex normally follows each P wave.

Notes

Normal Sinus Rhythm (NSR)

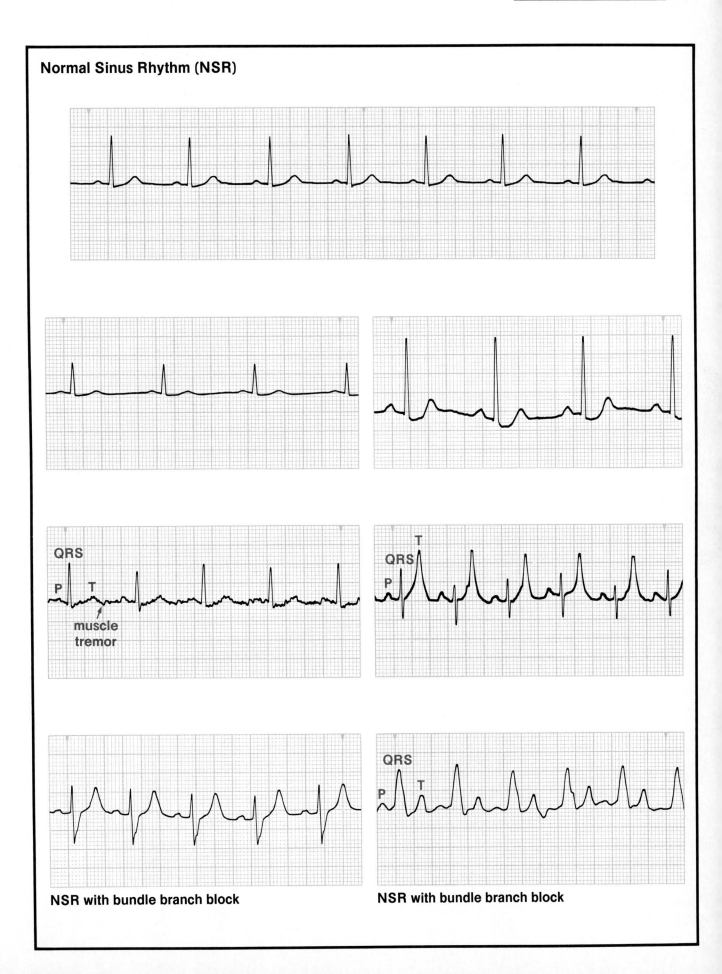

NSR with bundle branch block   NSR with bundle branch block

Sinus Arrhythmia

Heart Rate: The heart rate is 60 to 100 beats per minute. Occasionally, the heart rate may slow to less than 60 and increase to over 100 beats per minute. Commonly, the heart rate *increases* during inspiration and *decreases* during expiration.

Rhythm: The atrial and ventricular rhythms are irregularly irregular as the heart rate gradually increases and slows; the changes in rate occur in cycles.

Pacemaker Site: The pacemaker site is the SA node.

P Waves: The sinus P waves are identical and precede each QRS complex. They are positive (upright) in Lead II. **Sinus arrhythmia** is considered to be present when the difference between the longest and shortest P-P (or R-R) interval is greater than 0.16 second.

P-R Intervals: The P-R intervals are normal and constant.

R-R Intervals: The R-R intervals are unequal. The most common type of sinus arrhythmia is related to respiration in which the R-R intervals become shorter during inspiration as the heart rate increases and longer during expiration as the heart rate decreases. In the other type of sinus arrhyth-mia, the R-R intervals become shorter and longer without any relation to respiration. The difference between the longest and shortest R-R interval is greater than 0.16 second in sinus arrhythmia.

QRS Complexes: The QRS complexes are normal unless a preexisting bundle branch block is present. A QRS complex normally follows each P wave.

Cause of Arrhythmia: The most common type of sinus arrhythmia, the one related to respiration, is a normal phenomenon commonly seen in children, young adults, and elderly individuals and is caused by the inhibitory vagal (parasympathetic) effect of respiration on the SA node. The other, less common type of sinus arrhythmia, unrelated to respiration, may occur in healthy individuals but is more commonly found in adult patients with heart disease, especially following acute myocardial infarction, or in patients receiving certain drugs such as digitalis and morphine.

Clinical Significance: Sinus arrhythmia is usually of no clinical significance per se and does not require treatment. Marked sinus arrhythmia may cause palpitations, dizziness, and even syncope.

Notes

Sinus Arrhythmia

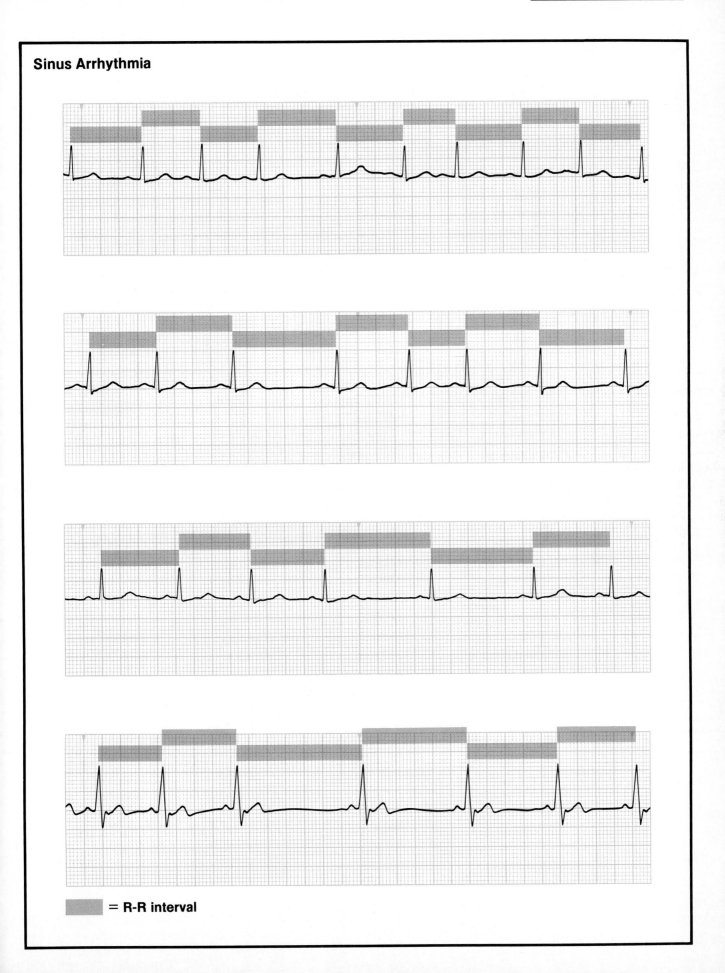

= R-R interval

Sinus Bradycardia

Heart Rate: The heart rate is less than 60 beats per minute.

Rhythm: The rhythm is essentially regular, but it may be irregular if sinus arrhythmia is also present.

Pacemaker Site: The pacemaker site is the SA node.

P Waves: The sinus P waves are identical and precede each QRS complex. They are positive (upright) in Lead II.

P-R Intervals: The P-R intervals are normal and constant. However, they tend to be at the upper limits of normal.

R-R Intervals: The R-R intervals are usually equal but may vary.

QRS Complexes: The QRS complexes are normal unless a preexisting bundle branch block is present. A QRS complex normally follows each P wave.

Cause of Arrhythmia: Sinus bradycardia may be caused by either an excessive inhibitory vagal (parasympathetic) tone or a decrease in sympathetic tone on the SA node, disease in the SA node, myxedema, hypothermia, hypoxia, or administration of digitalis, propranolol, or verapamil. Sinus bradycardia is not uncommon in acute myocardial infarction, especially in an inferior-wall myocardial infarction. Sinus bradycardia may be associated with vomiting and vasovagal syncope and follow carotid sinus stimulation. It is common during sleep and in trained athletes.

Clinical Significance: Sinus bradycardia with a heart rate between 50 to 59 beats per minute (**mild sinus bradycardia**) usually does not produce symptoms by itself. If the heart rate is 30 to 45 beats per minute or less (**marked sinus bradycardia**), hypotension with reduction in cardiac output and decreased perfusion of the brain and other vital organs may occur. This may result in dizziness, lightheadedness, near-syncope, or syncope.

In the presence of acute myocardial infarction, mild sinus bradycardia may actually be beneficial in some patients because of the decrease in the workload of the heart, which reduces the oxygen requirements of the heart, minimizes the extension of the infarction, and lessens the predisposition to certain arrhythmias. Marked sinus bradycardia, however, may result in hypotension with a marked reduction of cardiac output and lead to congestive heart failure, syncope, and shock and predispose the patient to more serious arrhythmias (i.e., premature ventricular contractions, ventricular tachycardia or fibrillation, or ventricular asystole).

Symptomatic or marked sinus bradycardia must be treated promptly to reverse the consequences of reduced cardiac output and to prevent the occurrence of serious ventricular arrhythmias.

Notes

Sinus Bradycardia

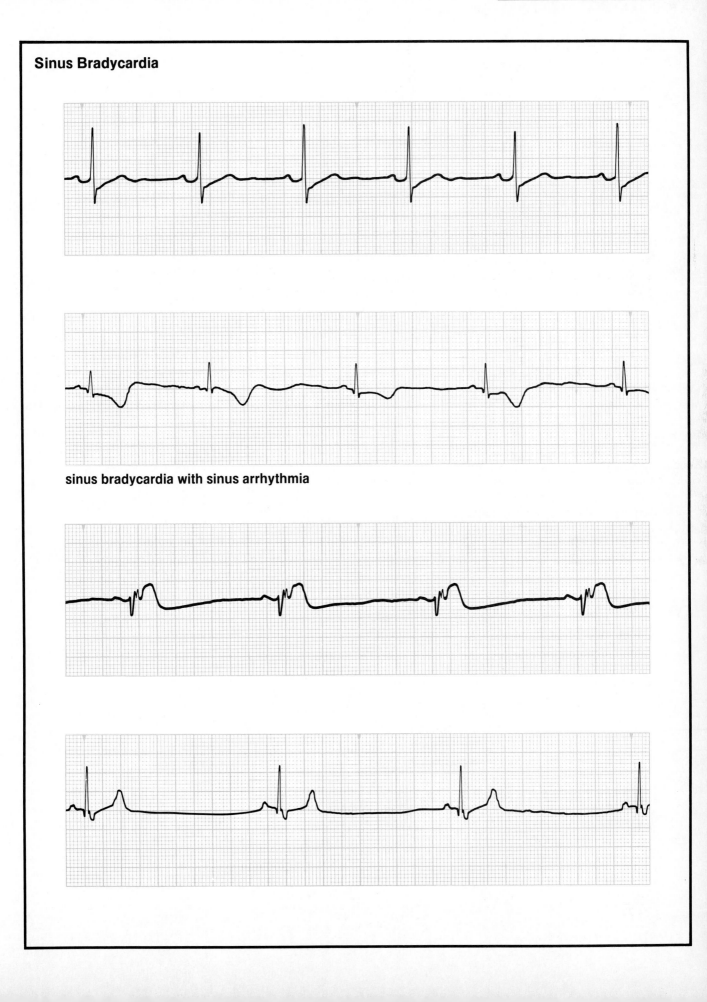

sinus bradycardia with sinus arrhythmia

Sinus Arrest and Sinoatrial (SA) Exit Block

Heart Rate: The heart rate is usually 60 to 100 beats per minute but may be less.

Rhythm: The rhythm is irregular when sinus arrest or SA exit block is present.

Pacemaker Site: The pacemaker site is the SA node.

P Waves: The sinus P waves of the underlying rhythm are identical and precede each QRS complex. If an electrical impulse is not generated by the SA node (**sinus arrest**) or if it is generated by the SA node but blocked from entering the atria (**sinoatrial [SA] exit block**), atrial depolarization does not occur and, consequently, neither does a P wave (**dropped P wave**). Often, it is difficult to distinguish sinus arrest from SA exit block when a dropped P wave occurs. Typically, an SA exit block is indicated by the absence of the normally expected sinus P wave(s) on the ECG. In addition, the long P-P interval caused by SA exit block is twice (or a multiple of) the P-P interval of the underlying rhythm since the underlying rhythm remains undisturbed. The long P-P interval caused by sinus arrest is, typically, not a multiple of the P-P interval of the underlying rhythm since the timing of the SA node is reset by the arrest.

P-R Intervals: The P-R intervals are those of the underlying rhythm and may be normal or abnormal.

R-R Intervals: The R-R intervals are unequal when sinus arrest or SA exit block is present.

QRS Complexes: The QRS complexes are normal unless a preexisting bundle branch block is present. A QRS complex normally follows each P wave.

A QRS complex is absent when a P wave does not occur.

Cause of Arrhythmia: Sinus arrest results from a marked depression in the automaticity of the SA node. SA exit block results from a block in the conduction of the electrical impulse from the SA node into the atria.

Sinus arrest or SA exit block may be precipitated by an increase in vagal (parasympathetic) tone on the SA node, hypoxia, an excessive dose of digitalis or propranolol, hyperkalemia, or damage to the SA node or adjacent atrium (acute myocardial infarction, acute myocarditis, degenerative forms of fibrosis).

Clinical Significance: Transient sinus arrest and SA exit block may have no clinical significance per se if an AV junctional or ventricular escape pacemaker takes over promptly. If an escape pacemaker does not take over, ventricular asystole may result and cause lightheadedness followed by syncope. The signs and symptoms, clinical significance, and management of sinus arrest and SA exit block with excessively slow heart rates are the same as those in symptomatic or marked sinus bradycardia.

Intermittent sinus arrest or SA exit block can, however, progress to prolonged sinus arrest (**atrial standstill**). If a junctional or ventricular escape pacemaker does not take over, ventricular asystole occurs and requires immediate treatment, including external or transvenous cardiac pacing.

Notes

Sinus Arrest and Sinoatrial (SA) Exit Block

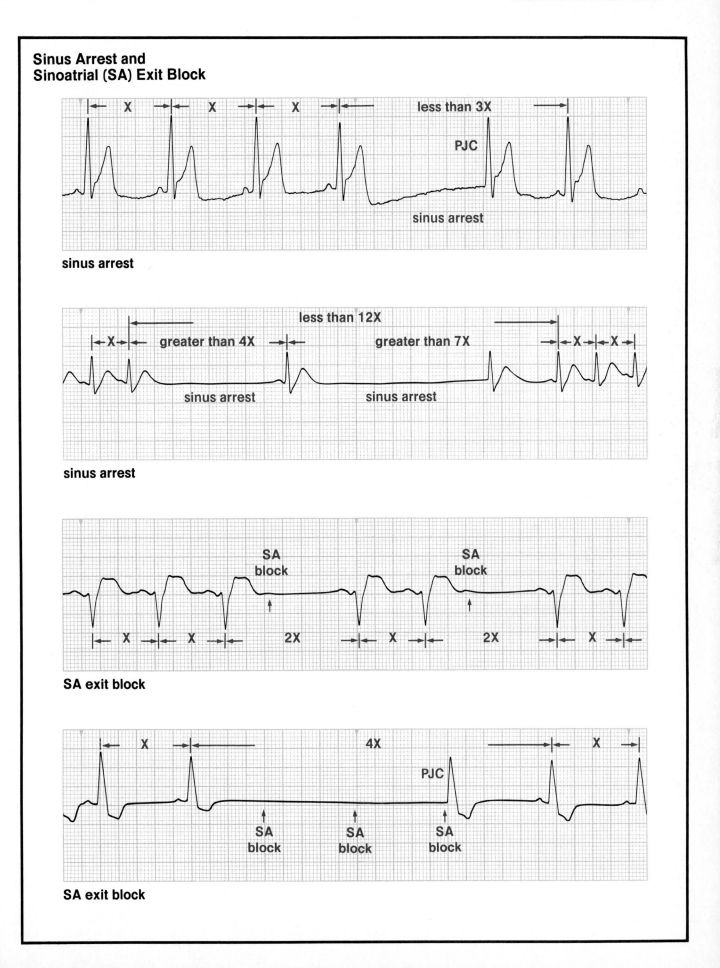

sinus arrest

sinus arrest

SA exit block

SA exit block

Sinus Tachycardia

Heart Rate: The heart rate is over 100 beats per minute and may be as high as 180 beats per minute or greater with extreme exertion. The onset and termination of **sinus tachycardia** are typically gradual. Vagal stimulation causes a gradual slowing of the heart rate, followed by a gradual return to the prestimulation rate.

Rhythm: The rhythm is essentially regular.

Pacemaker Site: The pacemaker site is the SA node.

P Waves: The sinus P waves are usually normal but may be slightly taller and more peaked than usual. The sinus P waves are identical and precede each QRS complex. They are positive (upright) in Lead II. When the heart rate is very rapid, the sinus P waves may be buried in the preceding T waves (**buried P waves**) and not be easily identified.

P-R Intervals: The P-R intervals are normal and constant. They are shorter when the heart rate is fast than when the rate is slow.

R-R Intervals: The R-R intervals may be equal but may vary slightly.

QRS Complexes: The QRS complexes are normal unless aberrant ventricular conduction or a pre-existing bundle branch block is present. A QRS complex normally follows each P wave. Sinus tachycardia with abnormal QRS complexes may resemble ventricular tachycardia (see Ventricular Tachycardia, page 138).

Cause of Arrhythmia: Sinus tachycardia in adults is a normal response of the heart to the demand for increased blood flow, as in exercise and exertion. It may also be caused by the ingestion of coffee, tea, and alcohol or by smoking, an increase in catecholamines and sympathetic tone, anxiety, pain, stress, fever, thyrotoxicosis, anemia. hypovolemia, hypoxia, congestive heart failure, pulmonary embolism, myocardial ischemia, acute myocardial infarction, hypotension or shock, or an excessive dose of atropine or a sympathomimetic drug, such as epinephrine, isoproterenol, and norepinephrine.

Clinical Significance: Sinus tachycardia per se in healthy individuals is a benign arrhythmia and does not require treatment. When its cause is removed or treated, sinus tachycardia resolves gradually and spontaneously. Because a rapid heart rate increases the workload of the heart, the oxygen requirements of the heart are increased. For this reason, sinus tachycardia in acute myocardial infarction may increase myocardial ischemia and the frequency and severity of chest pain, cause an extension of the infarct or even pump failure (e.g., congestive heart failure, hypotension, cardiogenic shock), or predispose the patient to more serious arrhythmias.

Treatment of sinus tachycardia should be directed to correcting the underlying cause of the arrhythmia.

Notes

Sinus Tachycardia

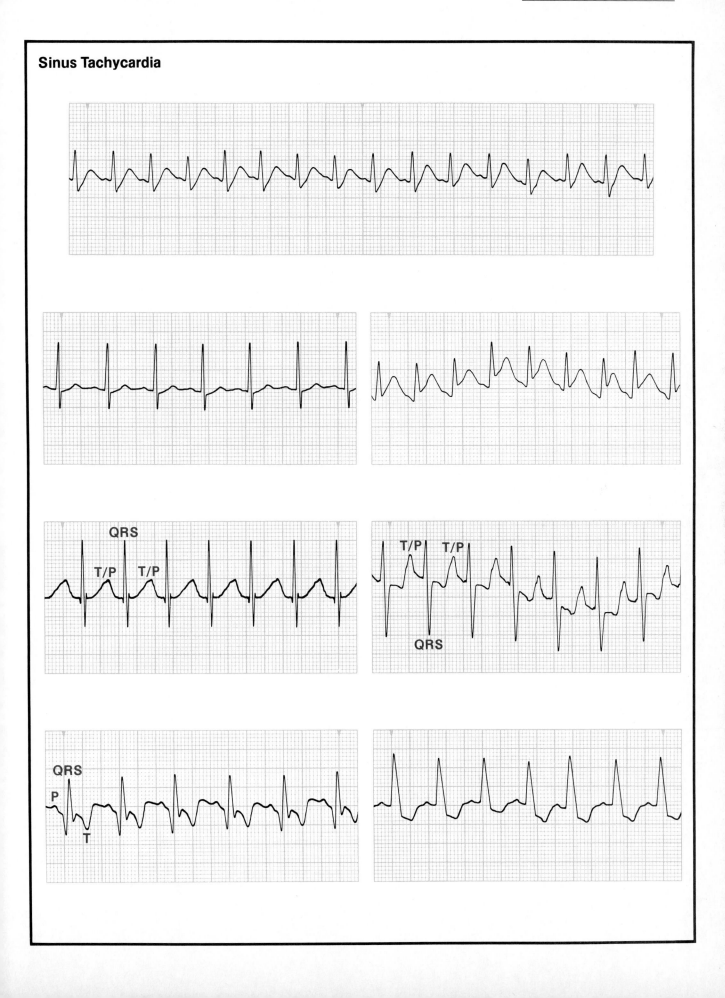

Wandering Atrial Pacemaker (WAP)

Heart Rate: The heart rate is usually 60 to 100 beats per minute but may be slower. Usually, the heart rate gradually slows slightly when the pacemaker site shifts from the SA node to the atria or AV junction and increases as the pacemaker site shifts back to the SA node.

Rhythm: The rhythm is usually irregular, but, rarely, it is regular.

Pacemaker Site: The pacemaker site shifts back and forth between the SA node and an ectopic pacemaker in the atria or AV junction.

P Waves: The P waves gradually change in size, shape, and direction over the duration of several beats. They vary in Lead II from normal, positive (upright) P waves to abnormal, negative (inverted) P waves or even become buried in the QRS complexes as the pacemaker site shifts from the SA node to the atria or AV junction. These changes occur in reverse as the pacemaker site shifts back to the SA node. The P waves other than those arising in the SA node are called ectopic P waves or P' waves.

P-R Intervals: The P-R intervals usually vary from about 0.20 second to about 0.12 second or less as the pacemaker site shifts from the SA node to the atria or AV junction. The duration of the intervals reverses as the pacemaker site shifts back to the SA node.

R-R Intervals: The R-R intervals are usually unequal, but they may be equal. They increase in duration as the pacemaker site shifts from the SA node to the atria or AV junction and decrease as the pacemaker shifts back to the SA node.

QRS Complexes: The QRS complexes are normal unless a preexisting bundle branch block is present. A QRS complex normally follows each P wave.

Cause of Arrhythmia: A **wandering atrial pacemaker** may be a normal phenomenon seen in the very young or the aged and in athletes. It is caused in the majority of cases by the inhibitory vagal (parasympathetic) effect of respiration on the SA node and AV junction. It may also be caused by the administration of digitalis.

Clinical Significance: A wandering atrial pacemaker is usually not clinically significant, and treatment is not indicated. When the heart rate slows excessively, the signs and symptoms, clinical significance, and management are the same as those in symptomatic or marked sinus bradycardia.

Notes

Wandering Atrial Pacemaker (WAP)

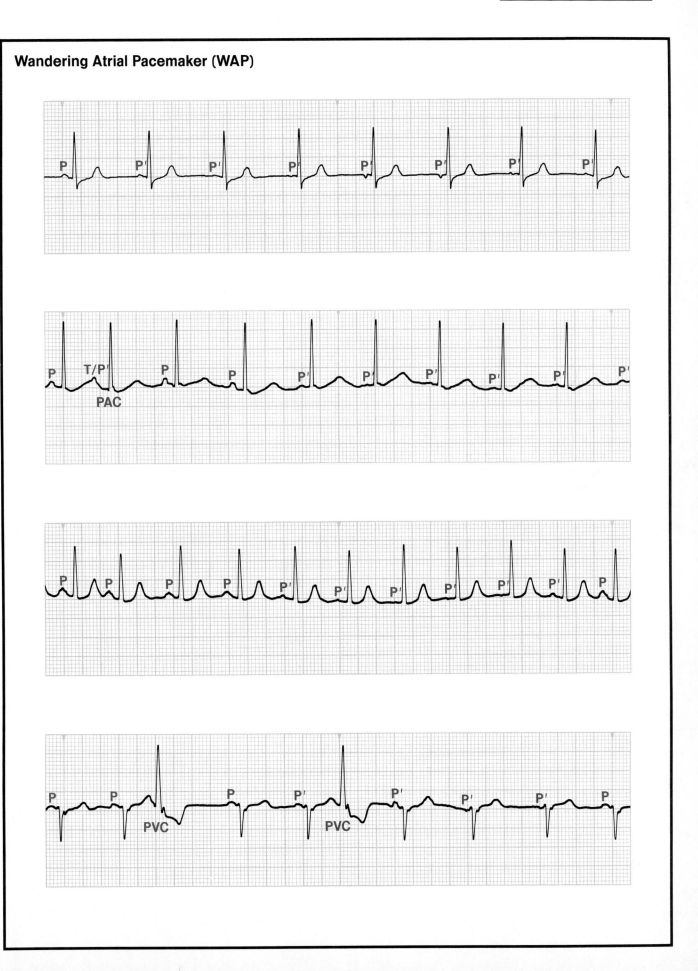

Premature Atrial Contractions (PACs)

Heart Rate: The heart rate is that of the underlying rhythm.

Rhythm: The rhythm is irregular when **premature atrial contractions** (also called premature atrial beats or complexes) are present.

Pacemaker Site: The pacemaker site of the **PAC** is an ectopic pacemaker in any part of the atria outside the SA node. Premature atrial contractions may originate from a single ectopic pacemaker site or from multiple sites in the atria.

P Waves: A premature atrial contraction is diagnosed when a P wave accompanied by a QRS complex appears earlier than the next expected sinus P wave. The premature P wave is called an ectopic P wave (P′). Although the P′ waves of the PACs may resemble the normal sinus P waves, they are generally different. The size, shape, and direction of the P′ waves depend on the location of the pacemaker site. For example, they may appear positive (upright) and quite normal in Lead II if the pacemaker site is near the SA node but negative (inverted) if the pacemaker site is near the AV junction. P′ waves originating in the same atrial ectopic pacemaker are usually identical. The P′ waves precede the QRS complexes and are frequently buried in the preceding T waves, distorting them and often making these T waves more peaked and pointed than the other non-affected ones. A P′ wave followed by a QRS complex is said to be a **conducted PAC.**

If the atrial ectopic pacemaker discharges too soon after the preceding QRS complex, i.e., early in diastole, the AV junction may not be repolarized sufficiently to conduct the premature electrical impulse into the ventricles normally. That is, the AV junction may still be refractory from the preceding beat causing AV conduction to be slowed, prolonging the P-R interval (first-degree AV block), or to be blocked completely (complete AV block). When complete AV block occurs, the P′ wave is not followed by a QRS complex. Such a PAC is called a **nonconducted** or **blocked PAC.** Nonconducted PACs are commonly the cause of unexpected pauses in the ECG, suggesting sinus arrest or sinoatrial (SA) exit block.

The interval between the P wave of the QRS complex preceding the PAC and the P′ wave of the PAC (the P-P′ interval) is typically shorter than the P-P interval of the underlying rhythm. Since the PAC usually depolarizes the SA node prematurely, the timing of the SA node is reset, causing the next cycle of the SA node to begin anew at this point. When this occurs, the next expected P wave of the underlying rhythm appears earlier than it would have if the SA node had not been disturbed. The resulting P′-P interval is called an **"incomplete compensatory pause"** or a **"noncompensatory pause."** This interval may be equal to the P-P interval of the underlying rhythm, or it may be slightly longer because of the depressing effect on the automaticity of the SA node brought on by its being depolarized prematurely **(overdrive suppression).** The interval between the P waves of the underlying rhythm preceding and following the PAC is less than twice the P-P interval of the underlying rhythm.

Less commonly, the SA node is not depolarized by the PAC so that its timing is not reset, and the next P wave of the underlying rhythm appears at the time expected. Such a P′-P interval is said to be **"fully compensatory"** or a **"full compensatory pause."** In this case, the interval between the P waves of the underlying rhythm occurring before and after the PAC is twice the P-P interval of the underlying rhythm. A full compensatory pause may also occur if the automaticity of the SA node is suppressed for a prolonged period following its premature depolarization.

P-R Intervals: The P-R intervals of the PACs may be normal, but they usually differ from those of the underlying rhythm. The P-R interval of a PAC varies from about 0.20 second when the pacemaker site is near the SA node to about 0.12 second when the pacemaker is near the AV junction. The PAC's P-R interval may be greater than 0.20 second if there is a delay in AV conduction (first-degree AV block).

Premature Atrial Contractions (PACs)

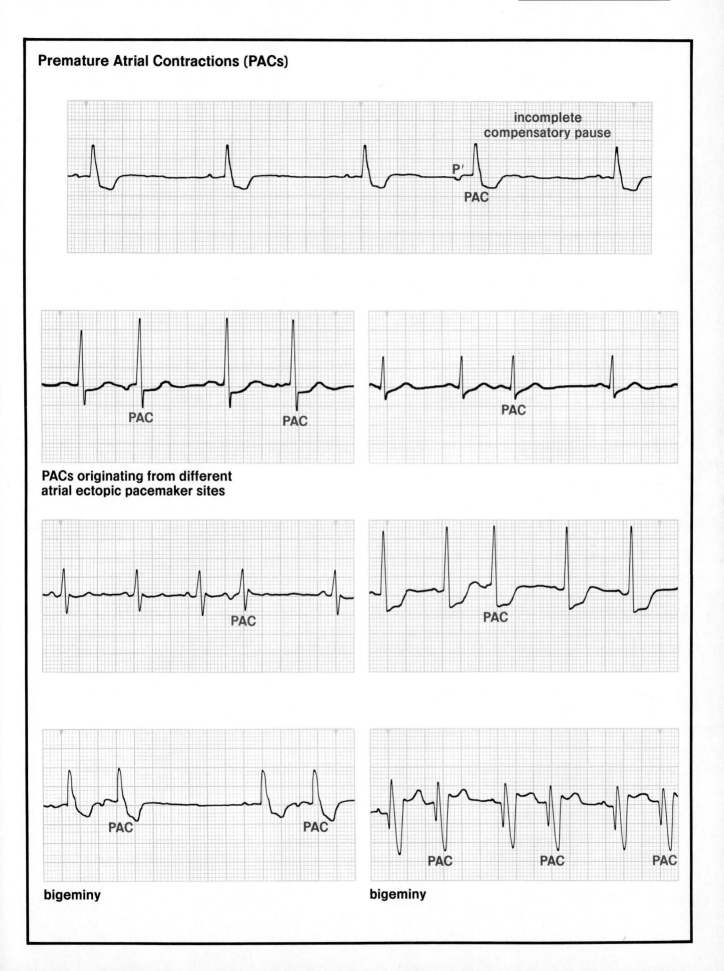

incomplete
compensatory pause

P'

PAC

PACs originating from different
atrial ectopic pacemaker sites

PAC

PAC

PAC

PAC

PAC

PAC

PAC

PAC

PAC

PAC

PAC

bigeminy

bigeminy

Premature Atrial Contractions (PACs)—Cont.

R-R and P-P Intervals: The R-R intervals are unequal when premature atrial contractions are present. The interval between the P wave of the underlying rhythm preceding a PAC and the P' wave of the PAC, the P-P' interval (**coupling interval**), varies depending on the location of the ectopic pacemaker site. The coupling intervals of PACs originating in the same ectopic pacemaker site are similar.

QRS Complexes: The QRS complex of the PAC usually resembles that of the underlying rhythm because the conduction of the electrical impulse through the bundle branches is usually unchanged. If the atrial ectopic pacemaker discharges very soon after the preceding QRS complex, the bundle branches may not be repolarized sufficiently to conduct the electrical impulse of the PAC normally. If this occurs, the electrical impulse may only be conducted down one bundle branch, usually the left one, and blocked in the other, the right,
producing a wide and bizarre-appearing QRS complex that resembles a right bundle branch block. Such a PAC, called a **premature atrial contraction with aberrancy** (or **aberrant ventricular conduction**), can mimic a premature ventricular contraction (see Premature Ventricular Contractions, page 134). Usually, a QRS complex follows each P' wave (**conducted PACs**), but a QRS complex may be absent because of a temporary complete AV block (**nonconducted PAC**).

Types of PACs: PACs may occur as **isolated beats** or consecutively as two or more beats (**group beats**). Two PACs in a row is called a "**couplet.**" When three or more PACs occur consecutively, **atrial tachycardia** is considered to be present. PACs may alternate with the QRS complexes of the underlying rhythm (**atrial bigeminy**) or occur after every two QRS complexes (**atrial trigeminy**) or after every three QRS complexes of the underlying rhythm (**atrial quadrigeminy**).

Cause of Arrhythmia: Common causes of PACs include an increase in catecholamines and sympathetic tone, infections, emotion, stimulants (e.g., alcohol, caffeine, tobacco), sympathomimetic drugs (e.g., epinephrine, isoproterenol, norepinephrine), electrolyte imbalance, hypoxia, or digitalis toxicity. PACs may also be associated with cardiovascular disease (such as myocardial ischemia, acute myocardial infarction, early congestive heart failure) or with dilated or hypertrophied atria resulting from increased atrial pressure commonly caused by mitral stenosis or an atrial septal defect. Often, however, PACs may occur without apparent cause. The electrophysiologic mechanism responsible for PACs is probably enhanced automaticity or a reentry mechanism.

Clinical Significance: Isolated premature atrial contractions may occur in persons with apparently healthy hearts and are not significant. In persons with heart disease, however, frequent premature atrial contractions may indicate enhanced automaticity of the atria or a reentry mechanism resulting from a variety of causes, such as congestive heart failure or acute myocardial infarction. In addition, such PACs may warn of or initiate (especially if digitalis excess is present) more serious supraventricular arrhythmias, such as atrial tachycardia, atrial flutter, atrial fibrillation, or paroxysmal supraventricular tachycardia.

If nonconducted premature atrial contractions are frequent and the heart rate is less than 50 beats per minute, the signs and symptoms, clinical significance, and management are the same as those of symptomatic or marked sinus bradycardia.

Because premature atrial contractions with aberrancy resemble premature ventricular contractions (see Premature Ventricular Contractions, page 134), such PACs must be correctly identified so that the patient is not treated inappropriately.

Notes

Atrial Tachycardia (AT)
(Nonparoxysmal Atrial Tachycardia,
Paroxysmal Atrial Tachycardia [PAT])

Heart Rate: The atrial rate is usually 160 to 240 beats per minute. The ventricular rate is usually the same as that of the atria, but it may be slower, often half the atrial rate because of a 2:1 AV block. **Atrial tachycardia** commonly starts and ends abruptly, occurring in paroxysms (**paroxysmal atrial tachycardia** or **PAT**) which may last from a few seconds to many hours and recur for many years. PAT is usually initiated by a premature atrial contraction. When atrial tachycardia does not start and end abruptly, it is called **nonparoxysmal atrial tachycardia.** By definition, three or more consecutive premature atrial contractions are considered to be atrial tachycardia. Vagal maneuvers, such as carotid sinus massage, by increasing the parasympathetic (vagal) tone, may slow the ventricular rate in nonparoxysmal atrial tachycardia, whereas, it may either terminate paroxysmal atrial tachycardia abruptly or slow it slightly during vagal stimulation.

Rhythm: The atrial rhythm is essentially regular. The ventricular rhythm is usually regular if the AV conduction ratio is constant, but it may be grossly irregular if a variable AV block is present.

Pacemaker Site: The pacemaker site is an ectopic pacemaker in any part of the atria outside the SA node. Atrial tachycardia may occasionally originate in more than one atrial ectopic pacemaker site; one originating in three or more different ectopic pacemaker sites is called **multifocal atrial tachycardia (MAT).** The activity of the SA node is completely suppressed by atrial tachycardia.

P Waves: The ectopic P waves in atrial tachycardia usually differ from normal sinus P waves. The size, shape, and direction of the P′ waves vary, depending on the location of the pacemaker site. They may appear positive (upright) and quite normal in Lead II if the pacemaker site is near the SA node but negative (inverted) if they originate near the AV junction. The P′ waves are usually identical (except in multifocal atrial tachycardia) and precede each QRS complex. In multifocal atrial tachycardia, the P′ waves vary in size, shape, and direction in each given lead. The P′ waves are often not easily identified because they are buried in the preceding T or U waves or QRS complexes. Normal sinus P waves are absent.

P′ Wave-QRS Complex Relationship: The AV conduction ratio in most untreated atrial tachycardias not caused by digitalis intoxication is 1:1 when the atrial rate is less than 200 per minute. When the atrial rate is greater than 200 per minute, a 2:1 AV conduction ratio is common. (A 2:1 AV conduction ratio indicates that for every two P′ waves, one is followed by a QRS complex.) When the AV block occurs only during the tachycardia, the arrhythmia is called **atrial tachycardia with block.** The cause of the AV block is the long refractory period of the AV junction which prevents the conduction of all the rapidly occurring atrial electrical impulses into the ventricles (**physiological AV block**).

If there is a preexisting AV block because of cardiac disease, if digitalis excess is the cause of the atrial tachycardia (e.g., nonparoxysmal atrial tachycardia), or if certain drugs (e.g., digitalis, propranolol, verapamil) have been administered, 2:1 AV block may occur at atrial rates less than 200 per minute. Higher-degree AV block (e.g., 3:1, 4:1, and so forth) or variable AV block may also occur, particularly in nonparoxysmal atrial tachycardia caused by digitalis toxicity.

P-R Intervals: The P-R intervals are usually normal and constant. However, occasionally, the P-R intervals are prolonged (greater than 0.20 second), particularly when the atrial rate is extremely rapid. This occurs when the atrial impulses reach the AV junction while it is in the relative refractory period thereby increasing the AV conduction time. In addition, a preexisting first-degree AV block may be present. A shorter than normal P-R interval may be present when atrial tachycardia is relatively slow or when it occurs in healthy young individuals. In multifocal atrial tachycardia, the P-R intervals usually vary in each given lead.

R-R Intervals: The R-R intervals are usually equal if the AV conduction ratio is constant (i.e., 2:1, 2:1, 2:1, and so forth). But, if the AV conduction ratio varies (as in **atrial tachycardia with varying AV block,** i.e., 3:1, 2:1, 4:1, and so forth), the R-R intervals will be unequal. The R-R intervals will also vary in each given lead if multifocal atrial tachycardia is present.

Atrial Tachycardia (AT)
(Nonparoxysmal Atrial Tachycardia, Paroxysmal Atrial Tachycardia [PAT])

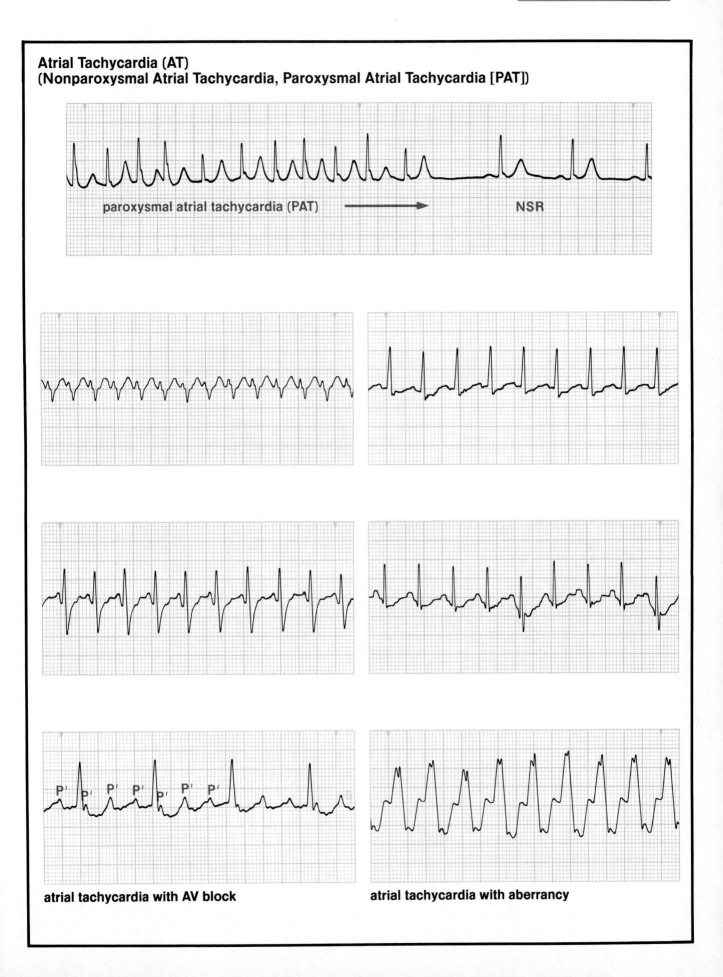

paroxysmal atrial tachycardia (PAT) ⟶ NSR

atrial tachycardia with AV block

atrial tachycardia with aberrancy

Atrial Tachycardia (AT)—Cont.

QRS Complexes: The QRS complexes are normal unless aberrant ventricular conduction or a pre-existing bundle branch block is present. If the QRS complexes are abnormal only during the tachycardia, the arrhythmia is called **atrial tachycardia with aberrancy** (or **aberrant ventricular conduction**). Atrial tachycardia with abnormal QRS complexes may resemble ventricular tachycardia (see Ventricular Tachycardia, page 138).

Cause of Arrhythmia: In general, the causes of atrial tachycardia are essentially the same as those of premature atrial contractions. Nonparoxysmal atrial tachycardia is most commonly caused by digitalis toxicity, in which case, it is often associated with a 2:1 or higher-degree AV block or a varying AV block at relatively slow atrial rates for atrial tachycardia (less than 200 per minute). Atrial tachycardia with AV block may also occur in patients with significant heart disease such as coronary artery disease or cor pulmonale. Multi-focal atrial tachycardia is most often associated with respiratory failure; it is rarely caused by digitalis excess. The electrophysiologic mechanism most likely responsible for nonparoxysmal atrial tachycardia is enhanced automaticity, whereas, for paroxysmal atrial tachycardia it is a reentry mechanism.

Clinical Significance: Atrial tachycardia may occur in persons with apparently healthy hearts. Most often it occurs in patients with rheumatic heart disease, coronary artery disease (especially following an acute myocardial infarction), digitalis toxicity, or preexcitation syndrome.

The signs and symptoms in atrial tachycardia depend upon the presence or absence of heart disease, the nature of the heart disease, the ventricular rate, and the duration of the arrhythmia. Frequently, atrial tachycardia is accompanied by feelings of palpitations, nervousness, or anxiety. When the ventricular rate is very rapid, the ventricles are unable to fill completely during diastole, resulting in a significant reduction of the cardiac output and a decrease in perfusion of the brain and other vital organs. This may cause confusion, dizziness, lightheadedness, near-syncope or syncope, and, in patients with coronary artery disease, angina, congestive heart failure, or myocardial infarction.

In addition, since a rapid heart rate increases the workload of the heart, the oxygen requirements of the heart are usually increased in atrial tachycardia. Because of this, in addition to the consequences of decreased cardiac output, atrial tachycardia in acute myocardial infarction may increase myocardial ischemia and the frequency and severity of chest pain, bring about the extension of the infarct, cause congestive heart failure, hypotension, or cardiogenic shock, or predispose the patient to serious ventricular arrhythmias.

Symptomatic atrial tachycardia must be treated promptly to reverse the consequences of the reduced cardiac output and increased workload of the heart and to prevent the occurrence of serious ventricular arrhythmias.

Note: Since it is often difficult to differentiate between paroxysmal atrial tachycardia and paroxysmal junctional tachycardia when the P′ waves are not clearly evident, the term **paroxysmal supraventricular tachycardia (PSVT)** is commonly used to indicate a paroxysmal tachycardia originating in the atria or AV junction without specifying the exact location of the ectopic pacemaker site.

Notes

Atrial Flutter (AF)

Heart Rate: Usually, the atrial rate is between 240 to 360 (average, 300) **flutter (F) waves** per minute, but it may be slower or faster. The ventricular rate is commonly about 150 beats per minute (half the atrial rate because of a 2:1 AV block) in an **uncontrolled (untreated) atrial flutter** and about 60 to 75 in a **controlled (treated)** one or one with a preexisting AV block. Rarely, the ventricular rate may be over 240 beats per minute, the same as the atrial rate, if the atrial rate is relatively slow and a 1:1 AV conduction ratio is present. Atrial flutter usually responds to vagal maneuvers, such as carotid sinus massage, with a decrease in ventricular rate in stepwise increments.

Rhythm: The atrial rhythm is typically regular, but it may be irregular. The ventricular rhythm is usually regular if the AV conduction ratio is constant, but it may be grossly irregular if a variable AV block is present.

Pacemaker Site: The pacemaker site is an ectopic pacemaker in part of the atria outside of the SA node. Commonly, it is located low in the atria near the AV node. The activity of the SA node is completely suppressed by atrial flutter.

Characteristics of Atrial Flutter Waves (F Waves):

1. Relationship to Cardiac Anatomy and Physiology: An atrial flutter wave represents depolarization of the atria in an abnormal direction followed by atrial repolarization. Depolarization of the atria commonly begins near the AV node and progresses across the atria in a retrograde direction. Normal P waves are absent.

2. Onset and End: The onset and end of the flutter waves cannot be determined with certainty.

3. Components: The flutter wave consists of an abnormal atrial depolarization wave corresponding to an ectopic P wave followed by an atrial T wave (Ta) of atrial repolarization.

4. Direction: The first part of the flutter wave, corresponding to an ectopic P wave, is commonly negative (inverted) in Lead II and followed by a positive (upright) atrial T wave.

5. Duration: The duration varies according to the rate of the flutter waves. At a flutter rate of 300 per minute, the duration of the F waves is 0.20 second.

6. Amplitude: The amplitude, measured from peak to peak of the flutter wave, varies greatly—from less than 1 mm to over 5 mm.

7. Shape: The F waves have a **saw-toothed** appearance. The typical atrial flutter wave consists of a negative (inverted), V-shaped ectopic atrial wave immediately followed by an upright, peaked atrial T wave in Lead II. An isoelectric line is seldom present between the waves. Typically, the first, downward part of the F wave is shorter and more abrupt than the second, upward part. Flutter waves are generally identical in shape and size in any given lead but may vary occasionally. If the flutter waves vary in shape and spacing and their rate is faster than usual, impure flutter (**flutter-fibrillation**) may be present, indicating the presence of atrial fibrillation in one atrium and atrial flutter in the opposite atrium.

8. F Wave-QRS Complex Relationship: The F waves precede, are buried in, and follow the QRS complexes and may be superimposed on the T waves or S-T segments. The AV conduction ratio in most untreated atrial flutters is commonly 2:1. This is because of the long refractory period of the AV junction which prevents the conduction of all the rapidly occurring atrial electrical impulses into the ventricles (**physiological AV block**). (A 2:1 AV conduction ratio, for example, indicates that for every two F waves, one is followed by a QRS complex.) Rarely, the AV conduction ratio in untreated atrial flutter is 1:1. The AV block may be greater (i.e., 3:1, 4:1, and so forth) or even variable because of disease of the AV node, increased vagal (parasympathetic) tone, and certain drugs (e.g., digitalis, propranolol, verapamil).

The AV conduction ratio is usually constant in any given lead, producing a regular ventricular rhythm. If the AV conduction ratio varies, the ventricular rhythm will be irregular. When there is 2:1 or 1:1 AV conduction ratio, the saw-toothed pattern of the F waves may be distorted by the QRS complexes and T waves, making them difficult to recognize. On rare occasions when a complete AV block is present and the atria and ventricles beat independently, there is no set relation between the F waves and the QRS complexes. When this occurs, **atrioventricular (AV) dissociation** is present.

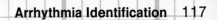

ATRIAL FLUTTER WAVES

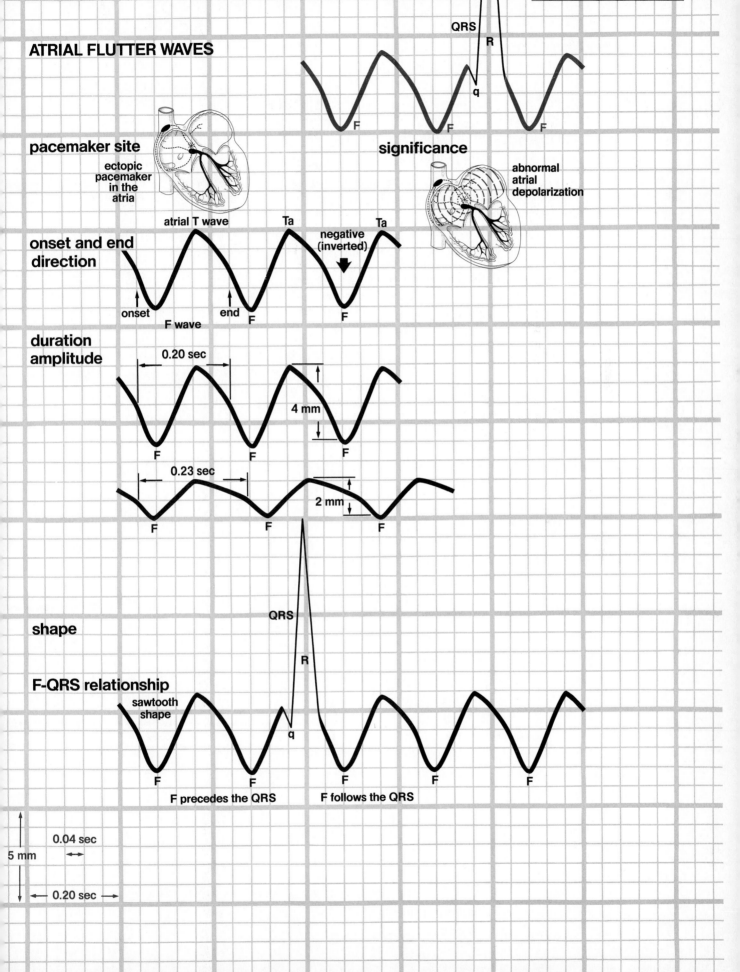

pacemaker site

ectopic pacemaker in the atria

significance

abnormal atrial depolarization

onset and end direction

atrial T wave

Ta

Ta

negative (inverted)

onset

end

F wave

F

F

duration amplitude

0.20 sec

4 mm

F   F   F

0.23 sec

2 mm

F   F   F

shape

QRS

R

q

F-QRS relationship

sawtooth shape

F   F   F   F   F

F precedes the QRS

F follows the QRS

QRS

R

q

F

F

F

0.04 sec

5 mm

0.20 sec

Atrial Flutter (AF)—Cont.

F-R Intervals: F-R intervals are usually equal but may vary.

R-R Intervals: The R-R intervals are equal if the AV conduction ratio is constant, but, if the AV conduction ratio varies, the R-R intervals are unequal.

QRS Complexes: The QRS complexes are normal unless aberrant ventricular conduction or a pre-existing bundle branch block is present. Atrial flutter with a rapid ventricular response and abnormal QRS complexes may resemble ventricular tachycardia (see Ventricular Tachycardia, page 138).

Cause of Arrhythmia: Chronic (persistent) atrial flutter is most commonly seen in middle-aged and elderly persons with advanced rheumatic heart disease, particularly if mitral or tricuspid valvular disease is present, and in those with coronary or hypertensive heart disease. **Transient (paroxysmal) atrial flutter** usually indicates the presence of cardiac disease; however, it may occasionally occur in apparently healthy persons. The arrhythmia may also be associated with the preexcitation syndrome, cardiomyopathy, thyrotoxicosis, digitalis toxicity (rarely), hypoxia, acute or chronic cor pulmonale, congestive heart failure, or damage to the SA node or atria (pericarditis and myocarditis). Atrial flutter may be initiated by a premature atrial contraction. The electrophysiologic mechanism responsible for atrial flutter is probably enhanced automaticity or a reentry mechanism.

Clinical Significance: The signs and symptoms and clinical significance of atrial flutter with a rapid ventricular response are the same as those of atrial tachycardia.

In addition, in 2:1 atrial flutter, in particular, the atria do not regularly contract and empty before each ventricular contraction, filling the ventricles during the last part of diastole, as they normally do. The loss of this **"atrial kick"** results in incomplete filling of the ventricles before they contract, causing a reduction of the cardiac output by as much as 25%.

Notes

Atrial Flutter (AF)

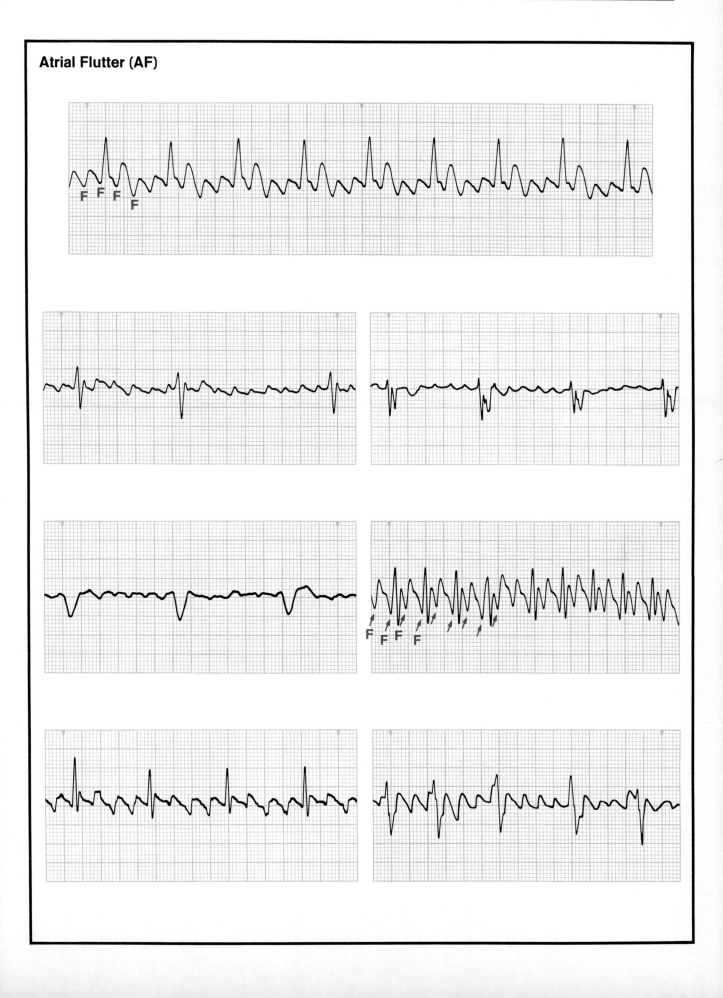

Atrial Fibrillation

Heart Rate: Typically, the atrial rate is 350 to 600 (average, 400) **fibrillation (f) waves** per minute, but it can be as high as 700. The ventricular rate is commonly about 160 to 180 (or as high as 200) beats per minute in an **uncontrolled (untreated) atrial fibrillation** and about 60 to 70 in a **controlled (treated)** one or one with a preexisting AV block. If the ventricular rate is greater than 100 per minute, atrial fibrillation is considered to be "**fast**," and, if it is less than 60, it is considered "**slow**." Carotid sinus massage usually slows the ventricular rate.

Rhythm: The atrial rhythm is grossly (or totally) irregular. The ventricular rhythm is almost always grossly (or totally) irregular.

Pacemaker Site: The pacemaker sites, multiple ectopic pacemakers in the atria outside of the SA node, generate electrical impulses chaotically. The activity of the SA node is completely suppressed by atrial fibrillation.

Characteristics of Atrial Fibrillation Waves (f Waves):

1. **Relationship to Cardiac Anatomy and Physiology:** Atrial fibrillation waves represent abnormal, chaotic, and incomplete depolarizations of small individual groups (or islets) of atrial muscle fibers. Since organized depolarizations of the atria are absent, P waves and organized atrial contractions are absent.

2. **Onset and End:** The onset and end of the f waves cannot be determined with certainty.

3. **Direction:** The direction of the f waves varies from positive (upright) to negative (inverted) at random.

4. **Duration:** The duration of the f waves varies greatly and cannot be determined with accuracy.

5. **Amplitude:** The amplitude varies from less than one millimeter to several millimeters. If the fibrillation waves are small (less than 1 mm), they are called "**fine**" **fibrillatory waves;** if they are large (1 mm or greater), they are called "**coarse**" **fibrillatory waves.** If the f waves are so small or "fine" that they are not recorded, the sections of the ECG between the QRS complexes may appear as a wavy or flat (isoelectric) line.

6. **Shape:** The f waves are irregularly shaped, rounded (or pointed), and dissimilar.

7. **f Wave-QRS Complex Relationship:** The f waves precede, are buried in, and follow the QRS complexes and are superimposed on the S-T segments and T waves. In atrial fibrillation, typically, fewer than one-half or one-third of the atrial electrical impulses are conducted through the AV junction into the ventricles, and these, at random, resulting in a grossly irregular ventricular rhythm. The main reason for this is the long refractory period of the AV junction which prevents the conduction of all the rapidly occurring atrial electrical impulses into the ventricles (**physiological AV block**).

ATRIAL FIBRILLATION WAVES

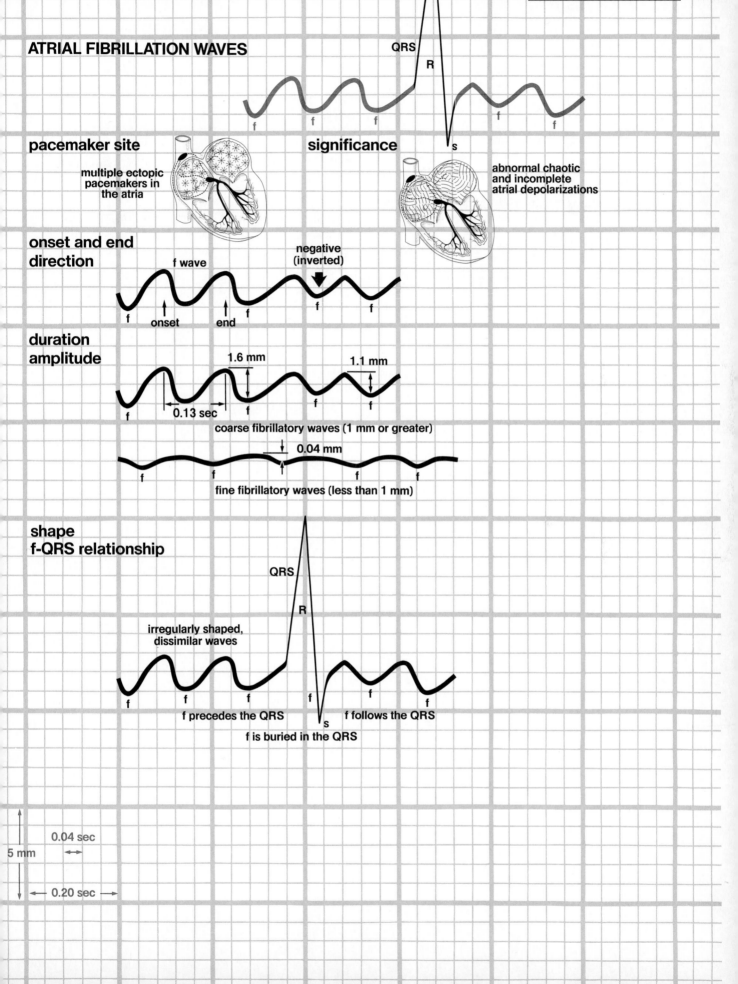

QRS

R

s

f f f f

pacemaker site

multiple ectopic
pacemakers in
the atria

significance

abnormal chaotic
and incomplete
atrial depolarizations

onset and end
direction

f wave

negative
(inverted)

f f f f

onset   end

duration
amplitude

1.6 mm

1.1 mm

f f f

0.13 sec

coarse fibrillatory waves (1 mm or greater)

0.04 mm

f f f f f

fine fibrillatory waves (less than 1 mm)

shape
f-QRS relationship

QRS

R

irregularly shaped,
dissimilar waves

f f f f f

f precedes the QRS   f follows the QRS

s

f is buried in the QRS

0.04 sec

5 mm

0.20 sec

Atrial Fibrillation—Cont.

R-R Intervals: The R-R intervals are typically unequal.

QRS Complexes: The QRS complexes are normal unless aberrant ventricular conduction or a pre-existing bundle branch block is present. Atrial fibrillation with a rapid ventricular response and 4bnormal QRS complexes may resemble ventricular tachycardia, except for the irregular rhythm (see Ventricular Tachycardia, page 138).

Cause of Arrhythmia: Atrial fibrillation is commonly associated with advanced rheumatic heart disease (particularly with mitral stenosis), hypertensive or coronary heart disease (with or without acute myocardial infarction), and thyrotoxicosis. Less commonly, atrial fibrillation may occur in cardiomyopathy, acute myocarditis and pericarditis, chest trauma, and the preexcitation syndrome; it is rarely caused by digitalis toxicity. Whatever the underlying form of heart disease, atrial fibrillation is commonly associated with congestive heart failure. In a small percentage of cases, atrial fibrillation may occur in apparently normal individuals following excessive ingestion of alcohol and caffeine, during emotional stress, and sometimes without any apparent cause. Atrial fibrillation may be intermittent, even occurring in paroxysms as does paroxysmal atrial tachycardia, or it may be chronic (persistent). The electrophysiologic mechanism responsible for atrial fibrillation is probably enhanced automaticity or a reentry mechanism.

Clinical Significance: The signs and symptoms and clinical significance of atrial fibrillation with a rapid ventricular response are the same as those of atrial tachycardia.

In addition, in atrial fibrillation, the atria do not regularly contract and empty, filling the ventricles during the last part of diastole, as they normally do. The loss of this **"atrial kick"** results in incomplete filling of the ventricles before they contract, causing a reduction of the cardiac output by as much as 25%.

Notes

Atrial Fibrillation

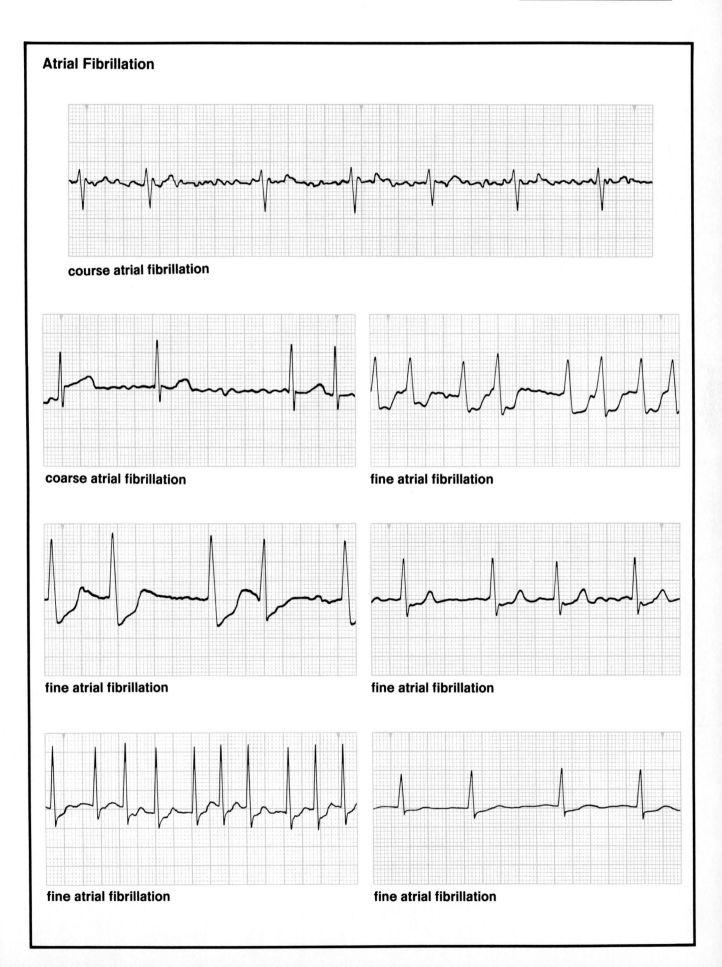

course atrial fibrillation

coarse atrial fibrillation

fine atrial fibrillation

fine atrial fibrillation

fine atrial fibrillation

fine atrial fibrillation

fine atrial fibrillation

Premature Junctional Contractions (PJCs)

Heart Rate: The heart rate is that of the underlying rhythm.

Rhythm: The rhythm is irregular when **premature junctional contractions** (also called premature junctional beats or complexes) are present.

Pacemaker Site: The pacemaker site of the **PJC** is an ectopic pacemaker in the AV junction.

P Waves: P waves may or may not be associated with the PJCs. If they are present, they are abnormal, varying in size, shape, and direction from normal P waves. The P′ waves may precede, be buried in, or, less commonly, follow the QRS complexes of the PJCs. A P′ wave that occurs before the QRS complex has most likely originated in the upper part of the AV junction, whereas one occurring during or after the QRS complex, in the middle or lower part of the AV junction, respectively. If the P′ waves precede the QRS complexes, they may be buried in the preceding T waves, distorting them. If the P′ waves follow the QRS complexes, they are usually found in the ST segments. Since atrial depolarization occurs in a retrograde fashion, the P′ waves that precede or follow the QRS complexes are negative (inverted) in Lead II. Absent P′ waves indicate that either (1) **retrograde atrial depolarizations** occurred during the QRS complexes or (2) atrial depolarizations have not occurred because of a **retrograde AV block** between the ectopic pacemaker site in the AV junction and the atria.

If the ectopic pacemaker in the AV junction discharges too soon after the preceding QRS complex, the premature P′ wave may not be followed by a QRS complex because the bundle of His or bundle branches may not be repolarized sufficiently to conduct an electrical wave into the ventricles (**nonconducted PJC**).

P-R Intervals: If the P′ waves of the PJCs precede the QRS complexes, the P′-R intervals are usually abnormal (less than 0.12 second). Rarely, the P′-R interval may be normal (0.12 to 0.20 second) or even prolonged (greater than 0.20 second) if there is a delay in the AV conduction (first-degree AV block) below the ectopic pacemaker site. If the P′ waves follow the QRS complexes, the R-P′ intervals are usually less than 0.20 second.

Premature Junctional Contractions (PJCs)

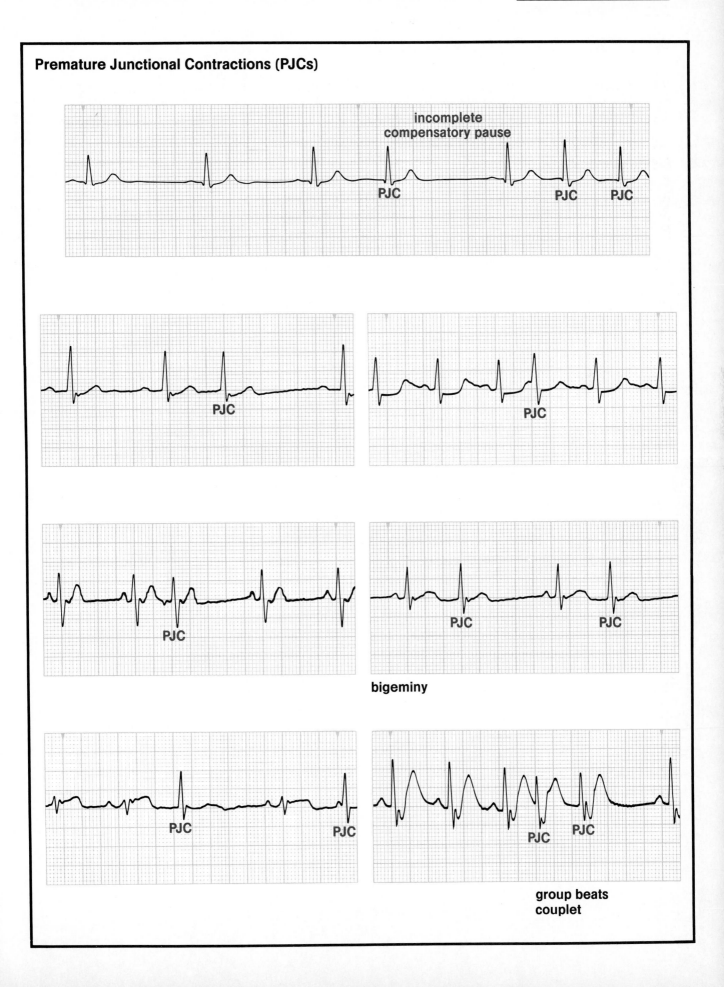

incomplete
compensatory pause

PJC

PJC PJC

PJC

PJC

PJC

PJC PJC

bigeminy

PJC PJC

PJC PJC

group beats
couplet

Premature Junctional Contractions (PJCs)—Cont.

R-R Intervals: The R-R intervals are unequal when premature junctional contractions are present. The interval between the PJC and the preceding QRS complex (the pre-PJC interval) is shorter than the R-R interval of the underlying rhythm. A **full compensatory pause** commonly follows a PJC since the SA node is usually not depolarized by the PJC. Less commonly, the SA node is depolarized by the PJC, resulting in an **incomplete compensatory pause.** (See the discussion of full and incomplete compensatory pause under Premature Atrial Contractions, page 108).

QRS Complexes: The QRS complex of the PJC usually resembles that of the underlying rhythm. If the ectopic pacemaker in the AV junction discharges too soon after the preceding QRS complex, the bundle branches may not be repolarized sufficiently to conduct the electrical impulse of the PJC normally. If this occurs, the electrical impulse may only be conducted down one bundle branch, usually the left one, and blocked in the other, the right, producing a wide and bizarre-appearing QRS complex that resembles a right bundle branch block. Such a premature junctional contraction, called a **premature junctional contraction with aberrancy** (or **aberrant ventricular conduction**), can mimic a premature ventricular contraction (see Premature Ventricular Contractions, page 134). Usually, a QRS complex follows each premature P′ wave (**conducted PJC**), but a QRS complex may be absent because of a transient complete AV block below the ectopic pacemaker site in the AV junction (**nonconducted PJC**).

Types of PJCs: PJCs may occur as **isolated beats** or consecutively as two or more beats (**group beats**). Two PJCs in a row is called a "**couplet.**" When three or more PJCs occur consecutively, **junctional tachycardia** is considered to be present. PJCs may alternate with the QRS complexes of the underlying rhythm (**bigeminy**) or occur after every two QRS complexes (**trigeminy**) or after every three QRS complexes (**quadrigeminy**) of the underlying rhythm.

Cause of Arrhythmia: Occasional PJCs may occur in a healthy person without apparent cause, but most commonly they are a result of digitalis toxicity and enhanced automaticity of the AV junction. Other causes are an increase in vagal (parasympathetic) tone on the SA node, an excessive dose of certain cardiac drugs (e.g., quinidine, procainamide) or sympathomimetic drugs (e.g., epinephrine, isoproterenol, norepinephrine), hypoxia, congestive heart failure, or damage to the AV junction. The electrophysiologic mechanism responsible for premature junctional contractions is probably enhanced automaticity or a reentry mechanism.

Clinical Significance: Isolated premature junctional contractions are not significant. However, if digitalis is being administered, premature junctional contractions may indicate digitalis toxicity and enhanced automaticity of the AV junction. Frequent premature junctional contractions, more than four to six per minute, may indicate an enhanced automaticity or a reentry mechanism in the AV junction and warn of the appearance of more serious junctional arrhythmias.

Because premature junctional contractions with aberrancy resemble premature ventricular contractions (see Premature Ventricular Contractions, page 134), such PJCs must be correctly identified so that the patient is not treated inappropriately.

Notes

Junctional Escape Rhythm

Heart Rate: The heart rate is typically 40 to 60 beats per minute, but it may be less.

Rhythm: The ventricular rhythm is essentially regular.

Pacemaker Site: The pacemaker site is an escape pacemaker in the AV junction.

P Waves: P waves may be present or absent. If P waves are present but have no relation to the QRS complexes of the **junctional escape rhythm,** appearing independently at a rate different (typically slower) from that of the junctional rhythm, the pacemaker site is the SA node or an ectopic pacemaker in the atria. These P waves are usually positive (upright) in Lead II. When the P waves occur independently of the QRS complexes, **atrioventricular (AV) dissociation** is present.

If the P waves regularly precede or follow the QRS complexes and are identical, the electrical impulses responsible for them have originated in the pacemaker site of the junctional escape rhythm. Such P′ waves differ from normal P waves in size, shape, and direction. Since the atria depolarize retrogradedly when the electrical impulses arise in the AV junction, the P′ waves are negative (inverted) in Lead II.

P′ waves are absent in junctional escape rhythm if the P′ waves occur during the QRS complexes or if atrial flutter or atrial fibrillation is the underlying atrial rhythm and an AV block is present.

P-R Intervals: If the P′ waves regularly precede the QRS complexes, the P′-R intervals are abnormal (less than 0.12 second). If the P′ waves regularly follow the QRS complexes, the R-P′ intervals are usually less than 0.20 second.

R-R Intervals: The R-R intervals are usually equal.

QRS Complexes: The QRS complexes are normal unless a preexisting bundle branch block is present. Junctional escape rhythm with abnormal QRS complexes may resemble ventricular escape rhythm.

Cause of Arrhythmia: Junctional escape rhythm is a normal response of the AV junction when the rate of impulse formation of the dominant pacemaker (usually the SA node) becomes less than that of the escape pacemaker in the AV junction or when the electrical impulses from the SA node or atria fail to reach the AV junction because of a sinus arrest, sinoatrial (SA) exit block, or third-degree (complete) AV block. Generally, when an electrical impulse fails to arrive at the AV junction within approximately 1.0 to 1.5 seconds, the escape pacemaker in the AV junction begins to generate electrical impulses at its inherent firing rate of 40 to 60 beats per minute.

Clinical Significance: The signs and symptoms and clinical significance of junctional escape rhythm are the same as those in symptomatic or marked sinus bradycardia. Symptomatic junctional escape rhythm must be treated promptly to reverse the consequences of the reduced cardiac output.

Notes

Junctional Escape Rhythm

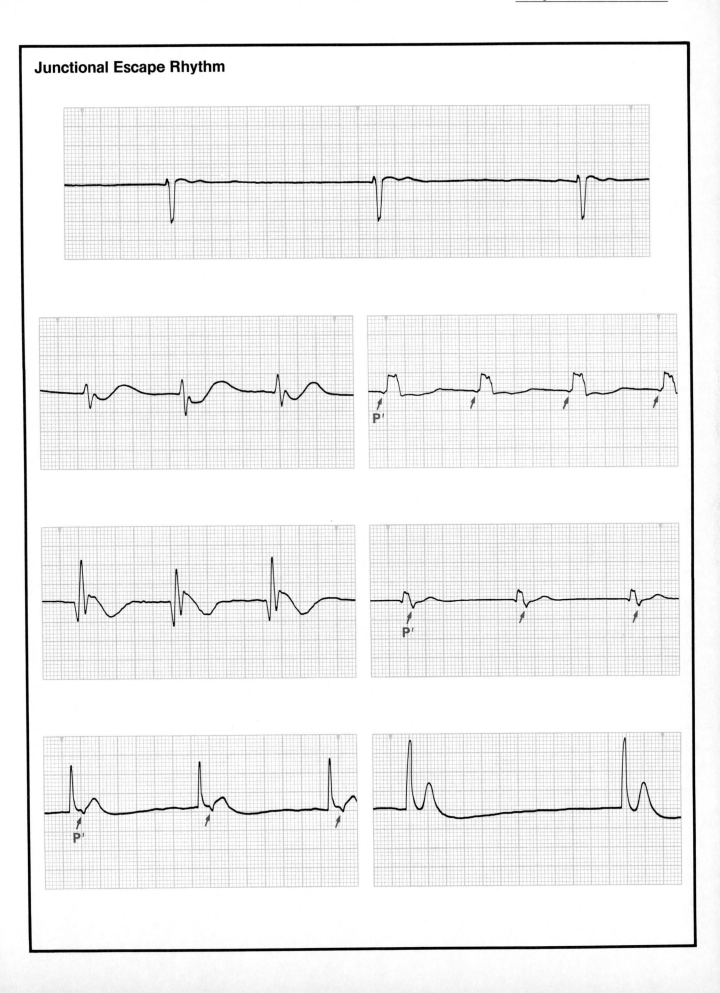

Nonparoxysmal Junctional Tachycardia (Accelerated Junctional Rhythm, Junctional Tachycardia)

Heart Rate: The heart rate is usually 60 to 130 beats per minute, but it may be greater than 130 beats per minute and as high as 150. **Nonparoxysmal junctional tachycardia** with a heart rate between 60 and 100 beats per minute is commonly called **accelerated junctional rhythm;** and one with a rate greater than 100 beats per minute, **junctional tachycardia.** The onset and termination of nonparoxysmal junctional tachycardia are usually gradual.

Rhythm: The rhythm is essentially regular.

Pacemaker Site: The pacemaker site is an ectopic pacemaker in the AV junction.

P Waves: P waves may be present or absent. If present, they may have no relation to the QRS complexes of the nonparoxysmal junctional tachycardia, appearing independently at a rate different from that of the junctional rhythm. The pacemaker site of such P waves is the SA node or an ectopic pacemaker in the atria. These P waves are usually positive (upright) in Lead II. When the P waves occur independently of the QRS complexes, **atrioventricular (AV) dissociation** is present.

If the P waves are identical and regularly precede or follow the QRS complexes, the electrical impulses responsible for them have originated in the pacemaker site of the nonparoxysmal junctional tachycardia. Such P′ waves differ from normal P waves in size, shape, and direction. Since the atria depolarize retrogradedly when the electrical impulses arise in the AV junction, the P′ waves are negative (inverted) in Lead II.

P waves are absent in nonparoxysmal junctional tachycardia if the P′ waves occur during the QRS complex or if atrial flutter or atrial fibrillation is the underlying atrial rhythm and an AV block is present.

P-R Intervals: If the P′ waves regularly precede the QRS complexes, the P′-R intervals are abnormal (less than 0.12 second). If the P′ waves regularly follow the QRS complexes, the R-P′ intervals are usually less than 0.20 second.

R-R Intervals: The R-R intervals are usually equal.

QRS Complexes: The QRS complexes are normal unless aberrant ventricular conduction or a preexisting bundle branch block is present. If abnormal QRS complexes occur only when junctional tachycardia is present, the arrhythmia is called **junctional tachycardia with aberrancy** (or **aberrant ventricular conduction**).

Nonparoxysmal junctional tachycardia with abnormal QRS complexes may resemble accelerated idioventricular rhythm if the heart rate is 60 to 100 beats per minute (accelerated junctional rhythm), or it may resemble ventricular tachycardia if the heart rate is over 100 beats per minute (junctional tachycardia).

Cause of Arrhythmia: Nonparoxysmal junctional tachycardia is usually due to enhanced automaticity of the AV junction, unlike paroxysmal junctional tachycardia (PJT), which results from a reentry mechanism. Nonparoxysmal junctional tachycardia is most commonly a result of digitalis toxicity Other common causes are excessive administration of catecholamines and damage to the AV junction from an inferior-wall myocardial infarction or rheumatic fever. The arrhythmia may begin with one or more PJCs.

Clinical Significance: Nonparoxysmal junctional tachycardia is clinically significant because it commonly indicates digitalis overdose. The signs and symptoms and clinical significance of rapid nonparoxysmal junctional tachycardia are the same as those of atrial tachycardia.

In addition, in nonparoxysmal junctional tachycardia, the atria do not regularly contract and empty before each ventricular contraction, filling the ventricles during the last part of diastole, as they normally do. The loss of this **"atrial kick"** results in incomplete filling of the ventricles before they contract, causing a reduction of the cardiac output by as much as 25%.

Notes

Nonparoxysmal Junctional Tachycardia
(Accelerated Junctional Rhythm, Junctional Tachycardia)

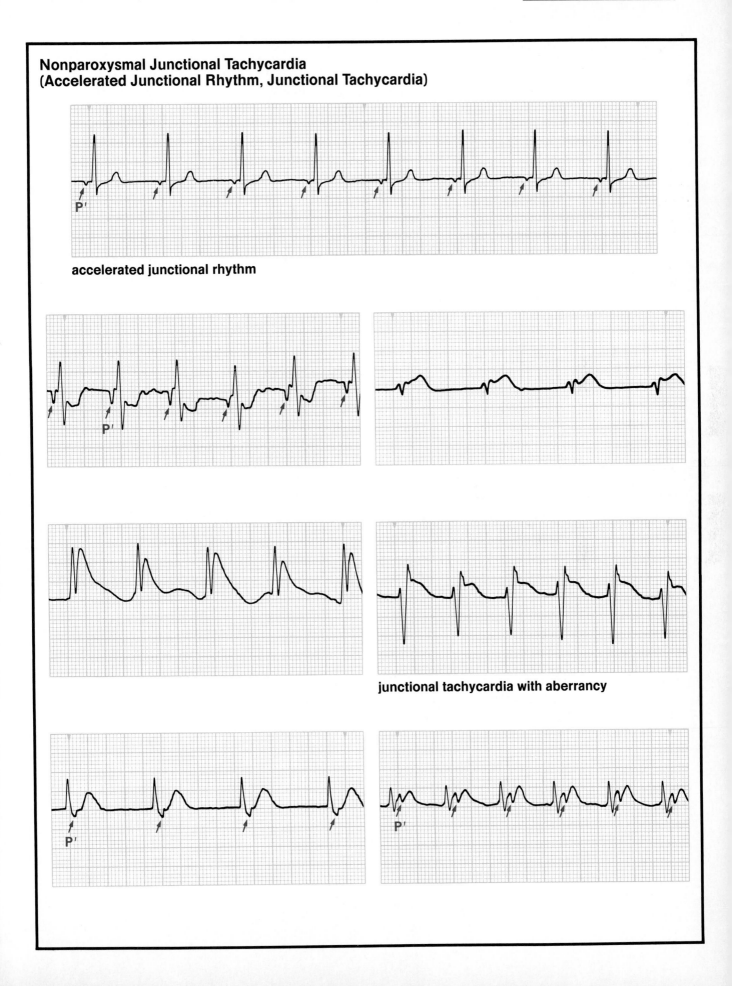

accelerated junctional rhythm

junctional tachycardia with aberrancy

Paroxysmal Junctional Tachycardia (PJT)

Heart Rate: The heart rate is usually 160 to 240 beats per minute and constant. Uncommonly, the heart rate may be as low as 110 beats per minute or exceed 240 per minute. The onset and termination of **paroxysmal junctional tachycardia** are typically abrupt, the onset often being initiated by a premature atrial contraction. A brief period of asystole may follow the termination of the arrhythmia. The rate may be slower during the few beats after onset and before termination. Paroxysmal junctional tachycardia is characterized by repeated episodes (paroxysms) of tachycardia that last from a few minutes to many hours and recur for many years. **Carotid sinus massage** usually results in the abrupt termination of paroxysmal junctional tachycardia.

Rhythm: The rhythm is essentially regular.

Pacemaker Site: The pacemaker site is an ectopic pacemaker in the AV junction.

P Waves: P′ waves are often absent, being buried in the QRS complex. If present, they are identical and typically follow the QRS complexes. Rarely, the P′ waves precede the QRS complexes. The P′ waves are generally abnormal, differing from normal P waves in size, shape, and direction. Since atrial depolarization occurs in a retrograde fashion, the P′ waves are negative (inverted) in Lead II.

P-R Intervals: If the P′ waves precede the QRS complexes, the P′-R intervals are abnormal (less than 0.12 second). If the P′ waves follow the QRS complexes, the R-P′ intervals are usually less than 0.20 second.

R-R Intervals: The R-R intervals are usually equal.

QRS Complexes: The QRS complexes are normal unless aberrant ventricular conduction or a pre-existing bundle branch block is present. If abnormal QRS complexes occur only with the tachycardia, the arrhythmia is called **paroxysmal junctional tachycardia with aberrancy** (or **aberrant ventricular conduction**). Paroxysmal junctional tachycardia with abnormal QRS complexes may resemble ventricular tachycardia.

Cause of Arrhythmia: Paroxysmal junctional tachycardia may occur without apparent cause in healthy persons of any age with no apparent underlying heart disease. In susceptible persons, it may be precipitated by an increase in catecholamines and sympathetic tone, overexertion, stimulants (e.g., alcohol, coffee, tobacco), electrolyte or acid-base abnormalities, hyperventilation, or emotional stress. The electrophysiologic mechanism responsible for paroxysmal junctional tachycardia is a reentry mechanism.

Clinical Significance: The signs and symptoms and clinical significance of paroxysmal junctional tachycardia are the same as those of paroxysmal atrial tachycardia. In addition, syncope may occur after the termination of paroxysmal junctional tachycardia because of the asystole that may follow its termination.

Note: Since it is often difficult to differentiate between paroxysmal atrial tachycardia and paroxysmal junctional tachycardia when the P′ waves are not clearly evident, the term **paroxysmal supraventricular tachycardia (PSVT)** is commonly used to indicate a paroxysmal tachycardia originating in the atria or AV junction without specifying the exact location of the ectopic pacemaker site.

Notes

Paroxysmal Junctional Tachycardia (PJT)

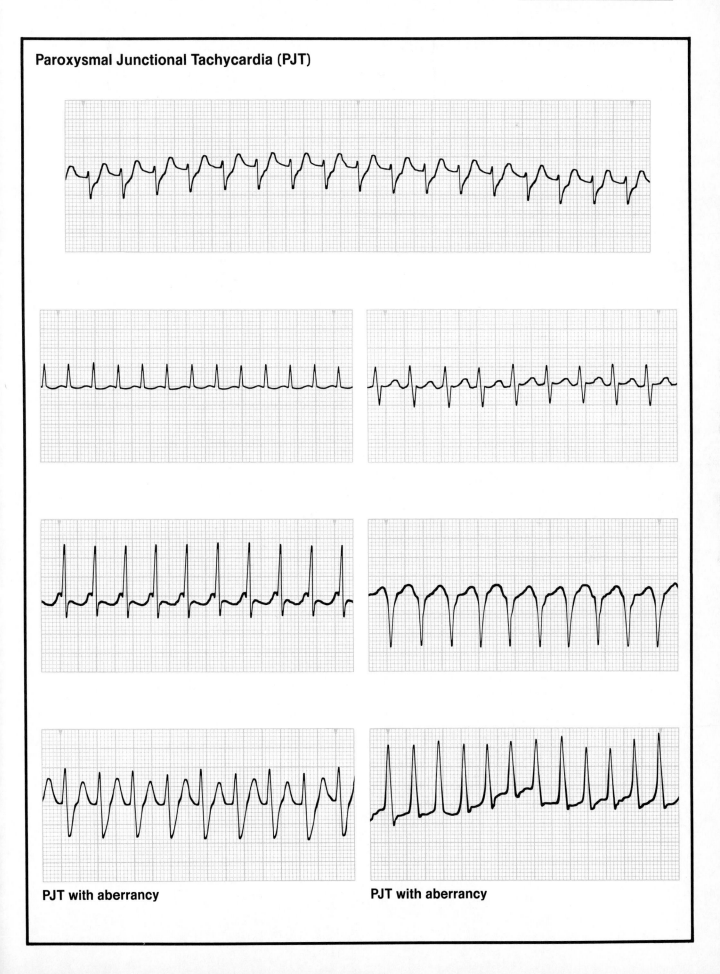

PJT with aberrancy

PJT with aberrancy

Premature Ventricular Contractions (PVCs)

Heart Rate: The heart rate is that of the underlying rhythm.

Rhythm: The rhythm is typically irregular when **premature ventricular contractions** are present.

Pacemaker Site: The pacemaker site of the **PVC** is an ectopic pacemaker in the ventricles, specifically in the bundle branches, Purkinje network or ventricular myocardium. Premature ventricular contractions may originate from a single ectopic pacemaker site (**unifocal PVCs**) or from multiple sites in the ventricles (**multifocal PVCs).**

P Waves: P waves may be present or absent. If present, they are usually of the underlying rhythm and have no relation to the PVCs. Typically, the PVCs do not disturb the P-P cycle of the underlying rhythm so that the P waves continue without disruption during and after the PVCs, occurring at their expected time. Uncommonly, the electrical impulse responsible for the PVC enters the atria, depolarizing them retrogradely. This results in a P wave that follows the QRS complex of the PVC at an R-P′ interval of about 0.20 second, but often the P′ wave is buried in the QRS complex. Since atrial depolarization occurs in a retrograde fashion, these P′ waves are negative (inverted) in Lead II. The electrical impulse of the PVC may also depolarize the SA node, momentarily suppressing it, so that the next P wave of the underlying rhythm appears later than expected.

Often the P waves of the underlying rhythm are obscured by the PVCs, but sometimes they appear as notches on the S-T segment or T wave of the PVCs. This provides a clue that the premature ectopic complex is a PVC and not a premature atrial contraction with aberrant ventricular conduction. In a premature atrial contraction, a P wave typically precedes the QRS complex (see Premature Atrial Contractions, page 108).

P-R Intervals: No P-R intervals are associated with the PVCs.

R-R Intervals: The R-R intervals are unequal when PVCs are present. The R-R interval between the PVC and the preceding QRS complex of the underlying rhythm is usually shorter than that of the underlying rhythm. This R-R interval is called the **coupling interval.** PVCs with the same coupling interval in a given ECG lead usually originate from the same ectopic pacemaker site.

A **full compensatory pause** commonly follows a PVC since the SA node is often not depolarized by the PVC (i.e., the P wave of the underlying rhythm that follows the PVC appears at the expected time). Consequently, the interval between the P waves of the underlying rhythm occurring before and after the PVC is twice the P-P interval of the underlying rhythm.

Rarely, when the SA node is depolarized by the PVC, an **incomplete compensatory pause** occurs. (See the discussion of full and incomplete compensatory pause under Premature Atrial Contractions, page 108).

A combination of a full compensatory pause and a P wave of the underlying rhythm superimposed on a premature ectopic beat with a wide and bizarre QRS complex helps to make a positive diagnosis of a PVC.

QRS Complexes: The QRS complex of the PVC typically appears prematurely (without a preceding ectopic P wave) before the next expected QRS complex of the underlying rhythm. The QRS complex is nearly always 0.12 second or greater in duration, and, because of the abnormal direction and sequence of ventricular depolarization, it is distorted and bizarre, often with notching, appearing different from the QRS complex of the underlying rhythm. It is usually followed by an abnormal S-T segment and a large T wave, opposite in direction to the major deflection of the QRS complex.

The shape of a PVC often resembles that of a right or left bundle branch block. For example, the QRS complex of a PVC originating from the left ventricle resembles that of right bundle branch block. Likewise, a PVC originating in the right ventricle has a QRS complex resembling that of left bundle branch block. However, the QRS complex of a PVC arising from a bundle branch appears only slightly bizarre (**fascicular PVC**). A PVC arising from the ventricles near the bifurcation of the bundle of His may appear relatively normal.

Premature Ventricular Contractions (PVCs)

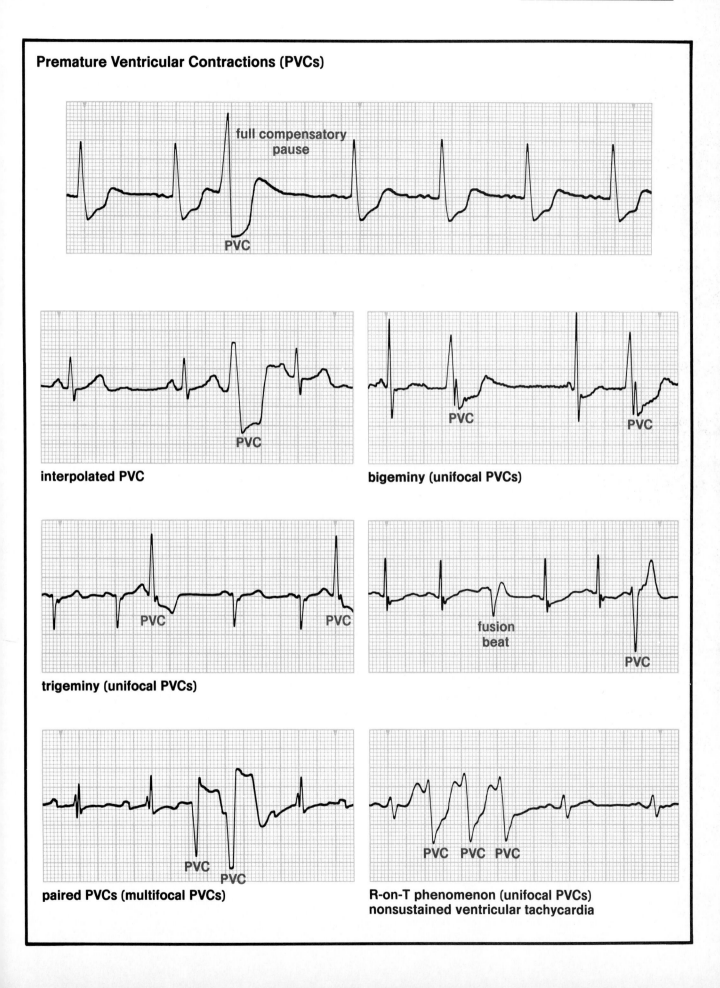

interpolated PVC

bigeminy (unifocal PVCs)

trigeminy (unifocal PVCs)

paired PVCs (multifocal PVCs)

R-on-T phenomenon (unifocal PVCs)
nonsustained ventricular tachycardia

Premature Ventricular Contractions (PVCs)—Cont.

The QRS complexes of PVCs that originate from the same ectopic pacemaker site (**unifocal or uniform PVCs**) are usually identical in each given lead. Such PVCs usually have a constant coupling interval. Occasionally, unifocal PVCs may differ from each other because of changing depolarization pathways within the ventricles—a common abnormality present in severely diseased myocardium. Such PVCs are called **multiform PVCs.** PVCs originating from two or more ectopic pacemaker sites (**multifocal PVCs**) characteristically have different coupling intervals and different QRS complexes in the same lead.

When a PVC occurs at about the same time that an electrical impulse of the underlying rhythm is activating the ventricles, depolarization of the ventricles occurs simultaneously in two directions. This results in a QRS complex which has the characteristics of both the PVC and the QRS complex of the underlying rhythm. Such a QRS complex is called a **ventricular fusion beat.** The presence of ventricular fusion beats provides evidence in favor of a premature ectopic contraction being ventricular in origin and not supraventricular with aberrant ventricular conduction.

Types of PVCs: The PVCs may be **infrequent** (less than five beats per minute) or **frequent** (five or more beats per minute). They may occur singly (**isolated**) or in groups of two or more in succession. Groups of two or more PVCs are called "**ventricular group beats**" or "**bursts**" or "**salvos**" of PVCs. Two PVCs in a row is called "**paired PVCs**" or a "**couplet.**" A group of three or more consecutive PVCs is considered to be **ventricular tachycardia.**

If PVCs alternate with the QRS complexes of the underlying rhythm, **ventricular bigeminy** is present. If, in ventricular bigeminy, the PVCs follow the QRS complexes of the underlying rhythm at precisely the same intervals, **coupling** is said to be present.

Ventricular trigeminy occurs when there is one PVC for every two QRS complexes of the underlying rhythm or one QRS complex of the underlying rhythm for every two PVCs.

The term "**R-on-T phenomenon**" is used to indicate that a PVC has occurred during the **vulnerable period of ventricular repolarization,** i.e., the relative refractory period of the ventricles (the **peak of the T wave**). During this period, the heart muscle is at its greatest electrical nonuniformity: some of the ventricular muscle fibers may be completely repolarized, others may be only partially repolarized, and still others may be completely refractory. Stimulation of the ventricles at this point by an intrinsic electrical impulse such as that generated by a PVC or by an extrinsic impulse from a cardiac pacemaker or a direct-current (DC) countershock may result in nonuniform conduction of the electrical impulse through the muscle fibers. Some of the fibers are able to conduct the electrical impulse, but others are only able to conduct slowly or not at all. Thus, a reentry mechanism is established that may precipitate repetitive ventricular contractions and result in ventricular tachycardia, flutter, or fibrillation. (See Chapter 1 for a discussion of the reentry mechanism, page 14).

A PVC that occurs at about the same time that ventricular depolarization of the underlying rhythm is expected to occur is called an **end-diastolic PVC.** This usually results in a **ventricular fusion beat.** End-diastolic PVCs tend to occur when the underlying rhythm is relatively rapid.

A PVC occurring between two normally conducted QRS complexes without greatly disturbing the underlying rhythm is called an **interpolated PVC.** This tends to occur when the underlying rhythm is relatively slow. The R-R interval that includes the PVC is often slightly greater than that of the underlying rhythm, but a full compensatory pause usually does not occur.

Cause of Arrhythmia: PVCs may occur in healthy persons with apparently healthy hearts and without apparent cause. PVCs, especially if they are frequent, may be caused by an increase in catecholamines and sympathetic tone (as in emotional stress), an increase in vagal (parasympathetic) tone, stimulants (e.g., alcohol, caffeine, tobacco), excessive administration of digitalis or sympathomimetic drugs (e.g., epinephrine, isoproterenol, norepinephrine), hypoxia, acidosis, hypokalemia, or congestive heart failure. PVCs frequently occur in acute myocardial infarction. The electrophysiologic mechanism responsible for PVCs in the above conditions is probably enhanced automaticity or a reentry mechanism.

Clinical Significance: Isolated premature ventricular contractions in patients with no underlying heart disease usually have no significance and require no treatment. Following an AMI, however, PVCs may indicate the presence of enhanced ventricular automaticity, a reentry mechanism, or both and may herald the appearance of such life-threatening arrhythmias as ventricular tachycardia, flutter, or fibrillation.

Although the so-called warning arrhythmias (i.e., an R-on-T phenomenon, frequent PVCs [more than five or six per minute], ventricular group beats [bursts or salvos of two, three, or more] and multiform PVCs) have been recognized as high-risk factors in triggering ventricular tachycardia, flutter, or fibrillation, any PVC can trigger these lethal arrhythmias in patients with an acute myocardial infarction or ischemic episode. For this reason, PVCs should be treated immediately when they occur under these conditions.

At times, premature atrial and junctional contractions with aberrant ventricular conduction may mimic PVCs.

Notes

Ventricular Tachycardia (VT)

Heart Rate: The heart rate is over 100 beats per minute, usually between 110 and 250 beats per minute. **Ventricular tachycardia** exists if three or more consecutive premature ventricular contractions are present, occurring at a rate greater than 100 beats per minute. The onset and termination of ventricular tachycardia may or may not be abrupt. Ventricular tachycardia may occur in paroxysms of three or more PVCs separated by the underlying rhythm (**nonsustained ventricular tachycardia** or **paroxysmal ventricular tachycardia**) or persist for a long period of time (**sustained ventricular tachycardia**).

Rhythm: The rhythm is usually regular, but it may be slightly irregular.

Pacemaker Site: The pacemaker site of ventricular tachycardia is an ectopic pacemaker in the bundle branches, Purkinje network, or ventricular myocardium.

P Waves: P waves may be present or absent. If present, they usually have no set relation to the QRS complexes of the ventricular tachycardia, appearing between the QRS complexes at a rate different from that of the ventricular tachycardia. The pacemaker site of such P waves is the SA node or an ectopic pacemaker in the atria or AV junction. These P waves may be positive (upright) or negative (inverted) in Lead II. P waves are often difficult to detect in ventricular tachycardia especially if it is rapid. When the P waves occur independently of the QRS complexes, **atrio-ventricular (AV) dissociation** is present. Rarely, identical P waves regularly follow the QRS complexes. The electrical impulses responsible for them have most likely originated in the ectopic pacemaker site of the ventricular tachycardia. Such P′ waves differ from normal P waves in size, shape, and direction. Since the atria depolarize retrogradedly when the electrical impulse enters the atria from the ventricles through the AV junction (**retrograde AV conduction**), the P′ waves are negative (inverted) in Lead II.

P-R Intervals: If P waves are present and occur independently of the QRS complexes, the P-R intervals vary widely. If P′ waves regularly follow the QRS complexes, the R-P′ intervals are usually less than 0.20 seconds.

R-R Intervals: The R-R intervals may be equal or vary slightly.

QRS Complexes: The QRS complexes exceed 0.12 second and are usually distorted and bizarre, often with notching. They are followed by large T waves, opposite in direction to the major deflection of the QRS complexes. Usually, the QRS complexes are identical, but, occasionally, one or more QRS complexes differ in size, shape, and direction, especially at the onset or end of ventricular tachycardia. These are most likely **fusion beats.** (See the discussion of fusion beats under Premature Ventricular Contractions, page 136). Occasionally. an electrical impulse of the underlying rhythm is conducted from the atria to the ventricles through the AV junction producing a normal-appearing QRS complex (0.10 second or less) amongst the QRS complexes of the ventricular tachycardia. Such a QRS complex is called a **capture beat.** The R-R interval between the QRS complex of the ventricular tachycardia preceding the capture beat and the QRS complex of the capture beat is usually less than that of the ventricular tachycardia. The presence of capture or ventricular fusion beats provides evidence that the tachycardia is most likely ventricular tachycardia and not a supra-ventricular tachycardia with aberrant ventricular conduction.

When there are two distinctly different forms of QRS complexes alternating with each other (indicating that there are two ventricular ectopic pacemakers), the arrhythmia is called **bidirectional ventricular tachycardia.** When the QRS complexes in a ventricular tachycardia differ markedly from beat to beat, the arrhythmia is called **multiform ventricular tachycardia.** Another form of ventricular tachycardia characterized by QRS complexes that gradually change back and forth from one shape and direction to another over a series of beats is called **torsades de pointes.** This term, literally translated from the French, means "twisting around a point."

Ventricular Tachycardia (VT)

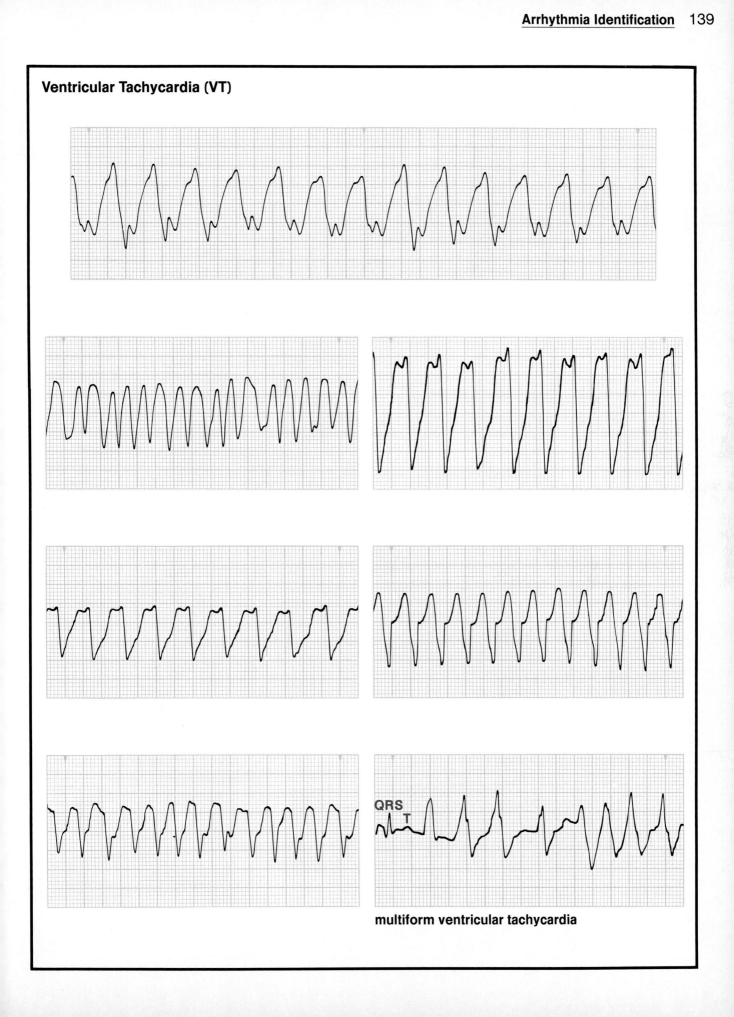

multiform ventricular tachycardia

Ventricular Tachycardia (VT)—Cont.

Cause of Arrhythmia: Ventricular tachycardia usually occurs in the presence of significant cardiac disease. Most commonly, it occurs in the setting of acute myocardial infarction and coronary artery disease, especially if hypoxia or acidosis is present. Digitalis toxicity is also a common cause of ventricular tachycardia. The arrhythmia also occurs in such cardiac conditions as cardiomyopathy, mitral valve prolapse, and congestive heart failure. The ventricles are particularly prone to ventricular tachycardia when the **QT interval*** is prolonged from various causes, including excess of certain drugs (e.g., quinidine, procainamide, disopyramide, phenothiazines, tricyclic antidepressants), brady-arrhythmias (e.g., severe sinus bradycardia, third-degree AV block with slow ventricular escape rhythm), electrolyte disturbances (e.g., hypo-kalemia), liquid protein diets, and central nervous system disorders (e.g., subarachnoid hemorrhage, intracranial trauma). The torsades de pointes form of ventricular tachycardia is particularly prone to occur following administration of such anti-arrhythmic agents as disopyramide, quinidine, or procainamide or other agents that prolong the QT interval. The electrophysiologic mechanism responsible for ventricular tachycardia is probably enhanced automaticity or a reentry mechanism.

A premature ventricular contraction can initiate ventricular tachycardia when the PVC occurs during the **vulnerable period** of ventricular repolarization coincident with the **peak of the T wave,** (i.e., the **R-on-T phenomenon**). (See the discussion of vulnerable period under Premature Ventricular Contractions, page 136). Often ventricular tachycardia may occur without preexisting or precipitating premature ventricular contractions.

Clinical Significance: The signs and symptoms of ventricular tachycardia are the same as those of atrial tachycardia, except that ventricular tachycardia is usually an ominous finding, indicating the presence of significant underlying cardiac disease.

In addition, in ventricular tachycardia, the atria do not regularly contract and empty before each ventricular contraction, filling the ventricles during the last part of diastole, as they normally do. The loss of this **"atrial kick"** results in incomplete filling of the ventricles before they contract, causing a reduction of the cardiac output by as much as 25%.

Because ventricular tachycardia often initiates or degenerates into ventricular fibrillation, ventricular tachycardia must be treated immediately.

At times, a supraventricular tachycardia (sinus and atrial tachycardia, atrial flutter, and paroxysmal junctional tachycardia) with aberrant ventricular conduction may mimic ventricular tachycardia.

Atrial fibrillation with aberrant ventricular conduction and a rapid ventricular rate may also mimic ventricular tachycardia, but, usually, the grossly irregular rhythm of atrial fibrillation provides a clue to its true identity. In addition, the presence of certain features common to ventricular tachycardia, namely, atrioventricular (AV) dissociation, a QRS complex duration greater than 0.14 second, and capture or ventricular fusion beats, help to differentiate ventricular tachycardia from a supraventricular tachycardia with aberrant ventricular conduction.

* The **QT Interval** is measured from the onset of the QRS complex to the end of the T wave. The QT interval represents the refractory period of the ventricles during which the ventricles depolarize and repolarize. It varies with heart rate, sex, and age. Usually, it is about 0.40 second or less at most heart rates but may be prolonged at slow rates.

Notes

Ventricular Fibrillation (VF)

Heart Rate: No coordinated ventricular beats are present. The ventricles contract from about 300 to 500 times a minute in an unsynchronized, uncoordinated, and haphazard manner.

Rhythm: The rhythm is grossly (totally) irregular.

Pacemaker Site: The pacemaker sites of **ventricular fibrillation** are multiple ectopic pacemakers in the Purkinje network and ventricular myocardium.

Characteristics of Ventricular Fibrillation Waves:

1. Relationship to Cardiac Anatomy and Physiology: Ventricular fibrillation waves represent abnormal, chaotic, and incomplete ventricular depolarizations caused by haphazard depolarization of small individual groups (or islets) of muscle fibers. Since organized depolarizations of the atria and ventricles are absent, distinct P waves, QRS complexes, ST segments, and T waves and organized atrial and ventricular contractions are absent.

2. Onset and End: The onset and end of the ventricular fibrillation waves cannot be determined with certainty.

3. Direction: The direction of the ventricular fibrillation waves varies at random from positive (upright) to negative (inverted).

4. Duration: The duration of ventricular fibrillation waves cannot be measured with certainty.

5. Amplitude: The amplitude varies from less than 1 mm to about 10 mm. Generally, if the ventricular fibrillation waves are small (less than 3 mm), the arrhythmia is called **"fine" ventricular fibrillation;** if the ventricular fibrillation waves are large (greater than 3 mm), it is called **"coarse" ventricular fibrillation.** If the ventricular fibrillation waves are so small or "fine" that they are not recorded, the ECG appears as a wavy or flat (isoelectric) line resembling ventricular asystole.

6. Shape: The ventricular fibrillation waves are of varying shape: bizarre, rounded or pointed, and markedly dissimilar.

VENTRICULAR FIBRILLATION WAVES

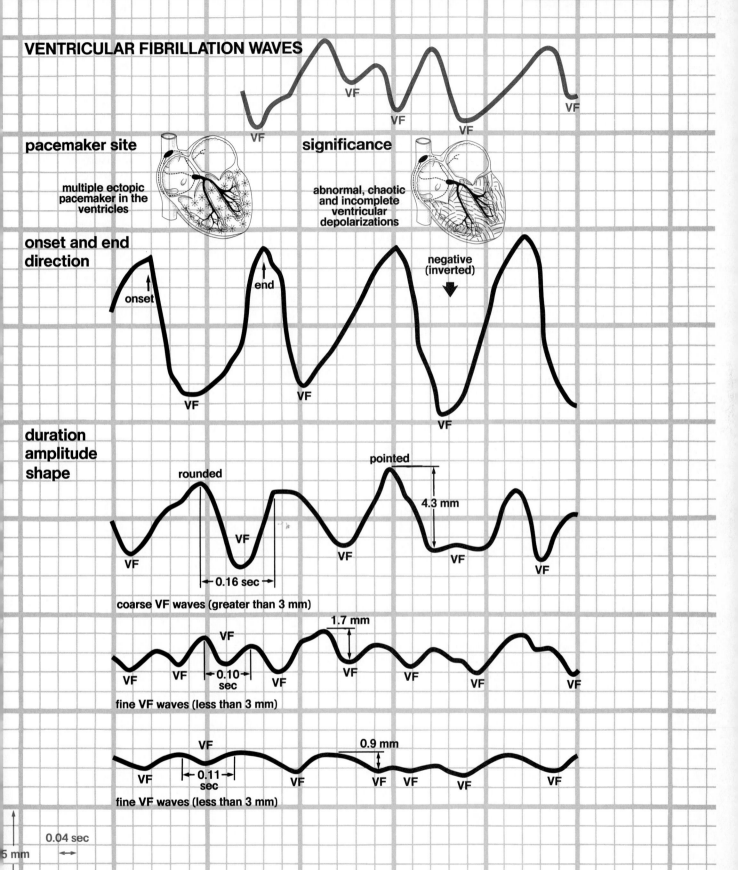

VF VF VF VF

pacemaker site

multiple ectopic pacemaker in the ventricles

significance

abnormal, chaotic and incomplete ventricular depolarizations

onset and end direction

onset

end

negative (inverted)

VF VF VF

duration amplitude shape

rounded

pointed

4.3 mm

VF

VF VF VF VF

← 0.16 sec →

coarse VF waves (greater than 3 mm)

VF

1.7 mm

VF VF ← 0.10 → sec VF VF VF VF VF VF

fine VF waves (less than 3 mm)

VF

0.9 mm

VF ← 0.11 → sec VF VF VF VF VF

fine VF waves (less than 3 mm)

0.04 sec

5 mm

← 0.20 sec →

Ventricular Fibrillation (VF)—Cont.

P-R Intervals: P-R intervals are absent.

R-R Intervals: R-R intervals are absent.

QRS Complexes: QRS complexes are absent.

Cause of Arrhythmia: Ventricular fibrillation, one of the most common causes of cardiac arrest, usually occurs in the presence of significant cardiac disease, most commonly in coronary artery disease, myocardial ischemia, acute myocardial infarction, and third-degree AV block with a slow ventricular escape rhythm. The arrhythmia occurs frequently as a terminal event in many cardiac conditions. It may also occur in cardiomyopathy, mitral valve prolapse, and cardiac trauma (penetrating or blunt). Digitalis toxicity is also a common cause of ventricular fibrillation. The arrhythmia may also be caused by an excessive dose of quinidine or procainamide, hypoxia, acidosis, or electrolyte imbalance (e.g., hypokalemia, hyperkalemia). Ventricular fibrillation may also occur during anesthesia, cardiac and noncardiac operations, cardiac catheterization, and cardiac pacing and following cardioversion or accidental electrocution. The electrophysiologic mechanism responsible for ventricular fibrillation is probably enhanced automaticity or a reentry mechanism.

A premature ventricular contraction can initiate ventricular fibrillation when the PVC occurs during the **vulnerable period** of ventricular repolarization, coincident with the **peak of the T wave** (i.e., the **R-on-T phenomenon**), particularly when electrical instability of the heart has been altered by ischemia and acute myocardial infarction. (See the discussion of vulnerable period under Premature Ventricular Contractions, page 136). Sustained ventricular tachycardia and ventricular flutter may also precipitate ventricular fibrillation. Often ventricular fibrillation may begin without preexisting or precipitating premature ventricular contractions or ventricular tachycardia or flutter.

Often ventricular fibrillation may begin without preexisting or precipitating premature ventricular contractions or ventricular tachycardia or flutter.

Clinical Significance: Organized ventricular depolarization and contraction and, consequently, cardiac output cease at the moment ventricular fibrillation occurs. Ventricular fibrillation results in faintness, followed within seconds by loss of consciousness, seizures, apnea, and, if the arrhythmia remains untreated, death. Ventricular fibrillation must be treated immediately.

The significance of coarse versus fine ventricular fibrillation is that coarse ventricular fibrillation, indicating a recent onset of the arrhythmia, is more apt to be reversed by direct-current (DC) shock than is fine ventricular fibrillation, which indicates that the arrhythmia has been present for a prolonged period of time.

Since fine ventricular fibrillation may resemble ventricular asystole, ventricular fibrillation must be correctly identified using at least two ECG leads so that the patient is not innapropriately treated for ventricular asystole.

In addition, ECG artifacts produced by loose or dry electrodes, broken ECG leads, or the patient's movements or muscle tremor may also resemble ventricular fibrillation. A rapid assessment of the patient, including a check of the patient's pulse, must be performed immediately upon the electrocardiographic onset of ventricular fibrillation to confirm the arrhythmia before treating the patient for cardiac arrest.

Notes

Ventricular Fibrillation (VF)

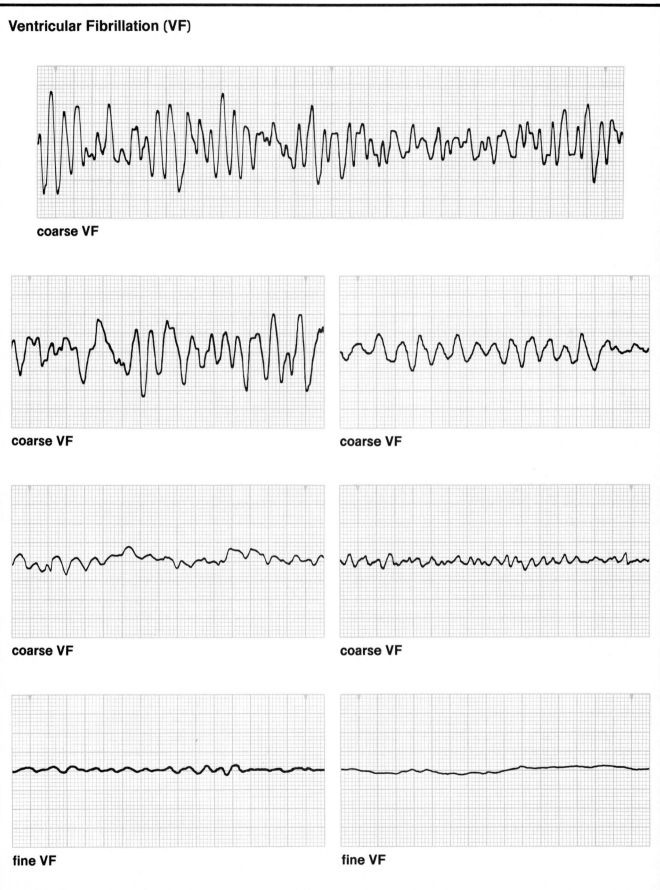

coarse VF

coarse VF

coarse VF

coarse VF

coarse VF

fine VF

fine VF

Accelerated Idioventricular Rhythm (AIVR)
(Accelerated Ventricular Rhythm, Idioventricular Tachycardia, Slow Ventricular Tachycardia)

Heart Rate: The heart rate is between 40 and 100 beats per minute. The onset and termination of **accelerated idioventricular rhythm** are usually gradual, but the arrhythmia may begin abruptly following a premature ventricular contraction.

Rhythm: The rhythm is essentially regular, but it may be irregular.

Pacemaker Site: The pacemaker site is an ectopic pacemaker in the bundle branches, Purkinje network, or ventricular myocardium.

P Waves: P waves may be present or absent. If present, they have no relation to the QRS complexes of the accelerated idioventricular rhythm, appearing independently at a rate different from that of the QRS complexes (**atrioventricular [AV] dissociation).**

The pacemaker site of such P waves is the SA node or an ectopic pacemaker in the atria or AV junction. These P waves may be positive (upright) or negative (inverted) in Lead II.

P-R Intervals: If P waves are present, the P-R intervals vary widely since the P waves and QRS complexes occur independently.

R-R Intervals: The R-R intervals may be equal or may vary.

QRS Complexes: The QRS complexes typically exceed 0.12 second and are bizarre, but they may be only slightly wider than normal (greater than 0.10 second but less than 0.12 second) if the pacemaker site is in the bundle branches. **Fusion beats** may be present if a supraventricular rhythm is present and particularly if its rate is about the same as that of the accelerated idioventricular rhythm. When this occurs, the cardiac rhythm alternates between the supraventricular rhythm and the accelerated idioventricular rhythm. The fusion beats most commonly appear at the onset and end of the arrhythmia. (See the discussion of fusion beats under Premature Ventricular Contractions, page 136).

Cause of Arrhythmia: Accelerated idioventricular rhythm is relatively common in acute myocardial infarction. It occurs when the firing rate of the dominant pacemaker (usually the SA node) or escape pacemaker in the AV junction becomes less than that of the ventricular ectopic pacemaker or when a sinus arrest, sinoatrial (SA) exit block, or AV block develops. Accelerated idioventricular rhythm may also result from digitalis toxicity. The electrophysiologic mechanism responsible for accelerated idioventricular rhythm is probably enhanced automaticity.

Clinical Significance: Accelerated idioventricular rhythm occurring in acute myocardial infarction usually requires no treatment since it is self-limited in most cases. Because it does not affect the course or prognosis of the myocardial infarction, it is considered relatively benign.

Notes

Accelerated Idioventricular Rhythm (AIVR)
(Accelerated Ventricular Rhythm, Idioventricular
Tachycardia, Slow Ventricular Tachycardia)

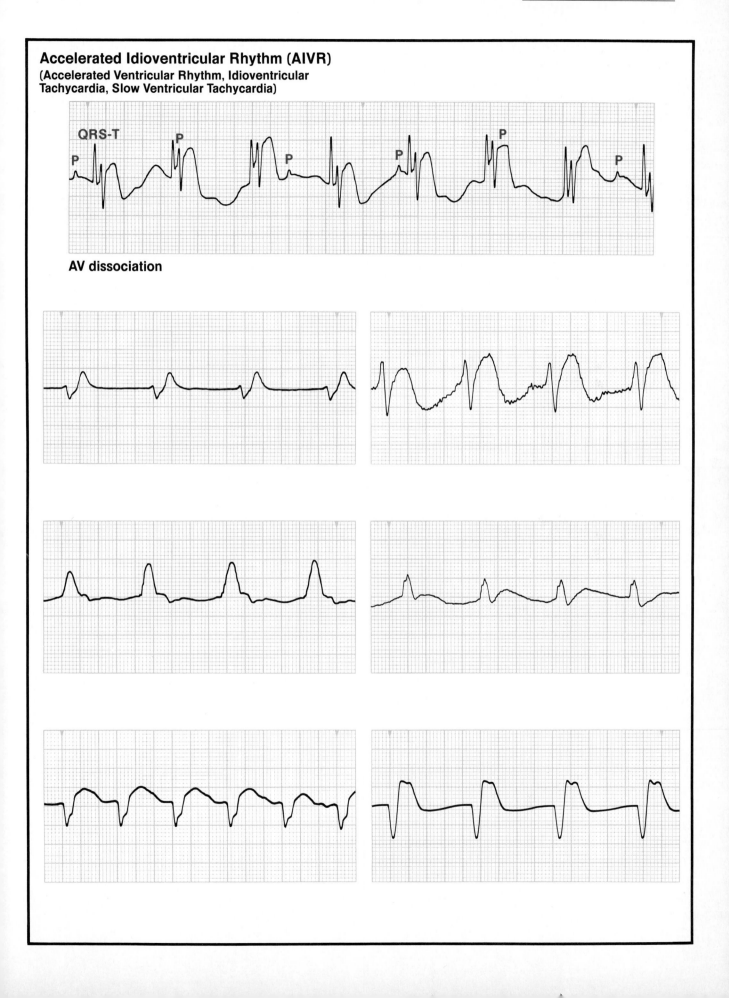

AV dissociation

Ventricular Escape Rhythm
(Idioventricular Rhythm)

Heart Rate: The heart rate is less than 40 beats per minute, usually between 30 and 40 beats per minute, but it may be less.

Rhythm: The ventricular rhythm is usually regular, but it may be irregular.

Pacemaker Site: The pacemaker site of **ventricular escape rhythm** is an escape pacemaker in the bundle branches, Purkinje network, or ventricular myocardium.

P Waves: P waves may be present or absent. If present, they have no set relation to the QRS complexes of the ventricular escape rhythm, appearing independently at a rate different from that of the QRS complexes. The pacemaker site of such P waves is the SA node or an ectopic pacemaker in the atria or AV junction. These P waves may be positive (upright) or negative (inverted) in Lead II.

They precede, are buried in, or follow the QRS complexes haphazardly. When the atria and ventricles thus beat independently, **atrioventricular (AV) dissociation** is present.

P-R Intervals: P-R intervals are absent.

R-R Intervals: The R-R intervals may be equal or may vary.

QRS Complexes: The QRS complexes exceed 0.12 second and are bizarre. Sometimes the shape of the QRS complexes vary in any given lead.

Cause of Arrhythmia: Ventricular escape rhythm usually occurs when the rate of impulse information of the dominant pacemaker (usually the SA node) and escape pacemaker in the AV junction becomes less than that of the escape pacemaker in the ventricles or when the electrical impulses from the SA node, atria, and AV junction fail to reach the ventricles because of a sinus arrest, sinoatrial (SA) exit block, or third-degree (complete) AV block. When this occurs, an escape pacemaker in the ventricles takes over at its inherent firing rate of 30 to 40 beats per minute. Ventricular escape rhythm also occurs in advanced heart disease and is often the cardiac arrhythmia that is present in a dying heart, the so-called **agonal rhythm,** just before the appearance of the final arrhythmia, ventricular asystole.

Clinical Significance: Ventricular escape rhythm is generally symptomatic. Hypotension with marked reduction in cardiac output and decreased perfusion of the brain and other vital organs may occur, resulting in syncope, shock, and congestive failure. Ventricular escape rhythm must be treated promptly to reverse the consequences of the reduced cardiac output.

Notes

Ventricular Escape Rhythm
(Idioventricular Rhythm)

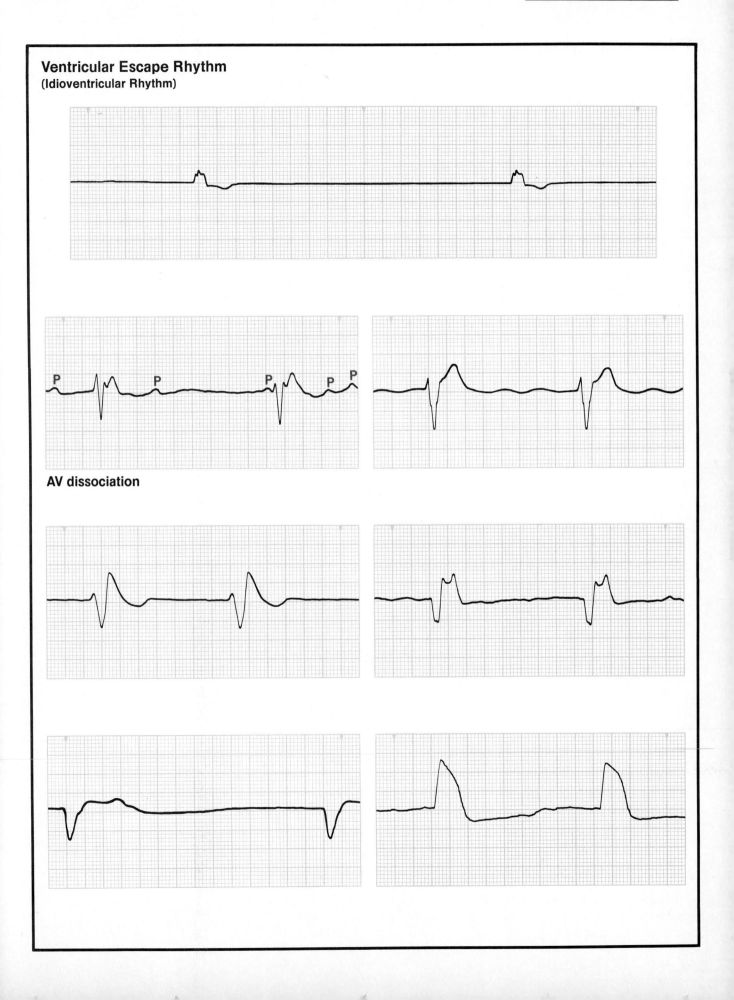

AV dissociation

Ventricular Asystole
(Cardiac Standstill)

Heart Rate: Heart rate is absent.

Rhythm: Rhythm is absent.

Pacemaker Site: A pacemaker site in the ventricles is absent. If P waves are present, their pacemaker site is the SA node or an ectopic pacemaker in the atria or AV junction.

P Waves: P waves may be present or absent.

P-R Intervals: P-R intervals are absent.

R-R Intervals: R-R intervals are absent.

QRS Complexes: QRS complexes are absent.

Cause of Arrhythmia: Ventricular asystole, one of the common causes of cardiac arrest, may occur in advanced cardiac disease as a primary event when electrical impulses fail to enter the ventricles and an escape pacemaker in the AV junction or the ventricles does not take over. In the dying heart, ventricular asystole is usually the final arrhythmia following ventricular tachycardia, ventricular flutter or fibrillation, electromechanical dissociation, or ventricular escape rhythm. Ventricular asystole may also follow the termination of tachyarrhythmias either by drugs or direct-current (DC) shock or countershock.

Clinical Significance: Organized ventricular depolarization and contraction and, consequently, cardiac output are absent in ventricular asystole. The occurrence of sudden ventricular asystole in a conscious person results in faintness, followed within seconds by loss of consciousness, seizures, and apnea **(Adams-Stokes syndrome),** and, if the arrhythmia remains untreated, death. Ventricular asystole must be treated immediately.

Notes

Ventricular Asystole
(Cardiac Standstill)

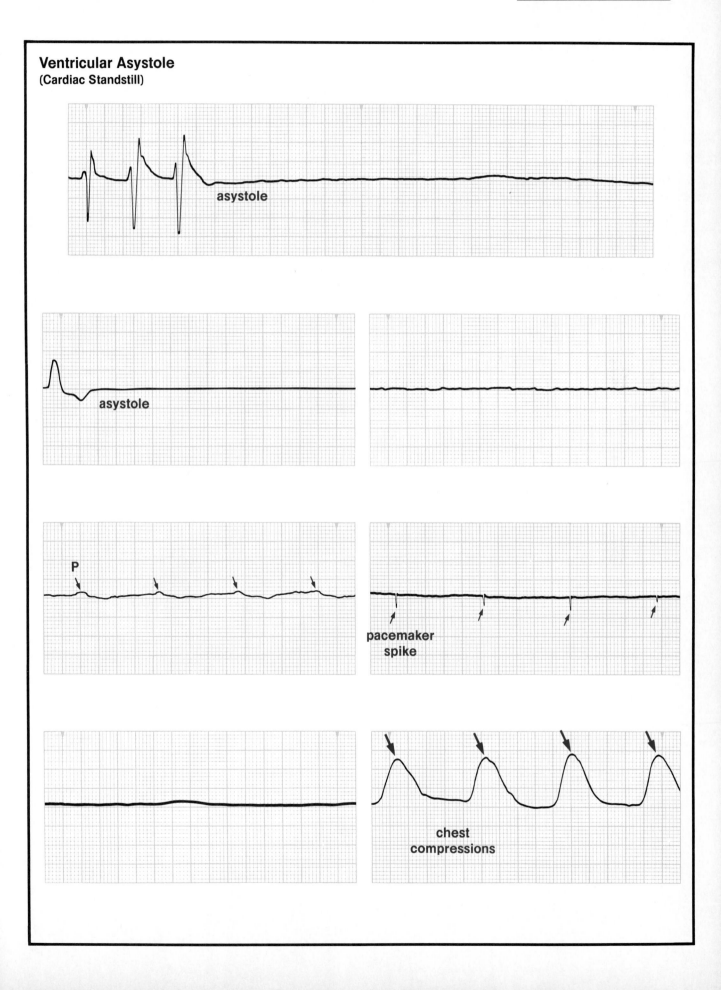

First-degree AV Block

Heart Rate: The heart rate is that of the underlying sinus or atrial rhythm. The atrial and ventricular rates are typically the same.

Rhythm: The rhythm is that of the underlying rhythm.

Pacemaker Site: The pacemaker site is that of the underlying rhythm.

P Waves: The P waves are identical and precede each QRS complex.

P-R Intervals: The P-R intervals are abnormal (greater than 0.20 second) and usually do not vary from beat to beat.

R-R Intervals: The R-R intervals are those of the underlying rhythm.

QRS Complexes: The QRS complexes are usually normal, but they may be abnormal (rarely) because of a preexisting bundle branch block. Typically, the AV conduction ratio is 1:1, that is, a QRS complex follows each P wave.

Cause of Arrhythmia: First-degree AV block usually represents a delay in the conduction of the electrical impulse through the AV node, and, thus, the QRS complex is typically normal—unless a preexisting bundle branch block is present. Infrequently, the AV block may occur below the AV node (infranodal) in the His-Purkinje system of the ventricles (i.e, bundle of His or bundle branches). Although first-degree AV block may occur without any apparent cause, it occurs most commonly in acute inferior-wall myocardial infarction or as the result of increased vagal (parasympathetic) tone or digitalis toxicity.

Clinical Significance: First-degree AV block produces no signs or symptoms but can progress to a higher-degree AV block. For this reason, the patient requires only observation and ECG monitoring.

Notes

First-degree AV Block

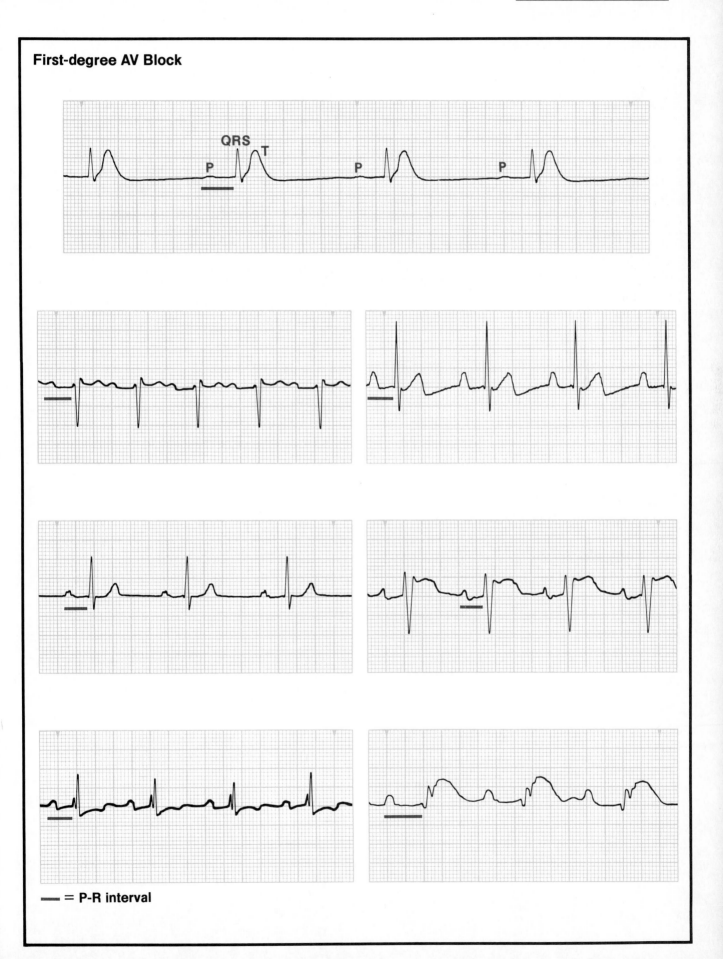

— = P-R interval

Second-degree AV Block
Type I AV Block (Wenckebach)

Heart Rate: The atrial rate is that of the underlying sinus or atrial rhythm. The ventricle rate is typically less than that of the atria.

Rhythm: The atrial rhythm is essentially regular. The ventricular rhythm is usually irregular.

Pacemaker Site: The pacemaker site is that of the underlying rhythm.

P Waves: The P waves are identical and precede the QRS complexes when they occur.

P-R Intervals: The P-R intervals gradually lengthen until a QRS complex fails to appear after a P wave (**nonconducted P wave** or **dropped beat**). Following the pause produced by the nonconducted P wave, the sequence begins again.

R-R and P-P Intervals: The R-R intervals are unequal. As the P-R intervals gradually lengthen, the R-R intervals typically decrease gradually until the P wave is not conducted. Rarely, the R-R interval may remain constant until the nonconduction of the P wave. The P-P interval that includes the nonconducted P wave is usually less than twice the P-P interval of the underlying rhythm.

QRS Complexes: The QRS complexes are typically normal, but they may be abnormal (rarely) because of a preexisting bundle branch block. Commonly, the AV conduction ratio is 5:4, 4:3, 3:2, or 3:1 but may be 6:5, 7:6, and so forth. An AV conduction ratio of 5:4, for example, indicates that for every five P waves, four are followed by QRS complexes. The repetitive sequence of two or more beats in a row followed by a dropped beat is called **group beating.** The AV conduction ratio may be fixed or may vary throughout any given lead.

Cause of Arrhythmia: Type I second-degree AV block most commonly represents defective conduction of the electrical impulse through the AV node, and, thus, the QRS is typically normal. The AV block may infrequently occur below the AV node (infranodal) in the His-Purkinje system of the ventricles (i.e., bundle of His or bundle branches). Type I second-degree AV block usually occurs in acute inferior-wall myocardial infarction or acute myocarditis or as the result of increased vagal (parasympathetic) tone, ischemia, drug toxicity (e.g., digitalis, propranolol, verapamil), or electrolyte imbalance.

Clinical Significance: Type I second-degree AV block is usually transient and reversible and produces no or very little symptoms, but it can progress to a higher-degree AV block. For these reasons, the patient usually requires only observation and ECG monitoring. Type I AV block does respond to atropine if it is necessary to increase the heart rate.

Notes

Second-degree AV Block
Type I AV Block (Wenckebach)

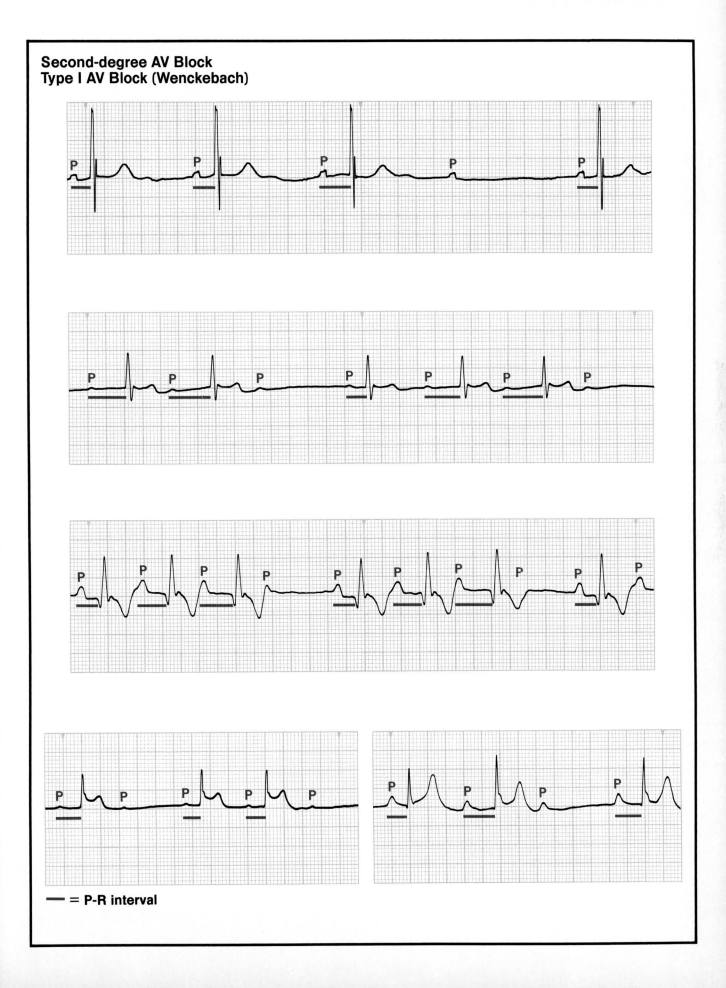

— = P-R interval

Second-degree AV Block
Type II AV Block

Heart Rate: The atrial rate is that of the underlying sinus, atrial or junctional rhythm. The ventricle rate is typically less than that of the atria.

Rhythm: The atrial rhythm is essentially regular. The ventricular rhythm is usually irregular.

Pacemaker Site: The pacemaker site is that of the underlying rhythm.

P Waves: The P waves are identical and precede the QRS complexes when they occur.

P-R Intervals: The P-R intervals may be normal or abnormal (greater than 0.20 second). They are usually constant.

R-R Intervals: The R-R intervals are equal except for those that include the **nonconducted P waves (dropped beats);** these are equal to or slightly less than twice the R-R interval of the underlying rhythm.

QRS Complexes: The QRS complexes are typically abnormal (greater than 0.12 second) because of a bundle branch block. Rarely, the QRS complex may be normal (0.10 second or less) if the AV block is at the level of the bundle of His and a preexisting bundle branch block is not present. Commonly, the AV conduction ratio is 4:3 or 3:2 but may be 5:4, 6:5, 7:6, and so forth. An AV conduction ratio of 4:3, for example, indicates that for every four P waves, three are followed by QRS complexes. The repetitive sequence of two or more beats in a row followed by a dropped beat is called **group beating.** The AV conduction ratio may be fixed, or it may vary throughout any given lead.

Cause of Arrhythmia: Type II second-degree AV block usually occurs below the bundle of His and represents an intermittent block of conduction of the electrical impulse through one bundle branch and a complete block in the other. This produces an intermittent AV block with an abnormally wide and bizarre QRS complex. Commonly, type II second-degree AV block is the result of extensive damage to the bundle branches following an anterior-wall myocardial infarction, and, unlike Type I second-degree AV block, not the result of increased vagal (parasympathetic) tone or drug toxicity. Rarely, the AV block occurs at the level of the bundle of His. When this occurs, the QRS complexes are normal (0.10 second or less) unless a preexisting bundle branch block is present.

Clinical Significance: The signs and symptoms of type II second-degree AV block with excessively slow heart rates are the same as those in symptomatic or marked sinus bradycardia. Because type II second-degree AV block is more serious than type I AV block, often progressing to a third-degree AV block and even ventricular asystole, an external or transvenous cardiac pacemaker is indicated immediately whether or not symptoms are present, especially in the setting of an acute anterior-wall myocardial infarction. Atropine is usually ineffective in reversing a type II AV block.

Notes

Second-degree AV Block
Type II AV Block

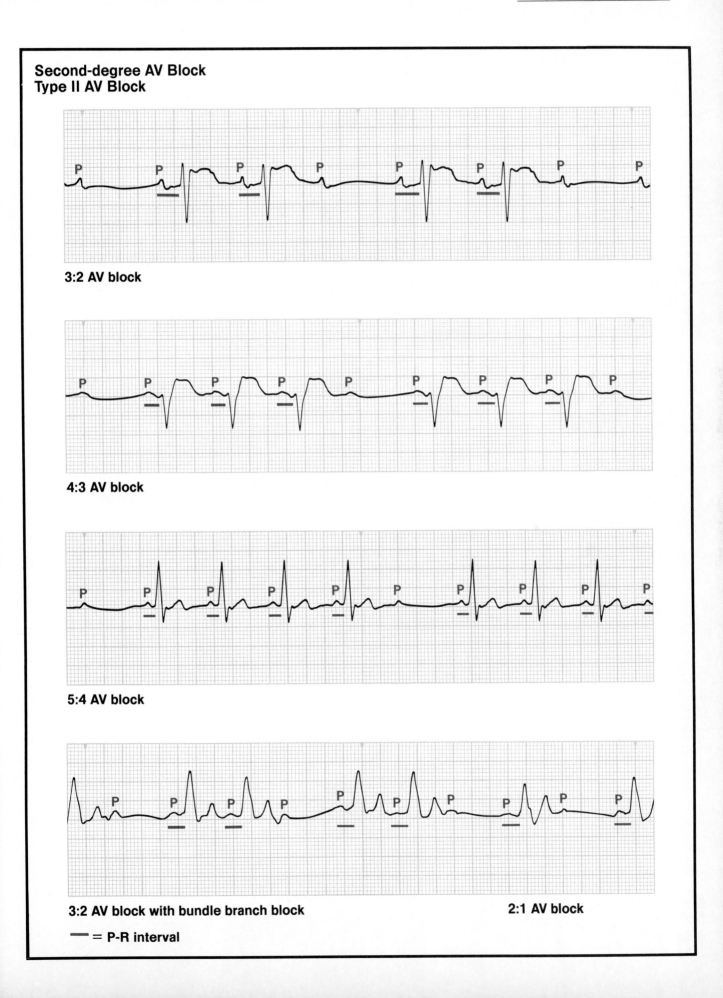

3:2 AV block

4:3 AV block

5:4 AV block

3:2 AV block with bundle branch block   **2:1 AV block**

━━ = P-R interval

Second-degree AV Block
2:1 and High-degree (Advanced) AV Block

Heart Rate: The atrial rate is that of the underlying sinus, atrial, or junctional rhythm. The ventricle rate is typically less than that of the atria.

Rhythm: The atrial rhythm is essentially regular. The ventricular rhythm may be regular or irregular. The ventricular rhythm is irregular when the AV block is intermittent or when the AV conduction ratio is variable.

Pacemaker Site: The pacemaker site is that of the underlying rhythm.

P Waves: The P waves are identical and precede the QRS complexes when they occur.

P-R Intervals: The P-R intervals may be normal or abnormal (greater than 0.20 second); they are constant.

R-R Intervals: The R-R intervals may be equal or may vary.

QRS Complexes: The QRS complexes may be normal or abnormal. Commonly, the AV conduction ratios are even numbers, such as 2:1, 4:1, 6:1, 8:1, and so forth. The AV block is identified by the AV conduction ratio present, e.g., 2:1, 3:1, 4:1, or 6:1 AV block. A 3:1 or higher AV block is called a **high-degree (or advanced) AV block.** An AV conduction ratio of 3:1, for example, indicates that for every three P waves, one is followed by a QRS complex. The AV conduction ratio may be fixed, or it may vary throughout any given lead.

Cause of Arrhythmia: Two-to-one and high-degree AV block with normal QRS complexes usually represent defective conduction of the electrical impulse through the AV node and are often associated with a second-degree type I AV block. They are commonly caused by an inferior-wall myocardial infarction, myocarditis, digitalis toxicity, or electrolyte imbalance.

Two-to-one and high-degree AV block with abnormal QRS complexes usually represent defective conduction of the electrical impulse through the bundle branches and are often associated with a second-degree type II AV block. These types of AV blocks are commonly caused by an anterior-wall myocardial infarction.

Clinical Significance: When the heart rate is excessively slow in 2:1 and high-degree AV block, the signs and symptoms are the same as those in symptomatic or marked sinus bradycardia. Two-to-one and high-degree AV block with normal QRS complexes may often be transient; however, 2:1 and high-degree AV block with abnormal QRS complexes frequently progress to a third-degree AV block.

An external or transvenous cardiac pacemaker is indicated in all symptomatic patients with 2:1 and high-degree AV block and in asymptomatic patients with abnormal QRS complexes, especially in the setting of an acute anterior-wall myocardial infarction. Two-to-one and high-degree AV block with normal QRS complexes usually respond to atropine.

Notes

Second-degree AV Block
2:1 and High-degree (Advanced) AV Block

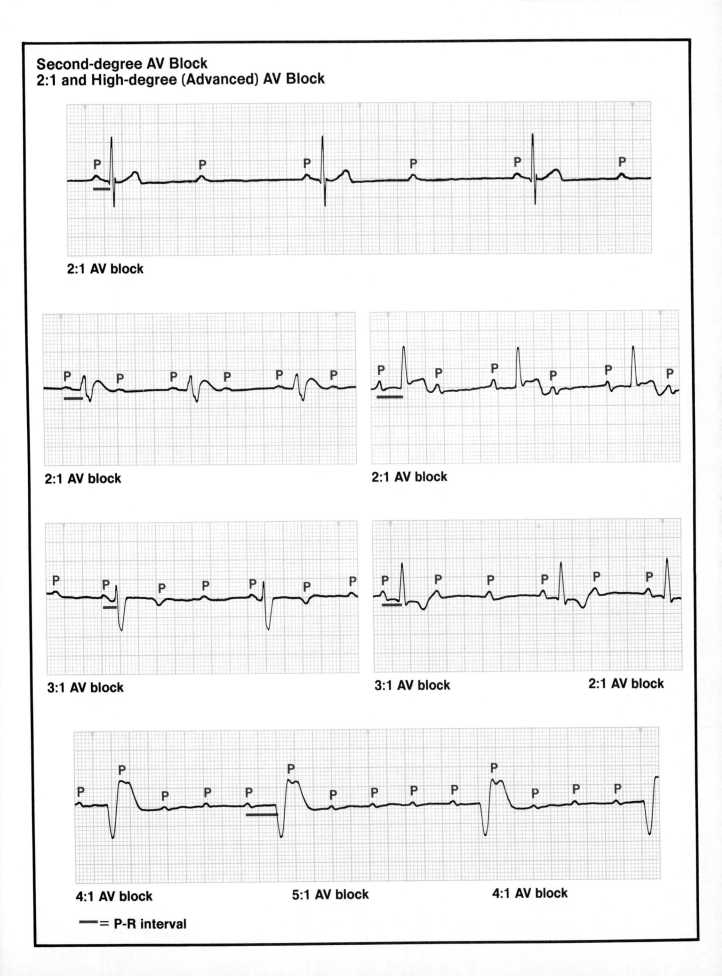

2:1 AV block

2:1 AV block

2:1 AV block

3:1 AV block

3:1 AV block   **2:1 AV block**

4:1 AV block   **5:1 AV block**   **4:1 AV block**

━━ = P-R interval

Third-degree AV Block
(Complete AV Block)

Heart Rate: The atrial rate is that of the underlying sinus or atrial rhythm. The ventricular rate is typically 40 to 60 beats per minute but may be as slow as 30 to 40 or less. Often, the ventricular rate is less than that of the atria.

Rhythm: The atrial rhythm may be regular or irregular, depending on the underlying atrial rhythm. The ventricular rhythm is essentially regular. The atrial and ventricular rhythms are independent of each other.

Pacemaker Site: If P waves are present, they may have originated in the SA node or an ectopic pacemaker in the atria. The pacemaker site of the QRS complexes is an escape pacemaker in the AV junction, bundle branches, or Purkinje network, below the AV block. Generally, if the third-degree AV block is at the level of the AV node, the escape pacemaker is usually infranodal, in the bundle of His. If the third-degree AV block is at the level of the bundle of His or bundle branches, the escape pacemaker is in the ventricles distal to the site of the AV block. If the escape pacemaker is in the AV junction (i.e., junctional escape rhythm), the heart rate is faster—40 to 60 beats per minute— than if the escape pacemaker were in the ventricles, i.e., bundle branches or Purkinje network (ventricular escape rhythm)—30 to 40 beats per minute or less.

P Waves: P waves or atrial flutter or fibrillation waves may be present. When present, they have no relation to the QRS complexes, appearing independently at a rate different from that of the QRS complexes (**atrioventricular [AV] dissociation).**

P-R Intervals: The P-R intervals vary widely since the P waves and QRS complexes occur independently.

R-R and P-P Intervals: The R-R intervals are usually equal and independent of the P-P intervals.

QRS Complexes: The QRS complexes typically exceed 0.12 second and are bizarre if the escape pacemaker site is in the ventricles or if the escape pacemaker site is in the AV junction and a pre-existing bundle branch block is present. But the QRS complexes may be normal (0.10 second or less) if the pacemaker site is above the bundle branches in the AV junction and no bundle branch block is present.

Cause of Arrhythmia: Third-degree AV block represents a complete block of the conduction of the electrical impulses from the atria to the ventricles at the level of the AV node, bundle of His, or bundle branches. It may be transient and reversible or permanent. **Transient** and **reversible third-degree AV block** is usually associated with normal QRS complexes and a heart rate of 45 to 60 beats per minute (i.e., junctional escape rhythm). It is commonly due to a complete block of conduction of the electrical impulse through the AV node, which can result from increased vagal (parasympathetic) tone associated with an acute inferior-wall myocardial infarction, from acute myocarditis, or from digitalis or propranolol toxicity or electrolyte imbalance. **Permanent** or **chronic third-degree AV block** is usually associated with wide and bizarre QRS complexes and a heart rate of 30 to 40 beats per minute or less (ventricular escape rhythm). It is commonly due to a complete block of conduction through both bundle branches, resulting from an anterior-wall myocardial infarction or chronic degenerative changes in the bundle branches in the elderly. It usually does not result from increased vagal (parasympathetic) tone or drug toxicity.

Clinical Significance: The signs and symptoms of third-degree AV block are the same as those in symptomatic or marked sinus bradycardia, except that third-degree AV block can be more ominous, especially when it is associated with wide and bizarre QRS complexes. If an AV junctional or ventricular escape pacemaker does not take over after a sudden onset of third-degree AV block, ventricular asystole will occur. This results in faintness, followed within seconds by loss of consciousness, seizures, and apnea (**Adams-Stokes syndrome),** and death if an escape pacemaker does not respond or ventricular asystole is not treated immediately.

An external or transvenous cardiac pacemaker is required immediately for the treatment of symptomatic third-degree AV block (regardless of cause) and for asymptomatic third-degree AV block with bundle branch block in a setting of an acute anterior-wall myocardial infarction. Third-degree AV block does respond to atropine occasionally.

Notes

Third-degree AV Block
(Complete AV Block)

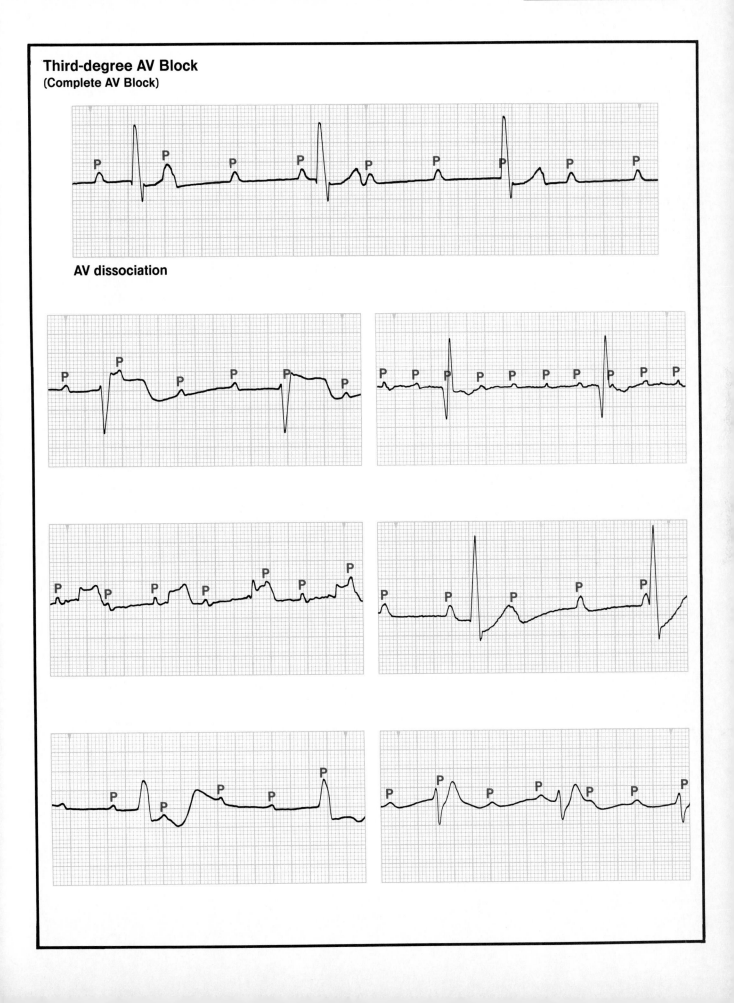

AV dissociation

Pacemaker Rhythm

Heart Rate: The ventricular rate per minute resulting from an **artificial pacemaker** is typically in the 60s or 70s.

Rhythm: The ventricular rhythm resulting from the pacemaker is regular.

Pacemaker Site: The pacemaker site of the pacemaker rhythm is the tip of the pacemaker wire, commonly positioned in the apex of the right ventricle (ventricular pacemaker), in the right atrium (atrial pacemaker), or in both (dual chamber pacemaker).

Types of Pacemakers: The major categories of pacemakers commonly used today include the **atrial and ventricular demand pacemakers** (pacemakers that pace either the atria or ventricles when there is no appropriate underlying spontaneous atrial or ventricular rhythm), the **atrial synchronous ventricular pacemakers** (pacemakers that are synchronized with the patient's atrial rhythm and pace the ventricles when an AV block occurs), **AV sequential pacemakers** (pacemakers that pace either the atria or ventricles or both sequentially when spontaneous ventricular activity is absent), and the **optimal sequential pacemakers** (pacemakers that pace the atria or ventricles or both sequentially when spontaneous atrial or ventricular activity is absent).

P Waves: P waves of the underlying rhythm may be present or absent. If present, they may be normal or abnormal. The relationship of the P waves to the pacemaker induced QRS complexes varies depending on the type of pacemaker present.

P-R Intervals: The presence and duration of the P-R intervals depend on the underlying rhythm and the type of pacemaker present.

R-R Intervals: The R-R intervals of the pacemaker rhythm are equal. When pacemaker induced QRS complexes are interspersed among the patient's normally occurring QRS complexes, the R-R intervals are unequal.

QRS Complexes: The QRS complexes resulting from a ventricular pacemaker typically exceed 0.12 second and are bizarre. Preceding each QRS complex is a narrow deflection, the pacemaker spike, representing the electrical discharge of the pacemaker. If only the atria are being paced, the QRS complexes are normal unless a preexisting bundle branch block is present.

Cause of Arrhythmia: A pacemaker rhythm indicates that the patient's heart is being artificially paced.

Clinical Significance: The presence of pacemaker spikes indicates that the patient's heart rate is being regulated by an artificial pacemaker. When every pacemaker spike is followed by a normal or wide and bizarre QRS complex, the pacemaker is functioning normally even if the patient's own P waves and QRS complexes are interspersed among the pacemaker spikes. Pacemaker spikes not followed by a QRS complex indicate a malfunctioning pacemaker, one whose electric impulse is unable to stimulate the heart to contract.

Notes

Pacemaker Rhythm

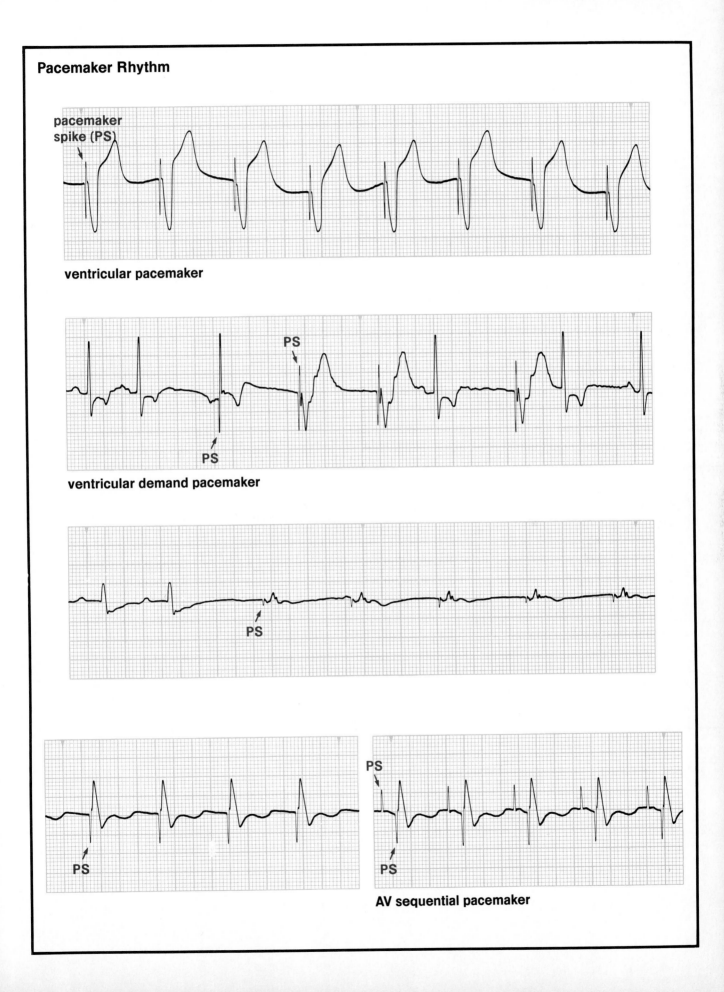

pacemaker spike (PS)

ventricular pacemaker

PS

PS

ventricular demand pacemaker

PS

PS

PS

PS

PS

AV sequential pacemaker

Chapter 6

Clinical Significance and Treatment of Arrhythmias

Bradycardias
- Sinus Bradycardia
- Sinus Arrest and Sinoatrial (SA) Exit Block
- Junctional Escape Rhythm
- Ventricular Escape Rhythm
- Second-degree AV Block Type I AV Block (Wenckebach)
- Second-degree AV Block Type II AV Block
- Second-degree AV Block 2:1 and High-degree (Advanced) AV Block
- Third-degree AV Block

Tachycardias
- Sinus Tachycardia
- Atrial Tachycardia (AT)
    - Nonparoxysmal Atrial Tachycardia without Block
    - Paroxysmal Atrial Tachycardia (PAT)
    - Atrial Tachycardia with Block
- Atrial Flutter (AF)
- Atrial Fibrillation
- Junctional Tachycardia
- Paroxysmal Junctional Tachycardia (PJT)
- Ventricular Tachycardia (VT)

Premature Ectopic Beats
- Premature Atrial Contractions (PACs)
- Premature Junctional Contractions (PJCs)
- Premature Ventricular Contractions (PVCs)

Ventricular Fibrillation (VF)

Ventricular Asystole

Electromechanical Dissociation (EMD)

The arrhythmia treatment protocols presented in this chapter are based on the recommendations of the 1985 National Conference on Standards and Guidelines for Cardiopulmonary Resuscitation (CPR) and Emergency Cardiac Care (ECC) sponsored by the American College of Cardiology, the American Heart Association, the American Red Cross, and the National Heart, Lung and Blood Institute.

These treatment protocols may be used as guidelines for the development of local or regional protocols for the management of arrhythmias during the prehospital and in-hospital phase of emergency cardiac care. Management may deviate from these treatment protocols or include additional treatment modalities when the physician in charge of the patients determines if such a deviation or addition is in the best interests of the patients.

The treatment sections have been color-coded to differentiate between prehospital and in-hospital emergency cardiac care. The drugs and techniques authorized for both prehospital and in-hospital emergency cardiac care are printed in black; those for in-hospital care only are in dark red. However, the scheme of authorization may be changed at the discretion of the medical control of the prehospital advanced life support system.

Bradycardias

Sinus Bradycardia

Sinus Arrest and
Sinoatrial (SA) Exit Block

Junctional Escape Rhythm

Ventricular Escape Rhythm

Second-degree AV Block
Type I AV Block (Wenckebach)

Second-degree AV Block
Type II AV Block

Second-degree AV Block
2:1 and High-degree (Advanced) AV Block

Third-degree AV Block

Clinical Significance of Bradycardias

A **bradycardia** with a heart rate between 50 to 59 beats per minute (**mild bradycardia**) usually does not produce symptoms by itself. If the heart rate slows to 30 to 45 beats per minute or less (**marked bradycardia**), the cardiac output may drop significantly, causing the systolic blood pressure to fall to 80 to 90 mm Hg or less and signs and symptoms of decreased perfusion of the body, especially of the vital organs, to appear. The skin may become pale, cold, and clammy; the pulse, weak or absent; and the patient, agitated, lightheaded, confused, or unconscious. The patient may experience chest pain and also become dyspneic.

In the presence of acute myocardial infarction, mild bradycardia may actually be beneficial in some patients because of the decrease in the workload of the heart, which reduces the oxygen requirements of the heart, minimizes the extension of the infarction, and lessens the predisposition to certain arrhythmias. Marked bradycardia, however, may result in hypotension with a marked reduction of cardiac output leading to congestive heart failure, loss of consciousness, and shock and predispose the patient to more serious arrhythmias (i.e., premature ventricular contractions, ventricular tachycardia or fibrillation, or ventricular asystole).

If sinus arrest or sinoatrial (SA) exit block is prolonged or second-degree AV block suddenly progresses to a third-degree AV block and if an escape pacemaker in the AV junction (junctional escape rhythm) or ventricles (ventricular escape rhythm) does not take over, ventricular asystole will occur.

Indications for Treatment of Bradycardias

Treatment as outlined below is usually not indicated if the heart rate is 60 beats per minute or greater.

Treatment of bradycardia—whatever its cause—is indicated if the heart rate is less than 60 beats per minute and one or more of the following are present (symptomatic or marked bradycardia):

- **Hypotension (systolic blood pressure, 80 to 90 mm Hg or less)**
- **Congestive heart failure**
- **Chest pain or dyspnea**
- **Signs and symptoms of decreased cardiac output (e.g., altered mental status)**
- **Premature ventricular contractions**

Treatment may not be indicated even if the heart rate falls below 60 beats per minute if the systolic blood pressure remains greater than 90 mm Hg and stable; if congestive heart failure, chest pain, and dyspnea are not present; if agitation, lightheadedness, confusion, and loss of consciousness are absent; and if premature ventricular contractions do not occur. Such an asymptomatic bradycardia may be considered a mild bradycardia.

Treatment

1. Consider the administration of a **precordial thump.**

If the bradycardia persists after the precordial thump and the indications for the treatment of the bradycardia are still present:

2. Administer a 0.5- to 1-mg bolus of **atropine** IV rapidly. Repeat every 5 minutes until the heart rate increases to 60 to 100 beats per minute or the maximum dose of 2.0 mg of atropine has been administered.

If the bradycardia persists after the maximum dose of atropine has been administered and the indications for the treatment of the bradycardia are still present:

3. Consider **external cardiac pacing.**

OR

Start an IV infusion of **isoproterenol** (1 mg of isoproterenol in 500 ml of 5% dextrose in water) at an initial rate of 2 to 10 μg per minute (1 to 5 ml of the diluted isoproterenol solution per minute), and adjust the infusion rate to maintain the heart rate at 60 to 70 beats per minute.

If the indications for the treatment of the brady-cardia are still present or if second-degree AV block (specifically, type II AV block and 2:1 or high-degree AV block with bundle branch block) or third-degree AV block with bundle branch block occurs in the setting of an acute anterior-wall myocardial infarction, even if asymptomatic:

4. Insert a **temporary transvenous cardiac pacemaker** immediately.

Notes

Tachycardias

Sinus Tachycardia

Atrial Tachycardia (AT)

Nonparoxysmal Atrial Tachycardia without Block

Paroxysmal Atrial Tachycardia (PAT)

Atrial Tachycardia with Block

Atrial Flutter (AF)

Atrial Fibrillation

Junctional Tachycardia

Paroxysmal Junctional Tachycardia (PJT)

Ventricular Tachycardia (VT)

Clinical Significance of Tachycardias

The signs and symptoms in a **tachycardia** depend upon the presence or absence of heart disease, the nature of the heart disease, the ventricular rate, and the duration of the tachycardia. Frequently, a tachycardia is accompanied by feelings of palpitations, nervousness, or anxiety.

A tachycardia with a heart rate over 120 to 140 beats per minute may cause the cardiac output to drop significantly because of the inability of the ventricles to fill completely during the extremely short diastole that results from the very rapid beating of the heart. Consequently, the systolic blood pressure may fall to 80 to 90 mm Hg or less and signs and symptoms of decreased perfusion of the body, especially of the brain and other vital organs, may occur. The skin may become pale, cold and clammy; the pulse may become weak or disappear; and the patient may become agitated, confused, lightheaded, or unconscious or may experience chest pain and also become dyspneic.

In addition, since a rapid heart rate increases the workload of the heart, the oxygen requirements of the heart are usually increased in a tachycardia. Because of this, in addition to the consequences of decreased cardiac output, a tachycardia in acute myocardial infarction may increase myocardial ischemia and the frequency and severity of chest pain, bring about the extension of the infarct, cause congestive heart failure, hypotension or cardiogenic shock, or predispose the patient to serious ventricular arrhythmias.

Another reason for low cardiac output in certain tachycardias (atrial flutter, atrial fibrillation, and junctional and ventricular tachycardias) is that because an atrial contraction does not precede each ventricular contraction, the so-called "atrial kick," as it normally does, the ventricles do not fill completely during diastole. Consequently, the cardiac output may drop by as much as 25%.

Indications for Treatment of Tachycardias

Specific treatment of nonparoxysmal atrial tachycardia without block, atrial flutter, atrial fibrillation, and paroxysmal atrial and junctional tachycardia is indicated if the heart rate is greater than 120 to 140 beats per minute (or even as low as 100 to 120 beats per minute) and, particularly, if signs and symptoms of decreased cardiac output or increased workload of the heart are associated with the tachycardia.

Treatment of ventricular tachycardia, however, is indicated immediately, whether or not signs and symptoms of decreased cardiac output are present, because of its potential of initiating or degenerating into ventricular fibrillation.

No specific treatment of sinus tachycardia, nonparoxysmal and paroxysmal atrial tachycardia with block, and junctional tachycardia is indicated.

Sinus Tachycardia

Treatment

No specific treatment of sinus tachycardia is indicated.

1. Treat the underlying cause of the tachycardia (anxiety, exercise, pain, fever, congestive heart failure, hypoxemia, hypovolemia, hypotension, or shock).

If excessive amounts of drugs, such as **atropine, epinephrine** or **isoproterenol,** have been administered:

2. Discontinue such drugs.

Notes

Atrial Tachycardia with Block and Junctional Tachycardia

Treatment

No specific treatment of atrial tachycardia with block or junctional tachycardia is indicated.

1. Treat the underlying cause of the tachycardia.

If an excessive dose of **digitalis** is suspected:

2. Discontinue **digitalis.**

CAUTION!

DO NOT ATTEMPT VAGAL MANEUVERS OR CARDIOVERSION!

Notes

Paroxysmal Atrial Tachycardia (PAT)

Paroxysmal Junctional Tachycardia (PJT)

Patient Hemodynamically Stable

Treatment

If the patient's condition is stable, that is, the patient is normotensive, without chest pain or congestive heart failure and not having an acute myocardial infarction or ischemic episode:

1. Attempt **vagal maneuvers,** such as **unilateral carotid sinus massage,** or have the patient perform the **Valsalva maneuver** or take a **deep breath while in a head-down tilt position.** ECG monitoring and an IV line must be in place and atropine and lidocaine immediately available before vagal maneuvers are performed. The technique of immersing the patient's face in ice water (**"diving reflex"**) may also be tried but only if ischemic heart disease is not present or suspected.

> **CAUTION!**
>
> **VERIFY THE ABSENCE OF KNOWN CAROTID ARTERY DISEASE OR CAROTID BRUITS BEFORE ATTEMPTING CAROTID SINUS MASSAGE!**

If the vagal maneuvers are unsuccessful and the patient remains stable:

2. Administer 5 mg of **verapamil** IV slowly over 2 minutes, and, if the initial dose is unsuccessful and no adverse effects (such as severe bradycardia, hypotension, and congestive heart failure) have occurred, administer 10 mg of verapamil IV slowly, in 15 to 30 minutes if needed.

> **CAUTION!**
>
> **VERAPAMIL IS CONTRAINDICATED IF HYPOTENSION, CONGESTIVE HEART FAILURE, OR A PREEXCITATION SYNDROME IS PRESENT, IF BETA BLOCKERS ARE BEING ADMINISTERED INTRAVENOUSLY, OR IF THERE IS A HISTORY OF BRADYCARDIA. VERAPAMIL SHOULD BE USED CAUTIOUSLY IN PATIENTS RECEIVING BETA BLOCKERS.**
>
> **THE PATIENT'S BLOOD PRESSURE AND PULSE MUST BE MONITORED FREQUENTLY DURING AND AFTER THE ADMINISTRATION OF VERAPAMIL. IF HYPOTENSION OCCURS WITH VERAPAMIL, ADMINISTER 0.5 TO 1.0 G OF CALCIUM CHLORIDE IV SLOWLY. IF BRADYCARDIA, AV BLOCK, OR ASYSTOLE OCCURS, REFER TO THE APPROPRIATE TREATMENT PROTOCOL.**

If the vagal maneuvers and verapamil are unsuccessful and if an excessive dose of digitalis is not suspected and the patient remains stable:

3. Deliver a **synchronized DC countershock** (75 to 100 joules*). If the patient is conscious, administer 5 to 15 mg of **diazepam** or 2 to 5 mg of **morphine sulfate** IV slowly to produce amnesia before cardioversion.

> **CAUTION!**
>
> **DO NOT ATTEMPT DC COUNTERSHOCK IF PAROXYSMAL ATRIAL OR JUNCTIONAL TACHYCARDIA RECURS AFTER INITIAL CONVERSION TO A SINUS RHYTHM AND ANY UNDERLYING CAUSES OF PAROXYSMAL ATRIAL OR JUNCTIONAL TACHYCARDIA (E.G., ELECTROLYTE AND ACID-BASE ABNORMALITIES) HAVE NOT BEEN CORRECTED!**

If paroxysmal atrial or junctional tachycardia persists and if an excessive dose of digitalis is not suspected:

4. Administer 0.5 mg of **digoxin** IV.

5. Repeat the **vagal maneuvers** and **electrical cardioversion.**

If paroxysmal atrial or junctional tachycardia persists:

6. Administer 1 mg of **propranolol,** diluted to 10 ml with 5% dextrose in water, IV slowly over 5 minutes. Repeat every 5 minutes if needed until the tachycardia is converted or a total dose of 0.1 mg/kg of propranolol has been administered.

> **CAUTION!**
>
> **PROPRANOLOL IS CONTRAINDICATED IN CARDIAC ARREST OR IN THE PRESENCE OF HYPOTENSION, BRADYCARDIA, CONGESTIVE HEART FAILURE, AV BLOCK, AND ASTHMA. PROPRANOLOL SHOULD BE ADMINISTERED CAUTIOUSLY IN ACUTE MYOCARDIAL INFARCTION.**
>
> **THE PATIENT'S BLOOD PRESSURE AND PULSE MUST BE MONITORED FREQUENTLY DURING AND AFTER THE ADMINISTRATION OF PROPRANOLOL. IF BRADYCARDIA OCCURS WITH PROPRANOLOL, ADMINISTER ATROPINE OR ISOPROTERENOL.**

Paroxysmal Atrial Tachycardia (PAT)

Paroxysmal Junctional Tachycardia (PJT)

Patient Hemodynamically Unstable

If paroxysmal atrial or junctional tachycardia persists:

7. Consider **external overdrive cardiac pacing.**

If an excessive dose of digitalis is suspected:

8. Withhold digitalis, and administer 40 mEq of **potassium chloride** in 500 ml of 0.9% saline IV at a rate of 10 to 15 mEq/hr (125 to 188 ml of the diluted potassium chloride solution per hour).

If paroxysmal atrial or junctional tachycardia persists:

9. Administer 1 mg of **propranolol,** diluted to 10 ml with 5% dextrose in water, IV slowly over 5 minutes. Repeat every 5 minutes if needed until the tachycardia is converted or a total dose of 0.1 mg/kg of propranolol has been administered. (See **CAUTION!** concerning the use of propranolol noted on page 172.)

* The energy delivered in direct-current (DC) countershock is indicated as joules (watt/seconds) of delivered energy. Generally, delivered energy is approximately 80% of the energy stored in the defibrillator.

If the patient's condition is unstable, that is, the patient is hypotensive with evidence of poor peripheral perfusion, has chest pain or congestive heart failure, or is having an acute myocardial infarction or ischemic episode:

1. Deliver a **synchronized DC countershock** (75 to 100 joules). If the patient is conscious and not hypotensive, consider the administration of 5 to 15 mg of **diazepam** or 2 to 5 mg of **morphine sulfate** IV slowly to produce amnesia before cardioversion.

ADMINISTRATION OF DIAZEPAM OR MORPHINE SULFATE SHOULD NOT DELAY CARDIOVERSION IF IT IS INDICATED IMMEDIATELY BY THE PATIENT'S CONDITION!

> **CAUTION!**
>
> **DO NOT ATTEMPT DC COUNTERSHOCK IF AN EXCESSIVE DOSE OF DIGITALIS IS SUSPECTED AS THE CAUSE OF PAROXYSMAL ATRIAL OR JUNCTIONAL TACHYCARDIA OR IF THE TACHYCARDIA RECURS AFTER INITIAL CONVERSION TO A SINUS RHYTHM AND ANY UNDERLYING CAUSES OF PAROXYSMAL ATRIAL OR JUNCTIONAL TACHYCARDIA (E.G., ELECTROLYTE AND ACID-BASE ABNORMALITIES) HAVE NOT BEEN CORRECTED!**

If the first DC countershock is unsuccessful:

2. Deliver a **second synchronized DC countershock** (200 joules).

If the second DC countershock is unsuccessful:

3. Deliver a **third synchronized DC countershock** (up to 360 joules).

If the third DC countershock is unsuccessful:

4. Correct any underlying causes of paroxysmal atrial or junctional tachycardia (e.g., electrolyte and acid-base abnormalities).

5. Consider the treatment protocol for **Hemodynamically Stable Paroxysmal Atrial or Junctional Tachycardia,** page 172.

Notes

Notes

Atrial Flutter (AF)
(Including Nonparoxysmal
Atrial Tachycardia without Block)

Treatment

If digitalis has not been administered previously:

1. Deliver a **synchronized, low-energy, DC countershock** (25 joules). If the patient is conscious, administer 5 to 15 mg of **diazepam** or 2 to 5 mg of **morphine sulfate** IV slowly to produce amnesia before cardioversion.

If cardioversion is unsuccessful and the indications for treatment of atrial flutter are still present:

2. Administer 0.5 to 1 mg of **digoxin** IV, and follow by full digitalization within 12 hours by administering 0.25 to 0.50 mg of digoxin IV every 2 to 4 hours until the ventricular rate is slowed or a total dose of 1 to 2.5 mg of digoxin has been administered.

If digitalis is unsuccessful in slowing the ventricular rate or in cardioverting the atrial flutter to normal sinus rhythm and the indications for treatment of atrial flutter are still present:

3. Repeat the **synchronized DC countershock** (50 joules or more).

If cardioversion is unsuccessful:

4. Administer 1 mg of **propranolol,** diluted to 10 ml with 5% dextrose in water, IV slowly over 5 minutes. Repeat every 5 minutes if needed until the ventricular rate is slowed or a total dose of 0.1 mg/kg of propranolol has been administered.

> **CAUTION!**
>
> **PROPRANOLOL IS CONTRAINDICATED IN CARDIAC ARREST OR IN THE PRESENCE OF HYPOTENSION, BRADYCARDIA, CONGESTIVE HEART FAILURE, AV BLOCK, AND ASTHMA. PROPRANOLOL SHOULD BE ADMINISTERED CAUTIOUSLY IN ACUTE MYOCARDIAL INFARCTION.**
>
> **THE PATIENT'S BLOOD PRESSURE AND PULSE MUST BE MONITORED FREQUENTLY DURING AND AFTER THE ADMINISTRATION OF PRO- PRANOLOL. IF BRADYCARDIA OCCURS WITH PROPRANOLOL, ADMINISTER ATROPINE OR ISOPROTERENOL.**

If atrial flutter persists:

5. Repeat the **synchronized DC countershock** (50 joules or more).

Notes

Atrial Fibrillation

Treatment

If digitalis has not been administered previously and the signs and symptoms of decreased cardiac output are not severe:

1. Administer 0.5 to 1 mg of **digoxin** IV, and follow by full digitalization within 12 hours by administering 0.25 to 0.50 mg of digoxin IV every 2 to 4 hours until the ventricular rate is slowed or a total dose of 1 to 2.5 mg of digoxin has been administered.

If the ventricular rate still fails to slow:

2. Administer 1 mg of **propranolol,** diluted to 10 ml with 5% dextrose in water, IV slowly over 5 minutes. Repeat every 5 minutes if needed until the ventricular rate is slowed or a total dose of 0.1 mg/kg of propranolol has been administered.

CAUTION!

PROPRANOLOL IS CONTRAINDICATED IN CARDIAC ARREST OR IN THE PRESENCE OF HYPOTENSION, BRADYCARDIA, CONGESTIVE HEART FAILURE, AV BLOCK, AND ASTHMA. PROPRANOLOL SHOULD BE ADMINISTERED CAUTIOUSLY IN ACUTE MYOCARDIAL INFARCTION.

THE PATIENT'S BLOOD PRESSURE AND PULSE MUST BE MONITORED FREQUENTLY DURING AND AFTER THE ADMINISTRATION OF PRO-PRANOLOL. IF BRADYCARDIA OCCURS WITH PROPRANOLOL, ADMINISTER ATROPINE OR ISOPROTERENOL.

If digitalis has not been administered previously and the signs and symptoms of decreased cardiac output are severe (e.g., hypotension and pulmonary edema):

1. Deliver a **synchronized DC countershock** (75 to 100 joules). If the patient is conscious, administer 5 to 15 mg of **diazepam** or 2 to 5 mg of **morphine sulfate** IV slowly to produce amnesia before cardioversion.

If digitalis has been administered previously:

1. Administer 1 mg of **propranolol,** diluted to 10 ml with 5% dextrose in water, IV slowly over 5 minutes. Repeat every 5 minutes if needed until the ventricular rate is slowed or a total dose of 0.1 mg/kg of propranolol has been administered. (See **CAUTION!** concerning the use of propranolol.)

Notes

Ventricular Tachycardia (with Pulse)

Patient Hemodynamically Stable

Treatment

If the patient's condition is hemodynamically stable—that is, the patient is conscious and has a pulse, the systolic blood pressure is greater than 90 mm Hg, and pulmonary edema and signs and symptoms of decreased cardiac output are absent:

1. Administer the highest concentration of oxygen possible.

2. Establish an **IV line.**

3. Administer a 1-mg/kg bolus of **lidocaine** IV slowly.

4. Repeat administration of a 0.5-mg/kg bolus of **lidocaine** IV slowly every 8 to 10 minutes if needed until the ventricular tachycardia is suppressed or a total dose of 3 mg/kg of lidocaine has been administered within 1 hour.

5. Start an IV infusion of **lidocaine** (1 g of lidocaine in 500 ml of 5% dextrose in water) as soon as possible at a rate of 2 mg of lidocaine per minute (1 ml of the diluted lidocaine solution per minute) to prevent the recurrence of ventricular tachycardia. If additional boluses of lidocaine are administered initially, increase the rate of the lidocaine infusion by 1-mg increments after each additional 1-mg/kg dose of lidocaine to a maximum rate of 4 mg of lidocaine per minute.

Initial Dose of Lidocaine	Rate of Lidocaine Infusion
1 mg/kg	2 mg/min
1-2 mg/kg	3 mg/min
2-3 mg/kg	4 mg/min

If lidocaine is unsuccessful in suppressing the ventricular tachycardia and the patient remains stable:

6. Discontinue the lidocaine infusion if it has been started, and administer 100 mg of **procainamide** IV slowly over 5 minutes at a rate of 20 mg of procainamide per minute.

7. Repeat the 100-mg dose of **procainamide** every 5 minutes until the ventricular tachycardia is suppressed, a total dose of 1,000 mg of procainamide has been administered, side effects from the procainamide (such as hypotension) appear, or the QRS complex widens by 50% of its original width.

8. Start an IV infusion of **procainamide** (1 g of procainamide in 500 ml of 5% dextrose in water) as soon as possible at a rate of 1 to 4 mg per minute (0.5 to 2 ml of the diluted procainamide solution per minute) to prevent the recurrence of ventricular tachycardia.

If lidocaine and procainamide are unsuccessful in suppressing the ventricular tachycardia and the patient remains stable:

9. Administer a dose of 5- to 10-mg/kg of **bretylium tosylate,** diluted to 50 ml with 5% dextrose in water, IV slowly over 8 to 10 minutes.

10. Start an IV infusion of **bretylium tosylate** (1 g of bretylium tosylate in 500 ml of 5% dextrose in water) at a rate of 1 to 2 mg per minute (0.5 to 1 ml of the diluted bretylium tosylate solution per minute) to prevent recurrence of ventricular tachycardia.

If lidocaine, procainamide, and bretylium tosylate are unsuccessful in suppressing the ventricular tachycardia and the patient remains stable:

11. Administer a **precordial thump.**

If ventricular tachycardia persists:

12. Administer a **synchronized DC countershock** (50 joules). In the conscious patient, consider the administration of 5 to 15 mg of **diazepam** or 2 to 5 mg of **morphine sulfate** IV slowly to produce amnesia before cardioversion.

If the first DC countershock is unsuccessful:

13. Deliver a **second synchronized DC countershock** (100 joules).

If the second DC countershock is unsuccessful:

14. Deliver a **third synchronized DC countershock** (200 joules).

If the third DC countershock is unsuccessful:

15. Deliver a **fourth synchronized DC countershock** (up to 360 joules).

If the patient with ventricular tachycardia becomes hemodynamically unstable (e.g., drowsy, stuporous, unconscious, or hypotensive [systolic blood pressure of 80 to 90 mm Hg or less]) or if signs and symptoms of decreased cardiac output (e.g., chest pain or dyspnea) appear:

16. Administer an **unsynchronized DC countershock** (50 joules). If the patient is still conscious, consider the administration of 5 to 15 mg of **diazepam** or 2 to 5 mg of **morphine sulfate** IV slowly to produce amnesia before cardioversion.

ADMINISTRATION OF DIAZEPAM OR MORPHINE SULFATE SHOULD NOT DELAY CARDIOVERSION IF IT IS INDICATED IMMEDIATELY BY THE PATIENT'S CONDITION!

If cardioversion is successful in terminating the ventricular tachycardia:

17. Administer a 1-mg/kg bolus of **lidocaine** IV slowly.

18. Start an IV infusion of **lidocaine,** if one has not already been started, (1 g of lidocaine in 500 ml of 5% dextrose in water) as soon as possible at a rate of 2 mg of lidocaine per minute (1 ml of the diluted lidocaine solution per minute) to prevent the recurrence of ventricular tachycardia.

Notes

Ventricular Tachycardia (with Pulse)

Patient Hemodynamically Unstable

Treatment

If the patient is conscious (or unconscious) and has a pulse, but with a hemodynamically unstable condition—that is, the patient is hypotensive (systolic blood pressure of 80 to 90 mm Hg or less) with evidence of poor peripheral perfusion, has congestive heart failure or symptoms (e.g., chest pain or dyspnea), or is having an acute myocardial infarction or ischemic episode:

1. Administer the highest concentration of oxygen possible.

2. Establish an **IV line.**

3. Deliver an **unsynchronized DC countershock** (50 joules). In the conscious patient, consider the administration of 5 to 15 mg of **diazepam** or 2 to 5 mg of **morphine sulfate** IV slowly to produce amnesia before cardioversion.

   ADMINISTRATION OF DIAZEPAM OR MORPHINE SULFATE SHOULD NOT DELAY CARDIOVERSION IF IT IS INDICATED IMMEDIATELY BY THE PATIENT'S CONDITION!

If the first DC countershock is unsuccessful:

4. Deliver a **second unsynchronized DC countershock** (100 joules).

If the second DC countershock is unsuccessful:

5. Deliver a **third unsynchronized DC countershock** (200 joules).

If the third DC countershock is unsuccessful:

6. Deliver a **fourth unsynchronized DC countershock** (up to 360 joules).

If cardioversion is successful in terminating the ventricular tachycardia:

7. Administer a 1-mg/kg bolus of **lidocaine** IV slowly.

8. Start an IV infusion of **lidocaine** (1 g of lidocaine in 500 ml of 5% dextrose in water) as soon as possible at a rate of 2 mg of lidocaine per minute (1 ml of the diluted lidocaine solution per minute) to prevent the recurrence of ventricular tachycardia.

If ventricular tachycardia persists (or recurs):

9. Administer a 1-mg/kg bolus of **lidocaine** IV slowly.

10. Repeat administration of a 0.5-mg/kg bolus of **lidocaine** IV slowly every 8 to 10 minutes if needed until the ventricular tachycardia is suppressed or a total dose of 3 mg/kg of lidocaine has been administered within 1 hour.

11. Start an IV infusion of **lidocaine** (1 g of lidocaine in 500 ml of 5% dextrose in water) at a rate of 2 to 4 mg of lidocaine per minute (1 to 2 ml of the diluted lidocaine solution per minute) or continue the IV infusion of lidocaine previously started to prevent the recurrence of ventricular tachycardia. The rate of lidocaine infusion is based on the dose of lidocaine administered as boluses to suppress ventricular tachycardia. The rate of the infusion is increased by 1-mg increments after each additional 1-mg/kg dose of lidocaine to a maximum rate of 4 mg of lidocaine per minute.

Initial Dose of Lidocaine	Rate of Lidocaine Infusion
1 mg/kg	2 mg/min
1-2 mg/kg	3 mg/min
2-3 mg/kg	4 mg/min

If ventricular tachycardia persists:

12. Deliver an **unsynchronized DC countershock** at the energy level at which cardioversion was previously effective, and repeat the **unsynchronized DC countershock** at progressively increasing energy levels if needed.

If lidocaine and DC countershock are unsuccessful in suppressing the ventricular tachycardia and the patient remains unstable:

13. Discontinue the lidocaine infusion if it has been started, and administer 100 mg of **procainamide** IV slowly over 5 minutes at a rate of 20 mg of procainamide per minute.

CAUTION!

DO NOT ADMINISTER PROCAINAMIDE IF HYPOTENSION OR PULMONARY EDEMA IS PRESENT OR IF THE PATIENT IS UNCONSCIOUS. ADMINISTER, INSTEAD, BRETYLIUM TOSYLATE AS IN STEP 17 BELOW.

---

14. Repeat the 100-mg dose of **procainamide** every 5 minutes until the ventricular tachycardia is suppressed, a total dose of 1,000 mg of procainamide has been administered, side effects from the procainamide (such as hypotension) appear, or the QRS complex widens by 50% of its original width.

15. Start an IV infusion of **procainamide** (1 g of procainamide in 500 ml of 5% dextrose in water) as soon as possible at a rate of 1 to 4 mg per minute (0.5 to 2 ml of the diluted procainamide solution per minute) to prevent the recurrence of ventricular tachycardia.

If ventricular tachycardia persists:

16. Deliver an **unsynchronized DC countershock** at the energy level at which cardioversion was previously effective, and repeat the **unsynchronized DC countershock** at progressively increasing energy levels if needed.

If lidocaine, procainamide and DC countershock are unsuccessful in suppressing the ventricular tachycardia and the patient remains unstable:

17. Administer a dose of 5- to 10-mg/kg of **bretylium tosylate,** diluted to 50 ml with 5% dextrose in water, IV slowly over 8 to 10 minutes.

18. Start an IV infusion of **bretylium tosylate** (1 g of bretylium tosylate in 500 ml of 5% dextrose in water) at a rate of 1 to 2 mg per minute (0.5 to 1 ml of the diluted bretylium tosylate solution per minute) to prevent recurrence of ventricular tachycardia.

If ventricular tachycardia persists:

19. Deliver an **unsynchronized DC countershock** at the energy level at which cardioversion was previously effective, and repeat the **unsynchronized DC countershock** at progressively increasing energy levels if needed, until the ventricular tachycardia is suppressed.

Notes

Ventricular Tachycardia (Pulseless)

Treatment

If the patient is unconscious and pulseless, the treatment is the same as that for ventricular fibrillation.

A. Witnessed Cardiac Arrest

If the cardiac arrest is witnessed by the rescuer or if cardiac arrest has been present for less than one or two minutes and CPR is being performed by someone other than the rescuer and the patient is not being monitored:

1. Verify cardiac arrest by checking the patient's pulse.

If the pulse is absent:

2. Administer a **precordial thump** immediately, and check the patient's pulse.

If the pulse remains absent:

3. Perform **CPR.**

4. Determine the rhythm by ECG monitor.

If ventricular tachycardia is present:

5. Deliver an **unsynchronized DC countershock** (200 joules) immediately, and check the patient's pulse and rhythm.

If ventricular tachycardia persists:

6. Deliver a **second unsynchronized DC countershock** (200 to 300 joules) immediately after the first DC countershock, and check the patient's pulse and rhythm.

If ventricular tachycardia persists:

7. Deliver a **third unsynchronized DC countershock** (up to 360 joules) immediately after the second DC countershock, and check the patient's pulse and rhythm.

If ventricular tachycardia persists:

8. Continue **CPR.**

9. Establish an **IV line.**

10. Administer 0.5 to 1.0 mg of **epinephrine** (5 to 10 ml of a 1:10,000 solution of epinephrine) IV, and repeat every 5 minutes if needed.

Note: If an intravenous line cannot be established, administer 1 mg of **epinephrine** (10 ml of a 1:10,000 solution of epinephrine) via the endotracheal tube, if one is in place. If both an intravenous line and an endotracheal tube are not in place, administer 0.5 mg of epinephrine (5 ml of a 1:10,000 solution of epinephrine) by intracardiac injection and repeat if needed.

11. Continue **CPR** for several minutes to circulate the drug.

12. Perform endotracheal intubation or, less preferably, insert an esophageal obturator airway.

13. Ventilate with the highest concentration of oxygen possible.

14. Deliver a **fourth unsynchronized DC countershock** (up to 360 joules), and check the patient's pulse and rhythm.

If ventricular tachycardia persists:

15. Administer a 1-mg/kg bolus of **lidocaine** IV slowly.

16. Continue **CPR** for several minutes to circulate the drug.

17. Deliver a **fifth unsynchronized DC countershock** (up to 360 joules), and check the patient's pulse and rhythm.

If ventricular tachycardia persists:

18. Administer a 5-mg/kg bolus of **bretylium tosylate** IV.

19. Continue **CPR** for several minutes to circulate the drug.

20. Consider administration of **sodium bicarbonate** at this point if it is indicated. The initial dose is 1 mEq/kg of sodium bicarbonate IV. Do not administer additional sodium bicarbonate until the patient's arterial blood pH and gases have been analyzed. If such a blood analysis is not feasible at this point, repeat the administration of half of the initial dose of sodium bicarbonate (0.5 mEq/kg of sodium bicarbonate) IV every 10 to 15 minutes for a total dose of 100 to 200 mEq of sodium bicarbonate.

21. Continue **CPR** for several minutes to circulate the drug.

22. Deliver a **sixth unsynchronized DC counter-shock** (up to 360 joules), and check the patient's pulse and rhythm.

If ventricular tachycardia persists:

23. Administer a 10-mg/kg bolus of **bretylium tosylate** IV.

24. Continue **CPR** for several minutes to circulate the drug.

25. Deliver a **seventh unsynchronized DC countershock** (up to 360 joules), and check the patient's pulse and rhythm.

If ventricular tachycardia persists:

26. Continue **CPR.**

27. Assess the effectiveness of ventilation and external chest compression.

28. Administer a 0.5-mg/kg bolus of **lidocaine** IV slowly.

OR

Administer a 10-mg/kg bolus of **bretylium tosylate** IV.

29. Continue **CPR** for several minutes to circulate the drug.

30. Deliver an **eighth unsynchronized DC countershock** (up to 360 joules), and check the patient's pulse and rhythm.

If ventricular tachycardia persists:

31. Continue **CPR.**

32. Reassess the effectiveness of ventilation and external chest compression.

33. Repeat administration of **epinephrine, lidocaine** (up to a total dose of 3 mg/kg), **bretylium tosylate** (up to a total dose of 30 mg/kg), **sodium bicarbonate** (if indicated), and **cardioversion,** and continue **CPR** until the ventricular tachycardia is terminated or a physician orders an end to the resuscitative efforts.

If ventricular tachycardia is terminated and a supraventricular rhythm is present:

34. Perform **CPR** until the patient's pulse is palpable and the systolic blood pressure is 90 mm Hg or greater.

IF LIDOCAINE HAS NOT BEEN ADMINISTERED PREVIOUSLY:

35. Administer a 1-mg/kg bolus of **lidocaine** IV slowly.

36. Start an IV infusion of **lidocaine** (1 g of lidocaine in 500 ml of 5% dextrose in water) as soon as possible at a rate of 2 mg of lidocaine per minute (1 ml of the diluted lidocaine solution per minute) to prevent the recurrence of ventricular tachycardia.

If ventricular tachycardia recurs:

37. Deliver an **unsynchronized DC countershock** immediately at the energy level at which cardioversion was previously effective, and check the patient's pulse and rhythm.

Notes

Ventricular Tachycardia (Pulseless)—Cont.

Treatment

B. Unwitnessed Cardiac Arrest

If the cardiac arrest is unwitnessed by the rescuer or if cardiac arrest has been present for more than one or two minutes and CPR is being performed by someone other than the rescuer and the patient is not being monitored:

1. Verify cardiac arrest by checking the patient's pulse.

2. Perform **CPR.**

3. Determine the rhythm by ECG monitor.

If ventricular tachycardia is present:

4. Deliver an **unsynchronized DC countershock** (200 joules) immediately, and check the patient's pulse and rhythm.

If ventricular tachycardia persists:

5. Deliver a **second unsynchronized DC countershock** (200 to 300 joules) immediately after the first DC countershock, and check the patient's pulse and rhythm.

If ventricular tachycardia persists:

6. Deliver a **third unsynchronized DC countershock** (up to 360 joules) immediately after the second DC countershock, and check the patient's pulse and rhythm.

If ventricular tachycardia persists:

7. Continue **CPR.**

8. Refer to **Step 9** in **A. Witnessed Cardiac Arrest** under **Ventricular Tachycardia (Pulseless),** page 180.

Notes

Treatment

C. Monitored Cardiac Arrest

If the patient is being monitored and ventricular tachycardia occurs:

1. Verify cardiac arrest by checking the patient's pulse.

2. Administer a **precordial thump** immediately, and check the patient's pulse and rhythm.

If ventricular tachycardia persists:

3. Deliver an **unsynchronized DC countershock** (200 joules) immediately, and check the patient's pulse and rhythm.

If ventricular tachycardia persists:

4. Deliver a **second unsynchronized DC countershock** (200 to 300 joules) immediately after the first DC countershock, and check the patient's pulse and rhythm.

If ventricular tachycardia persists:

5. Deliver a **third unsynchronized DC countershock** (up to 360 joules) immediately after the second DC countershock, and check the patient's pulse and rhythm.

If ventricular tachycardia persists:

6. Perform **CPR.**

7. Refer to **Step 9** in **A. Witnessed Cardiac Arrest** under **Ventricular Tachycardia (Pulseless),** page 180.

Notes

Premature Ectopic Beats

Premature Atrial Contractions (PACs)

Premature Junctional Contractions (PJCs)

Premature Ventricular Contractions (PVCs)

Premature Atrial Contractions (PACs)

Clinical Significance of Premature Atrial Contractions

Single isolated premature atrial contractions are not significant. Frequent PACs may indicate the presence of enhanced atrial automaticity, an atrial reentry mechanism or both and herald impending atrial arrhythmias (such as atrial tachycardia, atrial flutter, and atrial fibrillation) and paroxysmal atrial or junctional tachycardia.

Indications for Treatment of Premature Atrial Contractions

Treatment is indicated if the premature atrial contractions are frequent (eight to ten per minute), occur in groups of two or more, or alternate with the P-QRS-T complexes of the underlying rhythm (bigeminy).

Treatment

If stimulants (such as caffeine, tobacco, or alcohol) or excessive amounts of sympathomimetic drugs (such as epinephrine or isoproterenol) have been administered:

1. Discontinue the stimulants and sympatho-mimetic drugs.

If the premature atrial contractions continue and the indication for treatment is still present:

2. Administer 200 mg of **quinidine sulfate** by mouth.

If an excessive dose of **digitalis** is suspected:

3. Withhold **digitalis.**

Premature Junctional Contractions (PJCs)

Clinical Significance of Premature Junctional Contractions

Single isolated premature junctional contractions are not significant. Frequent PJCs may indicate the presence of enhanced AV junctional automaticity, an AV junctional reentry mechanism or both and herald an impending junctional tachycardia.

Indications for Treatment of Premature Junctional Contractions

Treatment is indicated if the premature junctional contractions are frequent (four to six per minute), occur in groups of two or more, or alternate with the QRS complexes of the underlying rhythm (bigeminy).

Treatment

Treatment of premature junctional contractions is the same as that of premature atrial contractions.

Premature Ventricular Contractions (PVCs)

Clinical Significance of Premature Ventricular Contractions

Single premature ventricular contractions, especially in patients who have no heart disease, are generally not significant. In patients with acute myocardial infarction or an ischemic episode, PVCs may indicate the presence of enhanced ventricular automaticity, a ventricular reentry mechanism, or both or herald the appearance of life-threatening arrhythmias, such as ventricular tachycardia, flutter, or fibrillation. Although these lethal arrhythmias may occur without warning, they are often initiated by premature ventricular contractions, especially if the PVCs are frequent (six or more per minute), occur in groups of two or more (group beats), arise from different ventricular ectopic pacemakers (multifocal), have different QRS configurations (multiform), are close coupled, or fall on the T wave (R-on-T phenomenon).

Premature Ventricular Contractions (PVCs)—Cont.

Indications for Treatment of Premature Ventricular Contractions

Treatment is indicated for all premature ventricular contractions in patients suspected of acute myocardial infarction or ischemic episode except for those that occur in conjunction with bradycardias. In such circumstances, the underlying bradycardia is treated first. Refer to page 169 for the treatment of bradycardias. If feasible, identify and correct any underlying causes of premature ventricular contractions (e.g., low serum potassium [hypokalemia], excessive administration of digitalis or sympathomimetic drugs [e.g., epinephrine, isoproterenol, and norepinephrine], hypoxia, acidosis, and congestive heart failure).

Treatment

1. Administer a 1-mg/kg bolus of **lidocaine** IV slowly.

2. Repeat administration of **lidocaine** as a 0.5-mg/kg bolus IV slowly every 8 to 10 minutes as necessary until the premature ventricular contractions are suppressed or a total dose of 3 mg/kg of lidocaine has been administered within 1 hour.

3. Start an IV infusion of **lidocaine** (1 g of lidocaine in 500 ml of 5% dextrose in water) as soon as possible at a rate of 2 mg of lidocaine per minute (1 ml of the diluted lidocaine solution per minute) to prevent the recurrence of premature ventricular contractions. If additional boluses of lidocaine are administered initially, increase the rate of the lidocaine infusion by 1-mg increments after each additional 1-mg/kg dose of lidocaine to a maximum rate of 4 mg of lidocaine per minute.

Initial Dose of Lidocaine	Rate of Lidocaine Infusion
1 mg/kg	2 mg/min
1-2 mg/kg	3 mg/min
2-3 mg/kg	4 mg/min

If lidocaine is unsuccessful in suppressing the premature ventricular contractions:

4. Discontinue the lidocaine infusion, and administer 100 mg of **procainamide** IV slowly over 5 minutes at a rate of 20 mg of procainamide per minute.

CAUTION!

DO NOT ADMINISTER PROCAINAMIDE IF HYPO-TENSION OR PULMONARY EDEMA IS PRESENT OR IF THE PATIENT IS UNCONSCIOUS. ADMINISTER, INSTEAD, BRETYLIUM TOSYLATE AS IN STEP 7 BELOW.

---

5. Repeat the 100-mg dose of **procainamide** every 5 minutes until the premature ventricular contractions are suppressed, a total dose of 1,000 mg of procainamide has been administered, side effects from the procainamide appear (such as hypotension), or the QRS complex widens by 50% of its original width.

6. Start an IV infusion of **procainamide** (1 g of procainamide in 500 ml of 5% dextrose in water) as soon as possible at a rate of 1 to 4 mg per minute (0.5 to 2 ml of the diluted procainamide solution per minute) to prevent the recurrence of premature ventricular contractions.

If lidocaine and procainamide are unsuccessful in suppressing the ventricular premature contractions and if bretylium tosylate is not contraindicated:

7. Administer a dose of 5- to 10-mg/kg of **bretylium tosylate,** diluted to 50 ml with 5% dextrose in water, IV slowly over 8 to 10 minutes.

8. Start an IV infusion of **bretylium tosylate** (1 g of bretylium tosylate in 500 ml of 5% dextrose in water) at a rate of 1 to 2 mg per minute (0.5 to 1 ml of the diluted bretylium tosylate solution per minute) to prevent recurrence of ventricular tachycardia.

If lidocaine, procainamide, and bretylium tosylate are unsuccessful in suppressing the ventricular premature contractions:

9. Consider **external overdrive cardiac pacing.**

Notes

Ventricular Fibrillation

Clinical Significance of Ventricular Fibrillation

Ventricular fibrillation is a life-threatening arrhythmia resulting in chaotic beating of the heart and the immediate end of organized ventricular contractions, cardiac output, and pulse. At the moment ventricular fibrillation occurs and cardiac output stops, **clinical death** is present. **Biological death** occurs within ten minutes unless cardiopulmonary resuscitation (CPR), direct-current (DC) shock, or both are administered within minutes.

Indications for Treatment of Ventricular Fibrillation

Treatment of ventricular fibrillation is indicated immediately.

Treatment

A. Witnessed Cardiac Arrest

If the cardiac arrest is witnessed by the rescuer or if cardiac arrest has been present for less than one or two minutes and CPR is being performed by someone other than the rescuer and the patient is not being monitored:

1. Verify cardiac arrest by checking the patient's pulse.

If the pulse is absent:

2. Administer a **precordial thump** immediately, and check the patient's pulse.

If the pulse remains absent:

3. Perform **CPR.**
4. Determine the rhythm by ECG monitor.

If ventricular fibrillation is present:

5. Deliver an **unsynchronized DC shock** (200 joules) immediately, and check the patient's pulse and rhythm.

If ventricular fibrillation persists:

6. Deliver a **second unsynchronized DC shock** (200 to 300 joules) immediately after the first DC shock, and check the patient's pulse and rhythm.

If ventricular fibrillation persists:

7. Deliver a **third unsynchronized DC shock** (up to 360 joules) immediately after the second DC shock, and check the patient's pulse and rhythm.

If ventricular fibrillation persists:

8. Continue **CPR.**
9. Establish an **IV line.**
10. Administer 0.5 to 1.0 mg of **epinephrine** (5 to 10 ml of a 1:10,000 solution of epinephrine) IV, and repeat every 5 minutes if needed.

Note: If an intravenous line cannot be established, administer 1 mg of **epinephrine** (10 ml of a 1:10,000 solution of epinephrine) via the endotracheal tube, if one is in place. If both an intravenous line and an endotracheal tube are not in place, administer 0.5 mg of epinephrine (5 ml of a 1:10,000 solution of epinephrine) by intracardiac injection, and repeat if needed.

11. Continue **CPR** for several minutes to circulate the drug.
12. Perform endotracheal intubation or, less preferably, insert an esophageal obturator airway.
13. Ventilate with the highest concentration of oxygen possible.
14. Deliver a **fourth unsynchronized DC shock** (up to 360 joules), and check the patient's pulse and rhythm.

If ventricular fibrillation persists:

15. Administer a 1-mg/kg bolus of **lidocaine** IV slowly.
16. Continue **CPR** for several minutes to circulate the drug.
17. Deliver a **fifth unsynchronized DC shock** (up to 360 joules), and check the patient's pulse and rhythm.

If ventricular fibrillation persists:

18. Administer a 5-mg/kg bolus of **bretylium tosylate** IV.
19. Continue **CPR** for several minutes to circulate the drug.

20. Consider administration of **sodium bicarbonate** at this point if it is indicated. The initial dose is 1 mEq/kg of sodium bicarbonate IV. Do not administer additional sodium bicarbonate until the patient's arterial blood pH and gases have been analyzed. If such a blood analysis is not feasible at this point, repeat the administration of half of the initial dose of sodium bicarbonate (0.5 mEq/kg of sodium bicarbonate) IV every 10 to 15 minutes for a total dose of 100 to 200 mEq of sodium bicarbonate.

21. Continue **CPR** for several minutes to circulate the drug.

22. Deliver a **sixth unsynchronized DC shock** (up to 360 joules), and check the patient's pulse and rhythm.

If ventricular fibrillation persists:

23. Administer a 10-mg/kg bolus of **bretylium tosylate** IV.

24. Continue **CPR** for several minutes to circulate the drug.

25. Deliver a **seventh unsynchronized DC shock** (up to 360 joules), and check the patient's pulse and rhythm.

If ventricular fibrillation persists:

26. Continue **CPR.**

27. Assess the effectiveness of ventilation and external chest compression.

28. Administer a 0.5-mg/kg bolus of **lidocaine** IV slowly.

OR

Administer a 10-mg/kg bolus of **bretylium tosylate** IV.

29. Continue **CPR** for several minutes to circulate the drug.

30. Deliver an **eighth unsynchronized DC shock** (up to 360 joules), and check the patient's pulse and rhythm.

If ventricular fibrillation persists:

31. Continue **CPR.**

32. Reassess the effectiveness of ventilation and external chest compression.

33. Repeat administration of **epinephrine, lidocaine** (up to a total dose of 3 mg/kg), **bretylium tosylate** (up to a total dose of 30 mg/kg), **sodium bicarbonate** (if indicated), and **defibrillation,** and continue **CPR** until ventricular fibrillation is terminated or a physician orders an end to the resuscitative efforts.

If ventricular fibrillation is terminated and a supraventricular rhythm is present:

34. Perform **CPR** until the patient's pulse is palpable and the systolic blood pressure is 90 mm Hg or greater.

IF LIDOCAINE HAS NOT BEEN ADMINISTERED PREVIOUSLY:

35. Administer a 1-mg/kg bolus of **lidocaine** IV slowly.

36. Start an IV infusion of **lidocaine** (1 g of lidocaine in 500 ml of 5% dextrose in water) as soon as possible at a rate of 2 mg of lidocaine per minute (1 ml of the diluted lidocaine solution per minute) to prevent the recurrence of ventricular fibrillation.

If ventricular fibrillation recurs:

37. Deliver an **unsynchronized DC shock** immediately at the energy level at which defibrillation was previously effective.

If a supraventricular rhythm is present and the patient's systolic blood pressure is 80 to 90 mm Hg or less:

38. Elevate the patient's legs 18 inches above the level of the heart, or apply and inflate an **antishock garment** (if pulmonary congestion and edema are absent) to increase the patient's systolic blood pressure to 90 to 100 mm Hg. If pulmonary congestion and edema are present, elevate the patient's head only.

If hypotension persists and epinephrine has not been administered previously:

39. Administer 0.5 to 1.0 mg of **epinephrine** (5 to 10 ml of a 1:10,000 solution of epinephrine) IV.

If hypotension persists:

40. Administer an inotropic and vasoconstrictive agent, such as **dopamine hydrochloride,** IV at a rate of 2 to 20 μg/kg per minute to increase the systolic blood pressure to 90 to 100 mm Hg.

OR

Administer a vasoconstrictive agent, such as **norepinephrine,** IV at a rate of 2 to 4 μg of norepinephrine base per minute to increase the systolic blood pressure to 90 to 100 mm Hg.

Notes

Ventricular Fibrillation—Cont.

Treatment

B. Unwitnessed and Unmonitored Cardiac Arrest

If the cardiac arrest is unwitnessed by the rescuer or if cardiac arrest has been present for more than one or two minutes and CPR is being performed by someone other than the rescuer and the patient is not being monitored:

1. Verify cardiac arrest by checking the patient's pulse.

2. Perform **CPR.**

3. Determine the rhythm by ECG monitor.

If ventricular fibrillation is present:

4. Deliver an **unsynchronized DC shock** (200 joules) immediately, and check the patient's pulse and rhythm.

If ventricular fibrillation persists:

5. Deliver a **second unsynchronized DC shock** (200 to 300 joules) immediately after the first DC shock, and check the patient's pulse and rhythm.

If ventricular fibrillation persists:

6. Deliver a **third unsynchronized DC shock** (up to 360 joules) immediately after the second DC shock, and check the patient's pulse and rhythm.

If ventricular fibrillation persists:

7. Continue **CPR.**

8. Refer to **Step 9** in **A. Witnessed Cardiac Arrest** under **Ventricular Fibrillation,** page 186.

Notes

Treatment

C. Monitored Cardiac Arrest

If the patient is being monitored and ventricular fibrillation occurs:

1. Verify cardiac arrest by checking the patient's pulse.

2. Administer a **precordial thump** immediately, and check the patient's pulse and rhythm.

If ventricular fibrillation persists:

3. Deliver an **unsynchronized DC shock** (200 joules) immediately, and check the patient's pulse and rhythm.

If ventricular fibrillation persists:

4. Deliver a **second unsynchronized DC shock** (200 to 300 joules) immediately after the first DC shock, and check the patient's pulse and rhythm.

If ventricular fibrillation persists:

5. Deliver a **third unsynchronized DC shock** (up to 360 joules) immediately after the second DC shock, and check the patient's pulse and rhythm.

If ventricular fibrillation persists:

6. Start **CPR.**

7. Refer to **Step 9** in **A. Witnessed Cardiac Arrest** under **Ventricular Fibrillation,** page 186.

Notes

Ventricular Asystole

Clinical Significance of Ventricular Asystole

Ventricular asystole is a life-threatening arrhythmia resulting in the absence of ventricular contractions, cardiac output, and a pulse. At the moment ventricular asystole occurs in a person with an adequate circulation, cardiac output stops and **clinical death** occurs. **Biological death** follows within ten minutes unless ventricular asystole is reversed.

Indications for Treatment of Ventricular Asystole

Treatment of ventricular asystole is indicated immediately.

Treatment

A. Witnessed Cardiac Arrest

If the cardiac arrest is witnessed by the rescuer or if cardiac arrest has been present for less than one or two minutes and CPR is being performed by someone other than the rescuer and the patient is not being monitored:

1. Verify cardiac arrest by checking the patient's pulse.

If the pulse is absent:

2. Administer a **precordial thump** immediately, and check the patient's pulse.

If the pulse remains absent:

3. Perform **CPR.**
4. Determine the rhythm by ECG monitor.

If ventricular asystole is present:

CONFIRM VENTRICULAR ASYSTOLE IN TWO ECG LEADS IF POSSIBLE SINCE FINE VENTRICULAR FIBRILLATION MAY MIMIC VENTRICULAR ASYSTOLE.

5. Consider the treatment protocol for **Witnessed Cardiac Arrest** under **Ventricular Fibrillation,** page 186, and deliver **three unsynchronized DC shocks** if ventricular asystole is not definitely confirmed.

6. Continue **CPR.**

7. Establish an **IV line.**

8. Administer 0.5 mg to 1.0 mg of **epinephrine** (5 to 10 ml of a 1:10,000 solution of epinephrine) IV bolus, and repeat every 5 minutes if needed.

Note: If an intravenous route cannot be established, administer 1.0 mg of **epinephrine** (10 ml of a 1:10,000 solution of epinephrine) via the endotracheal tube, if one is in place. If both an intravenous line and an endotracheal tube are not in place, administer 0.5 mg of epinephrine (5 ml of a 1:10,000 solution of epinephrine) by intracardiac injection, and repeat if needed.

9. Continue **CPR.**

10. Perform endotracheal intubation or, less preferably, insert an esophageal obturator airway.

11. Ventilate using the highest concentration of oxygen possible.

12. Continue **CPR.**

If ventricular asystole persists:

13. Consider administration of a 1-mg bolus of **atropine** IV rapidly, and repeat once in 5 minutes if ventricular asystole persists, for a total dose of 2 mg of atropine.

14. Continue **CPR.**

If ventricular asystole persists:

15. Consider administration of **sodium bicarbonate** at this point if it is indicated. The initial dose is 1 mEq/kg of sodium bicarbonate IV. Do not administer additional sodium bicarbonate until the patient's arterial blood pH and gases have been analyzed. If such a blood analysis is not feasible at this point, repeat the administration of half of the initial dose of sodium bicarbonate (0.5 mEq/kg of sodium bicarbonate) IV every 10 to 15 minutes for a total dose of 100 to 200 mEq of sodium bicarbonate.

16. Continue **CPR.**

If ventricular asystole persists:

17. Consider **external** or **transvenous cardiac pacing.**

18. Continue **CPR.**

If ventricular asystole persists:

19. Consider an IV infusion of **isoproterenol** (1 mg of isoproterenol in 500 ml of 5% dextrose in water) at an initial rate of 2 to 10 μg per minute (1 to 5 ml of the diluted isoproterenol solution per minute), and adjust the infusion rate to maintain the heart rate at 60 to 70 beats per minute.

20. Continue **CPR.**

If ventricular asystole persists:

21. Repeat administration of **epinephrine,** and continue the **isoproterenol** infusion, **CPR,** and attempts to **pace the heart** until ventricular asystole is terminated or a physician orders an end to the resuscitative efforts.

Notes

Ventricular Asystole—Cont

Treatment

B. Unwitnessed and Unmonitored Cardiac Arrest

If the cardiac arrest is unwitnessed by the rescuer or if cardiac arrest has been present for more than one or two minutes and CPR is being performed by someone other than the rescuer and the patient is not being monitored:

1. Verify cardiac arrest by checking the patient's pulse.

2. Perform **CPR.**

3. Determine the rhythm by ECG monitor.

If ventricular asystole is present:

CONFIRM VENTRICULAR ASYSTOLE IN TWO ECG LEADS IF POSSIBLE SINCE FINE VENTRICULAR FIBRILLATION MAY MIMIC VENTRICULAR ASYSTOLE.

4. Consider the treatment protocol for **Unwitnessed and Unmonitored Cardiac Arrest** under **Ventricular Fibrillation,** page 188, and deliver **three unsynchronized DC shocks** if ventricular asystole is not definitely confirmed.

5. Continue **CPR.**

6. Refer to **Step 7** in **A. Witnessed Cardiac Arrest** under **Ventricular Asystole,** page 190.

Notes

Treatment

C. Monitored Cardiac Arrest

If the patient is being monitored and ventricular asystole occurs:

1. Verify cardiac arrest by checking the patient's pulse.

2. Administer a **precordial thump** immediately, and check the patient's pulse and rhythm.

If ventricular asystole persists:

CONFIRM VENTRICULAR ASYSTOLE IN TWO ECG LEADS IF POSSIBLE SINCE FINE VENTRICULAR FIBRILLATION MAY MIMIC VENTRICULAR ASYSTOLE.

3. Consider the treatment protocol for **Monitored Cardiac Arrest** under **Ventricular Fibrillation,** page 189, and deliver **three unsynchronized DC shocks** if ventricular asystole is not definitely confirmed.

4. Continue **CPR.**

5. Refer to **Step 7** in **A. Witnessed Cardiac Arrest** under **Ventricular Asystole,** page 190.

Notes

Electromechanical Dissociation (EMD)

Clinical Significance of Electromechanical Dissociation

Electromechanical dissociation—the absence of effective ventricular contractions, cardiac output, and pulse in the presence of an ECG—is a life-threatening condition. At the moment electromechanical dissociation occurs in a person with an adequate circulation, cardiac output ceases and **clinical death** occurs. **Biological death** follows within ten minutes unless electromechanical dissociation is reversed.

Electromechanical dissociation is commonly the result of inadequate myocardial perfusion, which can occur in patients with acute blood loss (hemorrhagic shock due to trauma or other causes, such as ruptured abdominal aortic aneurysm or gastrointestinal hemorrhage) and in patients with obstruction of blood flow to the heart (tension pneumothorax or severe pulmonary embolization). Hypoxemia, severe acidosis, pericardial tamponade, and myocardial rupture can also cause EMD. Whenever CPR is unsuccessful in producing a palpable peripheral or carotid pulse, electromechanical dissociation must be suspected.

Indications for Treatment of Electromechanical Dissociation

Treatment of electromechanical dissociation is indicated immediately.

Treatment

A. Witnessed Cardiac Arrest

If the cardiac arrest is witnessed by the rescuer or if cardiac arrest has been present for less than one or two minutes and CPR is being performed by someone other than the rescuer and the patient is not being monitored:

1. Verify cardiac arrest by checking the patient's pulse.

If the pulse is absent:

2. Administer a **precordial thump** immediately, and check the patient's pulse.

If the pulse remains absent:

3. Perform **CPR.**

4. Determine the rhythm by ECG monitor.

If electromechanical dissociation is present, as indicated by the presence of an ECG and the absence of a pulse:

5. Continue **CPR.**

6. Establish an **IV line.**

7. Administer 0.5 to 1.0 mg of **epinephrine** (5 to 10 ml of a 1:10,000 solution of epinephrine) IV bolus. Repeat every 5 minutes if needed until pulse and blood pressure are established.

Note: If an intravenous route cannot be established, administer 1.0 mg of **epinephrine** (10 ml of a 1:10,000 solution of epinephrine) via the endotracheal tube, if one is in place. If both an intravenous line and an endotracheal tube are not in place, administer 0.5 mg of epinephrine (5 ml of a 1:10,000 solution of epinephrine) by intracardiac injection, and repeat if needed.

8. Continue **CPR.**

9. Perform endotracheal intubation or, less preferably, insert an esophageal obturator airway.

10. Ventilate the patient with the highest concentration of oxygen possible.

11. Continue **CPR.**

If electromechanical dissociation persists:

12. Consider administration of **sodium bicarbonate** at this point if it is indicated. The initial dose is 1 mEq/kg of sodium bicarbonate IV. Do not administer additional sodium bicarbonate until the patient's arterial blood pH and gases have been analyzed. If such a blood analysis is not feasible at this point, repeat the administration of half of the initial dose of sodium bicarbonate (0.5 mEq/kg of sodium bicarbonate) IV every 10 to 15 minutes for a total dose of 100 to 200 mEq of sodium bicarbonate.

13. Continue **CPR.**

If electromechanical dissociation persists and hypovolemia is suspected:

14. Consider elevating the patient's legs 30 degrees above the level of the heart.

15. Consider the application and inflation of an **antishock garment.**

16. Consider the administration of IV fluids

(**0.9% saline** or **Ringer's lactate solution**) in 100 to 200 ml aliquots IV while monitoring the pulse and blood pressure and auscultating the lungs for pulmonary edema.

17. Continue **CPR.**

If electromechanical dissociation or idioventricular rhythm persists:

18. Consider the presence of cardiac tamponade, tension pneumothorax, hypoxemia, acidosis, or pulmonary embolism. Treat the underlying condition.

19. Continue **CPR.**

If electromechanical dissociation or idioventricular rhythm persists:

20. Consider the treatment protocol for **Bradycardias,** page 169, including **external** or **transvenous cardiac pacing** and administration of **atropine** and **isoproterenol.**

Notes

Electromechanical Dissociation (EMD)—Cont.

Treatment

B. Unwitnessed and Unmonitored Cardiac Arrest

If the cardiac arrest is unwitnessed by the rescuer or if cardiac arrest has been present for more than one or two minutes and CPR is being performed by someone other than the rescuer and the patient is not being monitored:

1. Verify cardiac arrest by checking the patient's pulse.

2. Perform **CPR.**

3. Determine the rhythm by ECG monitor.

If electromechanical dissociation is present, as indicated by the presence of an ECG and the absence of a pulse:

4. Continue **CPR.**

5. Refer to **Step 6** in **A. Witnessed Cardiac Arrest** under **Electromechanical Dissociation,** page 194.

Notes

Treatment

C. Monitored Cardiac Arrest

If the patient is being monitored and cardiac arrest occurs:

1. Verify cardiac arrest by checking the patient's pulse.

2. Perform **CPR.**

If electromechanical dissociation is present, as indicated by the presence of an ECG and the absence of a pulse:

3. Continue **CPR.**

4. Refer to **Step 6** in **A. Witnessed Cardiac Arrest** under **Electromechanical Dissociation,** page 194.

Notes

Chapter 7

Arrhythmia Interpretation: Self-assessment

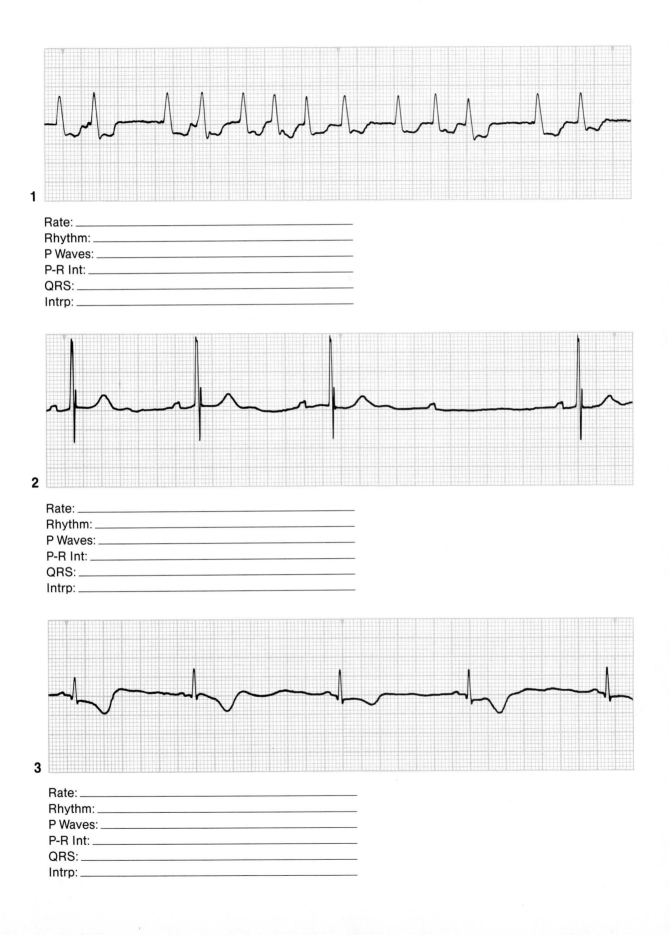

1

Rate: _____

Rhythm: _____

P Waves: _____

P-R Int: _____

QRS: _____

Intrp: _____

2

Rate: _____

Rhythm: _____

P Waves: _____

P-R Int: _____

QRS: _____

Intrp: _____

3

Rate: _____

Rhythm: _____

P Waves: _____

P-R Int: _____

QRS: _____

Intrp: _____

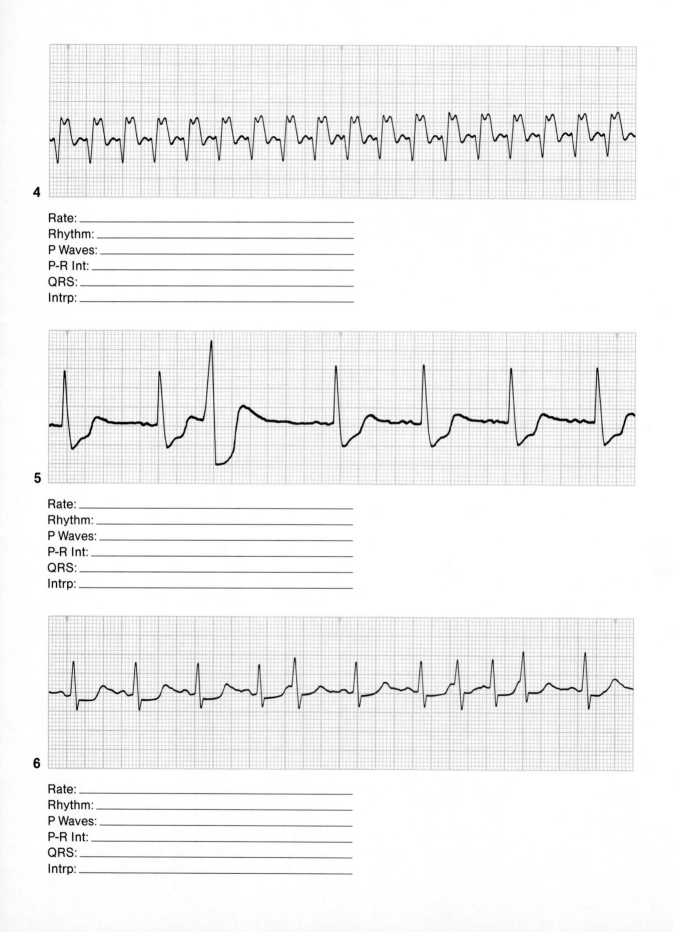

4

Rate: _____
Rhythm: _____
P Waves: _____
P-R Int: _____
QRS: _____
Intrp: _____

5

Rate: _____
Rhythm: _____
P Waves: _____
P-R Int: _____
QRS: _____
Intrp: _____

6

Rate: _____
Rhythm: _____
P Waves: _____
P-R Int: _____
QRS: _____
Intrp: _____

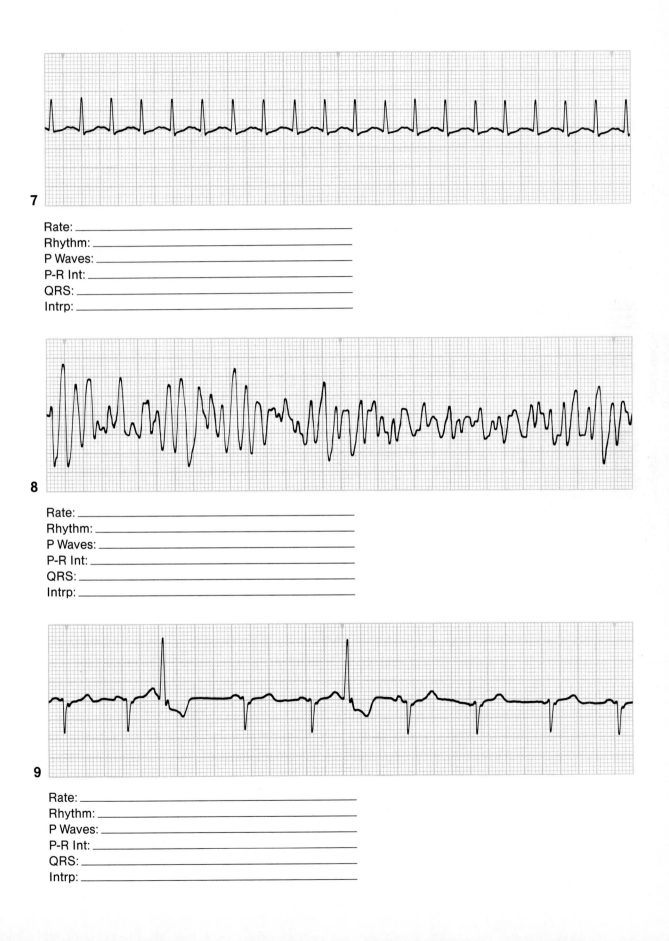

7

Rate: _____

Rhythm: _____

P Waves: _____

P-R Int: _____

QRS: _____

Intrp: _____

8

Rate: _____

Rhythm: _____

P Waves: _____

P-R Int: _____

QRS: _____

Intrp: _____

9

Rate: _____

Rhythm: _____

P Waves: _____

P-R Int: _____

QRS: _____

Intrp: _____

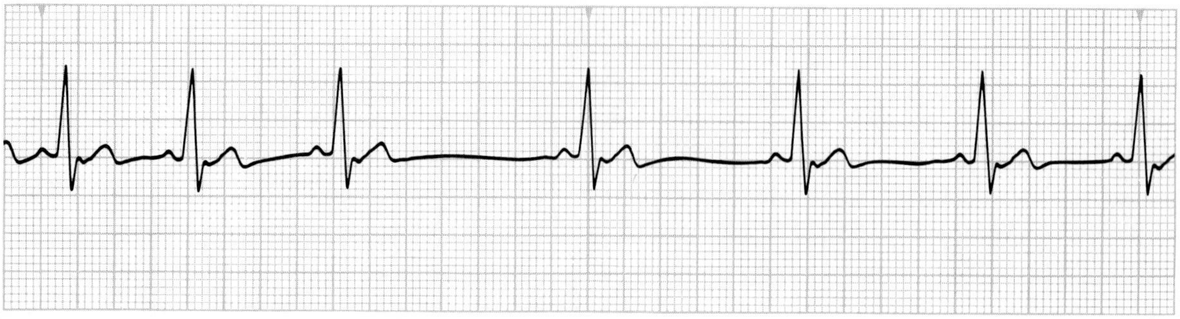

10

Rate: _____

Rhythm: _____

P Waves: _____

P-R Int: _____

QRS: _____

Intrp: _____

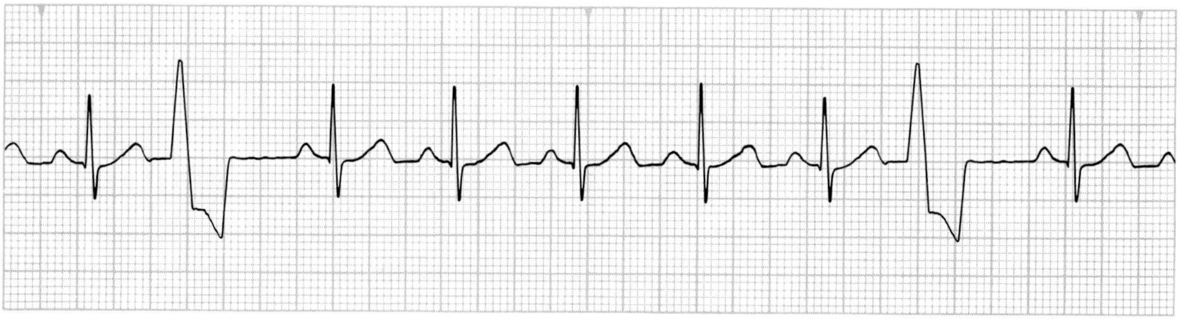

11

Rate: _____

Rhythm: _____

P Waves: _____

P-R Int: _____

QRS: _____

Intrp: _____

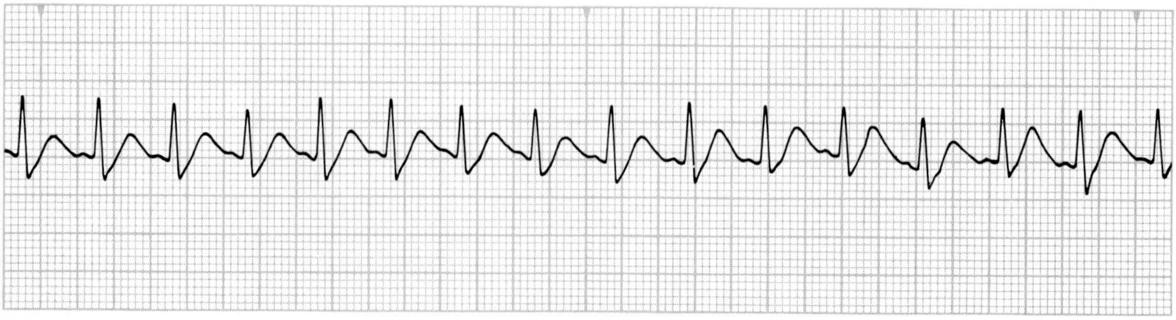

12

Rate: _____

Rhythm: _____

P Waves: _____

P-R Int: _____

QRS: _____

Intrp: _____

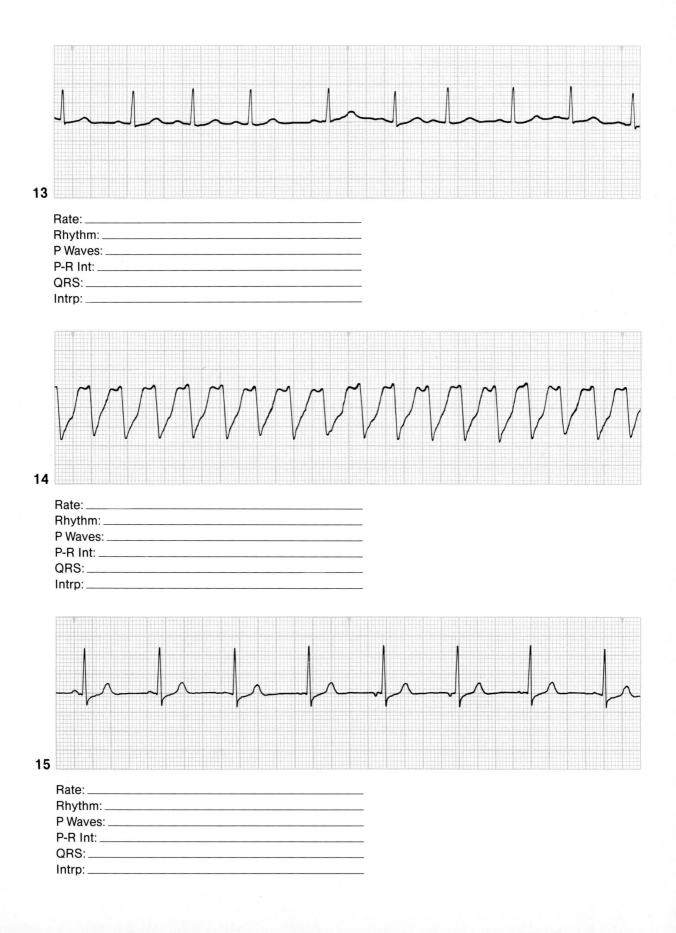

13

Rate: _____

Rhythm: _____

P Waves: _____

P-R Int: _____

QRS: _____

Intrp: _____

14

Rate: _____

Rhythm: _____

P Waves: _____

P-R Int: _____

QRS: _____

Intrp: _____

15

Rate: _____

Rhythm: _____

P Waves: _____

P-R Int: _____

QRS: _____

Intrp: _____

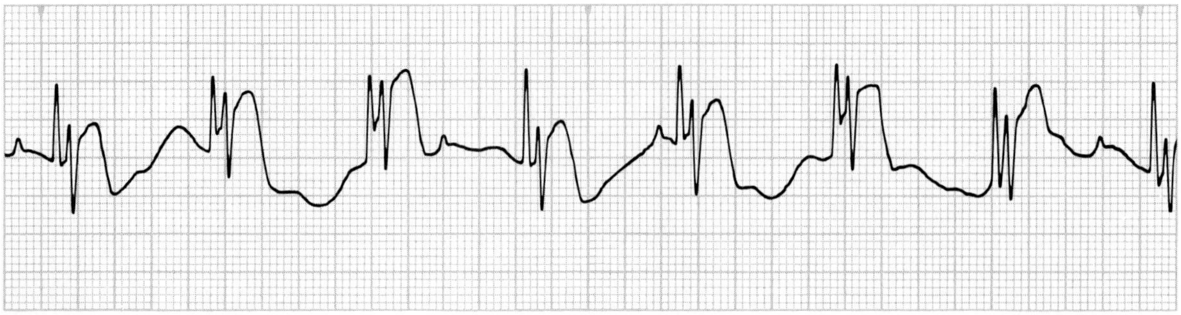

16

Rate: _____

Rhythm: _____

P Waves: _____

P-R Int: _____

QRS: _____

Intrp: _____

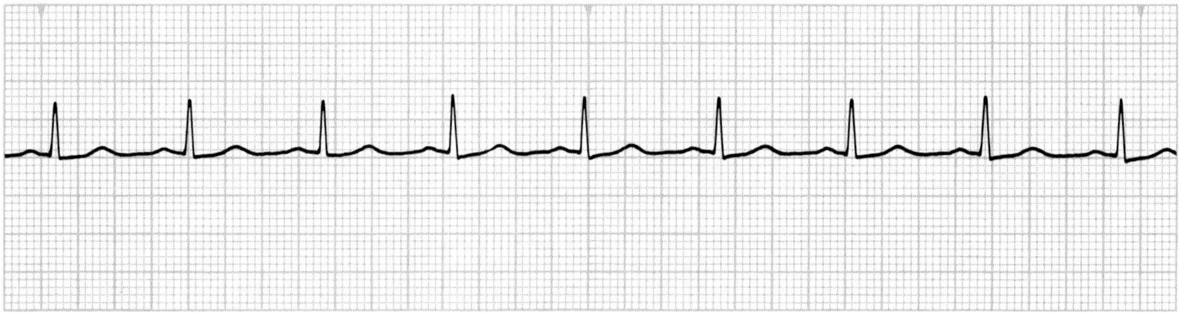

17

Rate: _____

Rhythm: _____

P Waves: _____

P-R Int: _____

QRS: _____

Intrp: _____

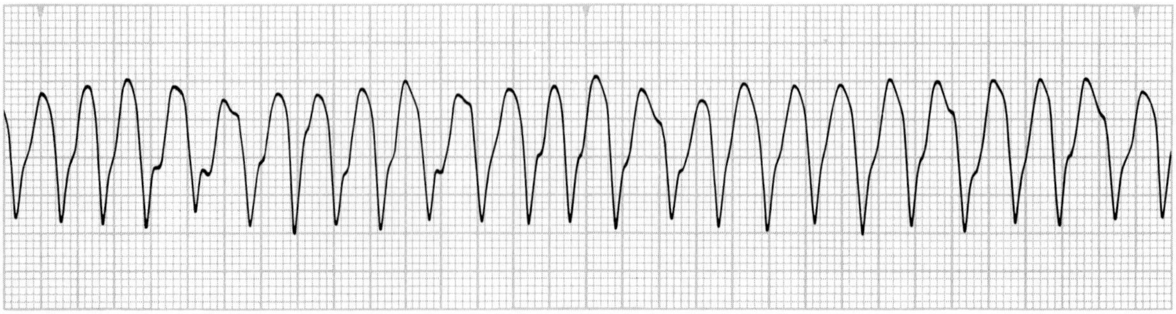

18

Rate: _____

Rhythm: _____

P Waves: _____

P-R Int: _____

QRS: _____

Intrp: _____

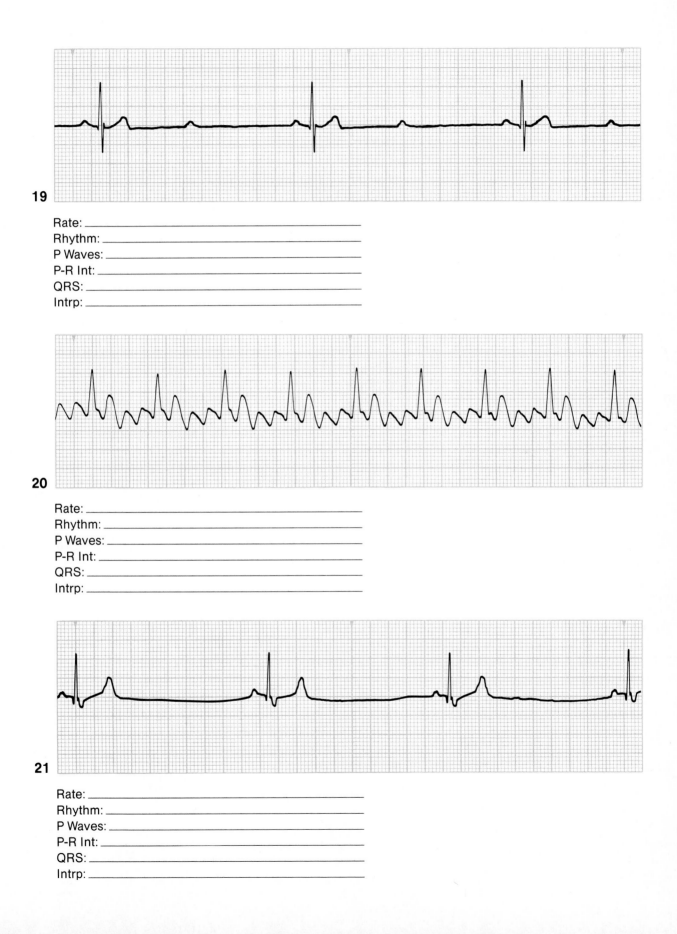

19

Rate: _____

Rhythm: _____

P Waves: _____

P-R Int: _____

QRS: _____

Intrp: _____

20

Rate: _____

Rhythm: _____

P Waves: _____

P-R Int: _____

QRS: _____

Intrp: _____

21

Rate: _____

Rhythm: _____

P Waves: _____

P-R Int: _____

QRS: _____

Intrp: _____

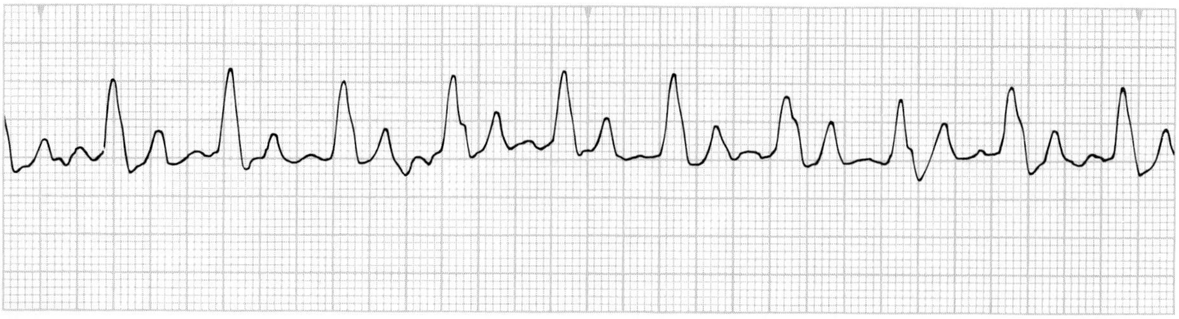

22

Rate: _____

Rhythm: _____

P Waves: _____

P-R Int: _____

QRS: _____

Intrp: _____

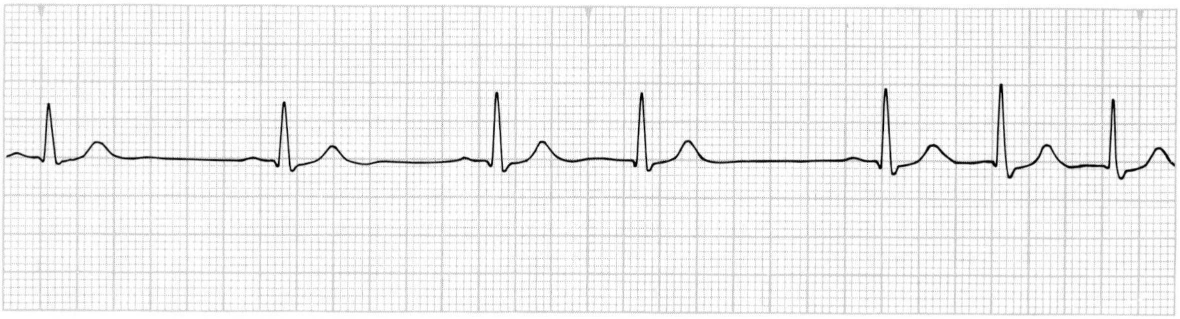

23

Rate: _____

Rhythm: _____

P Waves: _____

P-R Int: _____

QRS: _____

Intrp: _____

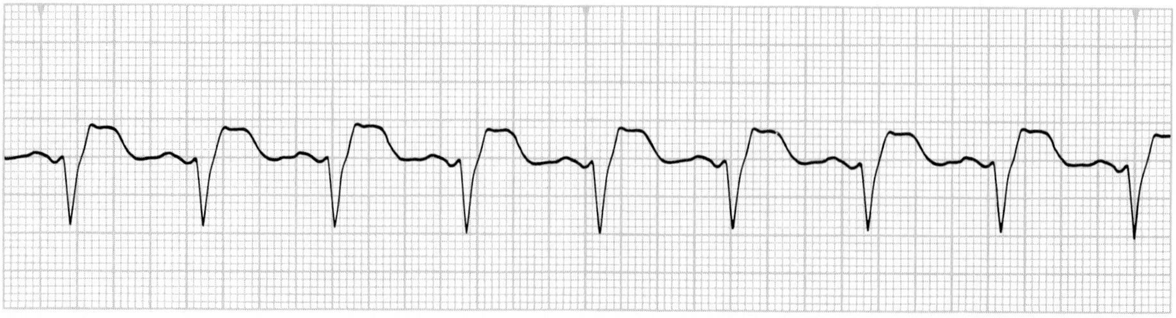

24

Rate: _____

Rhythm: _____

P Waves: _____

P-R Int: _____

QRS: _____

Intrp: _____

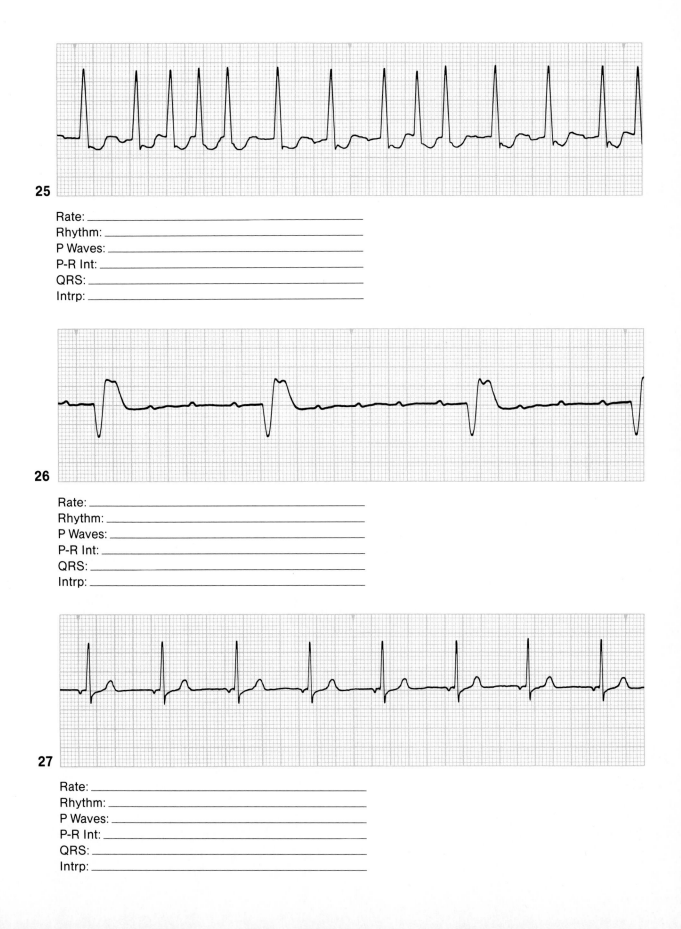

25

Rate: _____

Rhythm: _____

P Waves: _____

P-R Int: _____

QRS: _____

Intrp: _____

26

Rate: _____

Rhythm: _____

P Waves: _____

P-R Int: _____

QRS: _____

Intrp: _____

27

Rate: _____

Rhythm: _____

P Waves: _____

P-R Int: _____

QRS: _____

Intrp: _____

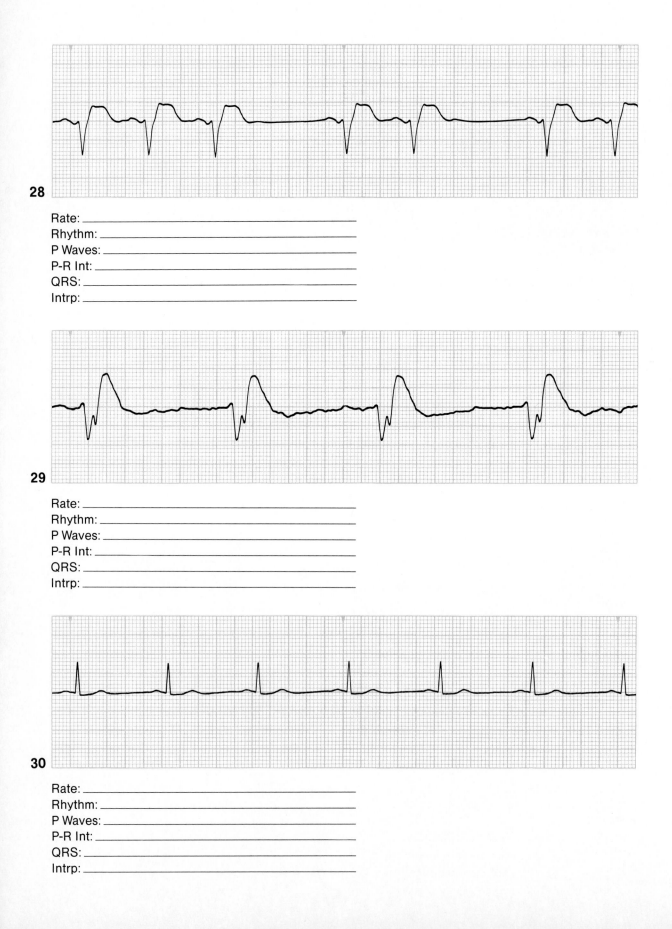

28

Rate: _____

Rhythm: _____

P Waves: _____

P-R Int: _____

QRS: _____

Intrp: _____

29

Rate: _____

Rhythm: _____

P Waves: _____

P-R Int: _____

QRS: _____

Intrp: _____

30

Rate: _____

Rhythm: _____

P Waves: _____

P-R Int: _____

QRS: _____

Intrp: _____

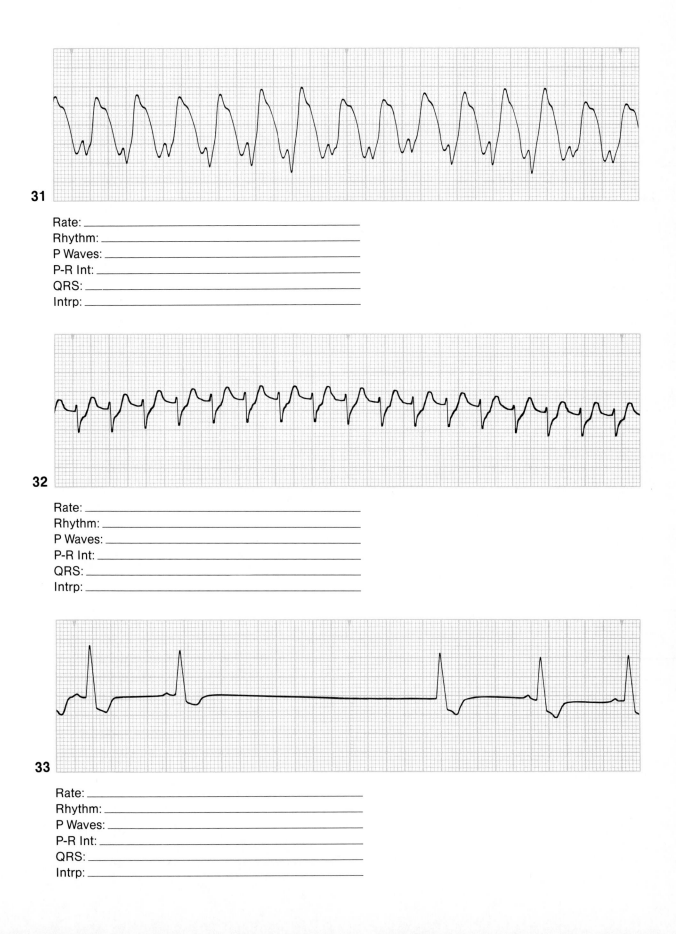

31

Rate: _____
Rhythm: _____
P Waves: _____
P-R Int: _____
QRS: _____
Intrp: _____

32

Rate: _____
Rhythm: _____
P Waves: _____
P-R Int: _____
QRS: _____
Intrp: _____

33

Rate: _____
Rhythm: _____
P Waves: _____
P-R Int: _____
QRS: _____
Intrp: _____

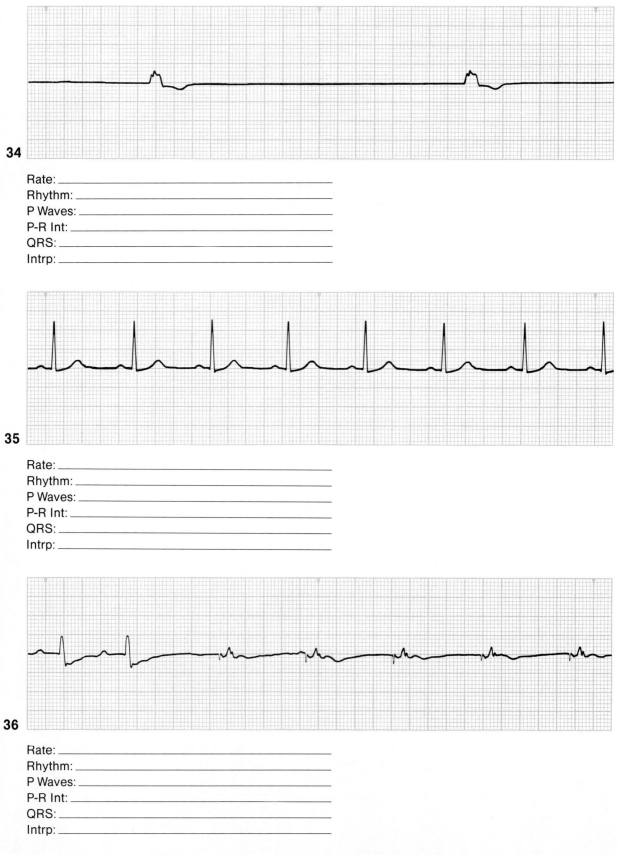

34

Rate: _____

Rhythm: _____

P Waves: _____

P-R Int: _____

QRS: _____

Intrp: _____

35

Rate: _____

Rhythm: _____

P Waves: _____

P-R Int: _____

QRS: _____

Intrp: _____

36

Rate: _____

Rhythm: _____

P Waves: _____

P-R Int: _____

QRS: _____

Intrp: _____

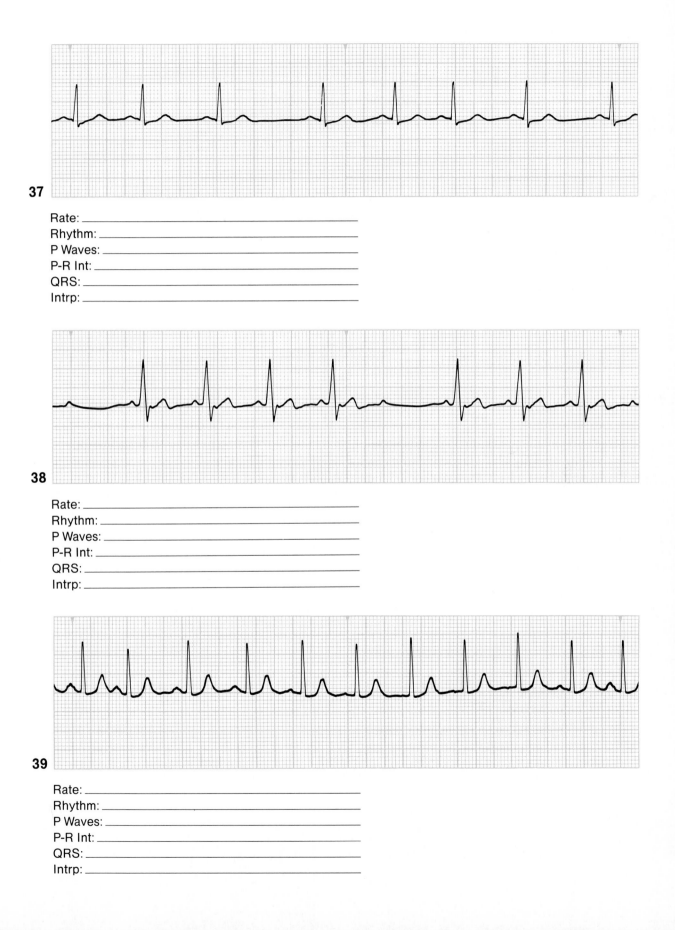

37

Rate: _____

Rhythm: _____

P Waves: _____

P-R Int: _____

QRS: _____

Intrp: _____

38

Rate: _____

Rhythm: _____

P Waves: _____

P-R Int: _____

QRS: _____

Intrp: _____

39

Rate: _____

Rhythm: _____

P Waves: _____

P-R Int: _____

QRS: _____

Intrp: _____

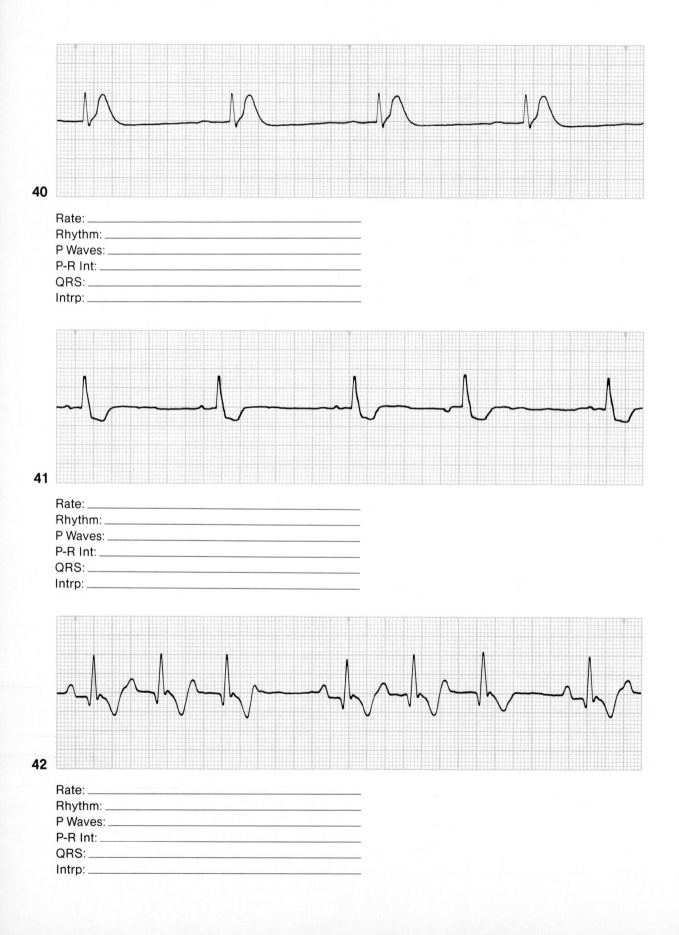

40

Rate: _____
Rhythm: _____
P Waves: _____
P-R Int: _____
QRS: _____
Intrp: _____

41

Rate: _____
Rhythm: _____
P Waves: _____
P-R Int: _____
QRS: _____
Intrp: _____

42

Rate: _____
Rhythm: _____
P Waves: _____
P-R Int: _____
QRS: _____
Intrp: _____

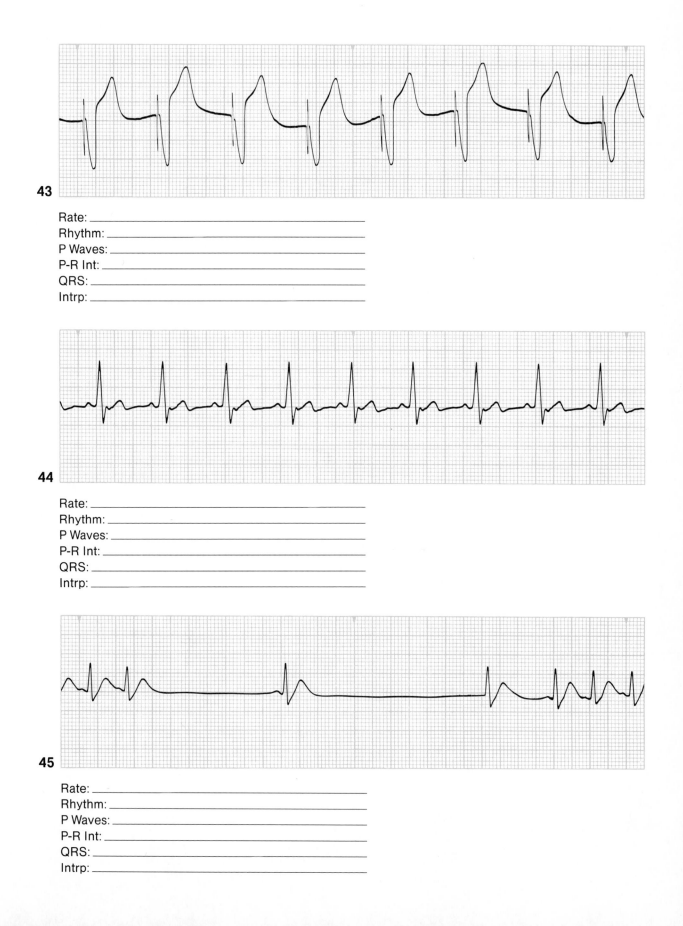

43

Rate: _____

Rhythm: _____

P Waves: _____

P-R Int: _____

QRS: _____

Intrp: _____

44

Rate: _____

Rhythm: _____

P Waves: _____

P-R Int: _____

QRS: _____

Intrp: _____

45

Rate: _____

Rhythm: _____

P Waves: _____

P-R Int: _____

QRS: _____

Intrp: _____

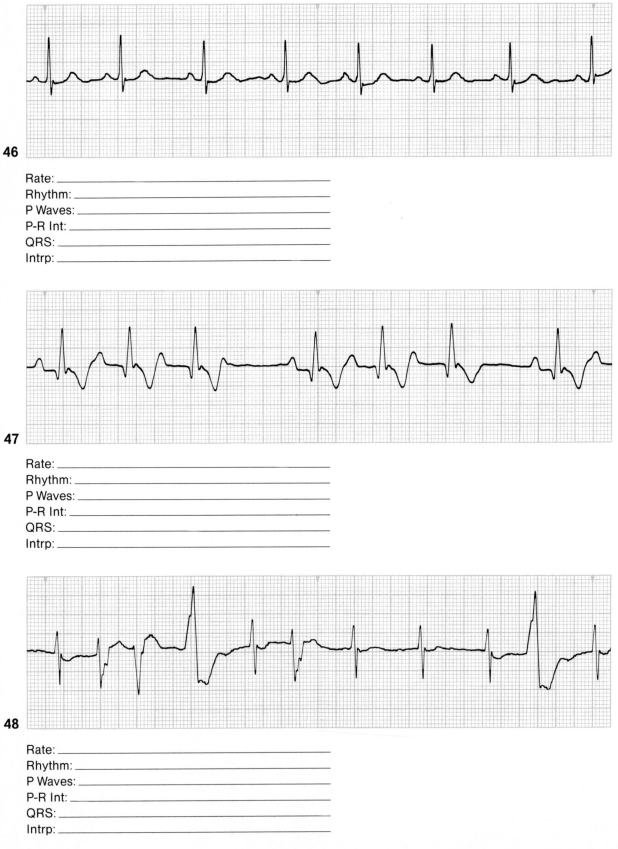

46

Rate: _____

Rhythm: _____

P Waves: _____

P-R Int: _____

QRS: _____

Intrp: _____

47

Rate: _____

Rhythm: _____

P Waves: _____

P-R Int: _____

QRS: _____

Intrp: _____

48

Rate: _____

Rhythm: _____

P Waves: _____

P-R Int: _____

QRS: _____

Intrp: _____

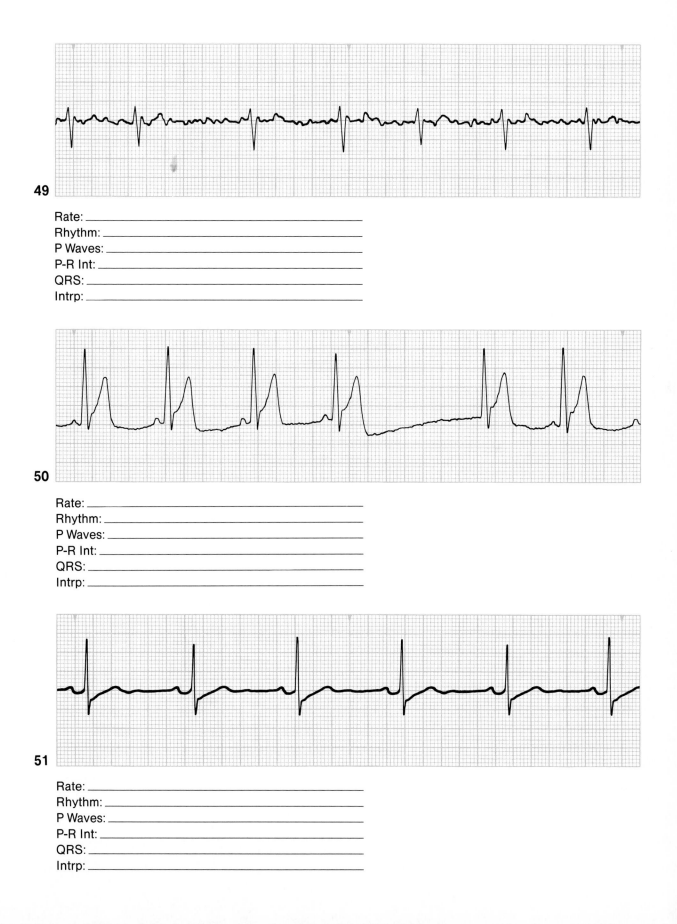

49

Rate: _____

Rhythm: _____

P Waves: _____

P-R Int: _____

QRS: _____

Intrp: _____

50

Rate: _____

Rhythm: _____

P Waves: _____

P-R Int: _____

QRS: _____

Intrp: _____

51

Rate: _____

Rhythm: _____

P Waves: _____

P-R Int: _____

QRS: _____

Intrp: _____

52

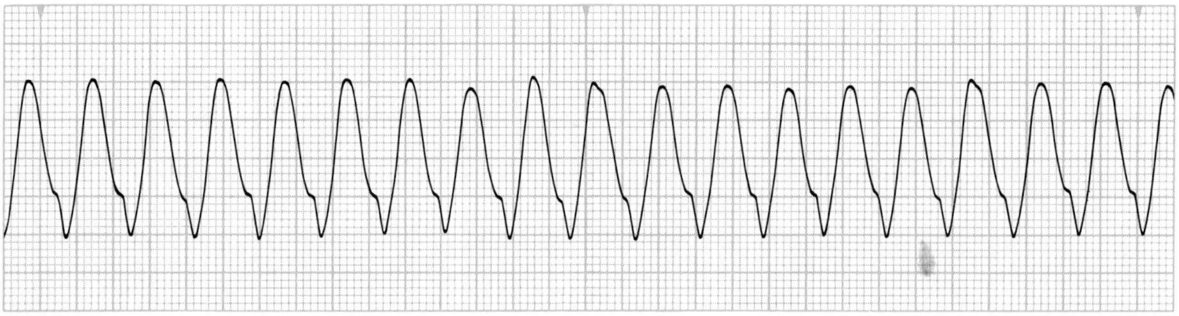

Rate: _____
Rhythm: _____
P Waves: _____
P-R Int: _____
QRS: _____
Intrp: _____

53

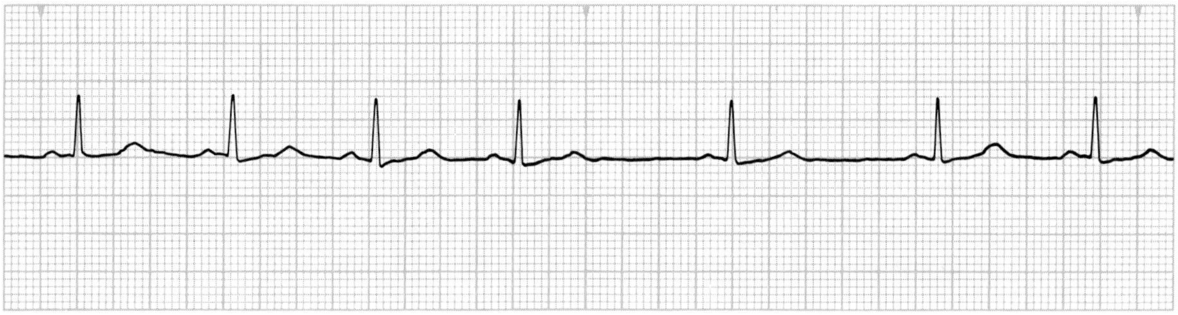

Rate: _____
Rhythm: _____
P Waves: _____
P-R Int: _____
QRS: _____
Intrp: _____

54

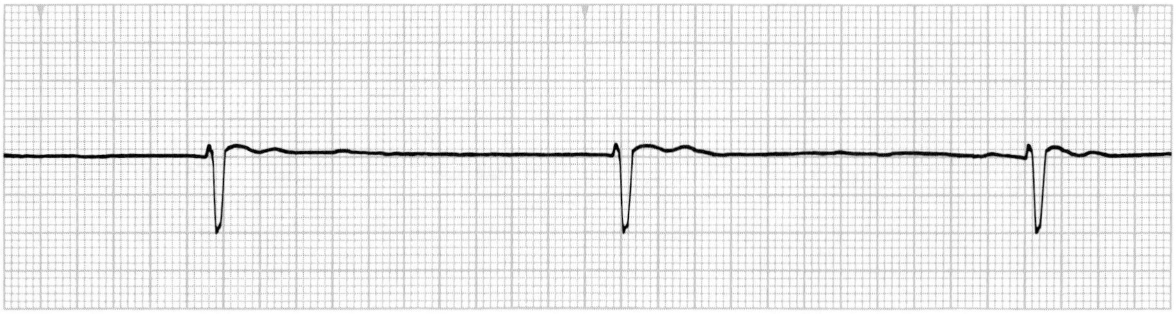

Rate: _____
Rhythm: _____
P Waves: _____
P-R Int: _____
QRS: _____
Intrp: _____

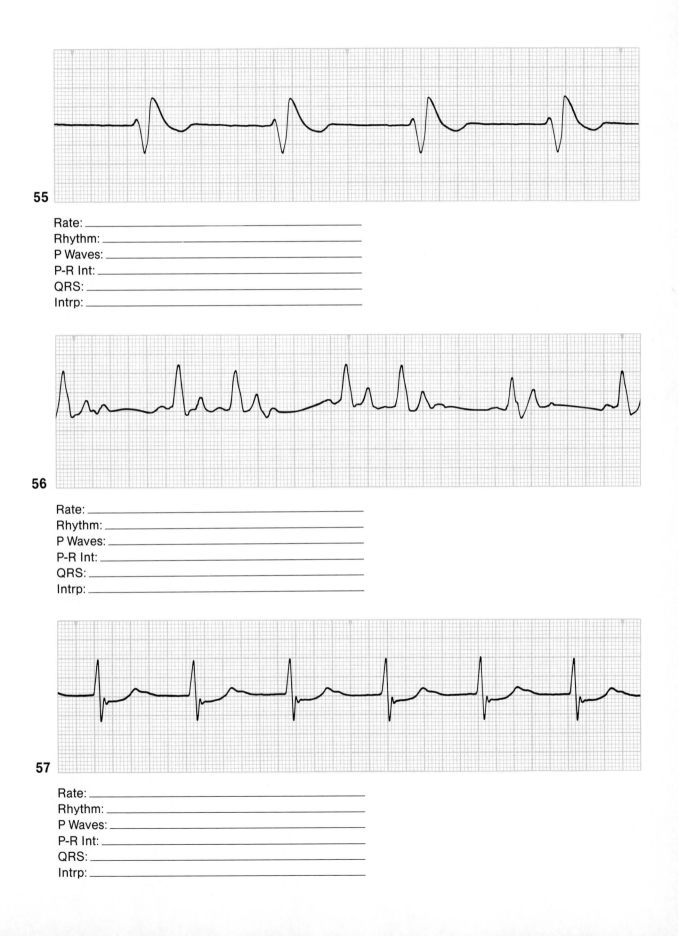

55

Rate: _____
Rhythm: _____
P Waves: _____
P-R Int: _____
QRS: _____
Intrp: _____

56

Rate: _____
Rhythm: _____
P Waves: _____
P-R Int: _____
QRS: _____
Intrp: _____

57

Rate: _____
Rhythm: _____
P Waves: _____
P-R Int: _____
QRS: _____
Intrp: _____

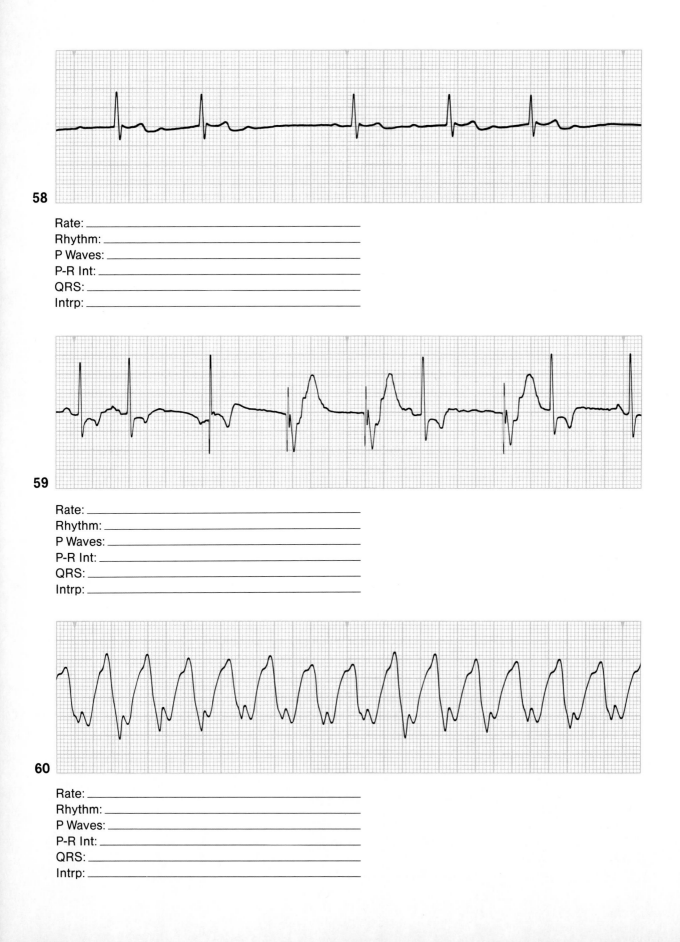

58

Rate: _____

Rhythm: _____

P Waves: _____

P-R Int: _____

QRS: _____

Intrp: _____

59

Rate: _____

Rhythm: _____

P Waves: _____

P-R Int: _____

QRS: _____

Intrp: _____

60

Rate: _____

Rhythm: _____

P Waves: _____

P-R Int: _____

QRS: _____

Intrp: _____

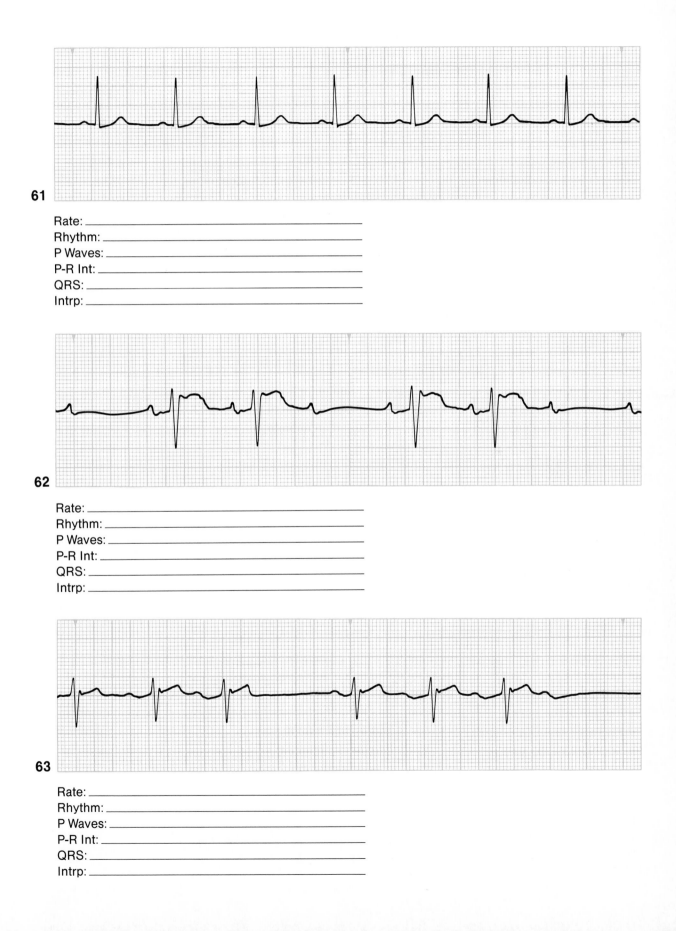

61

Rate: _____

Rhythm: _____

P Waves: _____

P-R Int: _____

QRS: _____

Intrp: _____

62

Rate: _____

Rhythm: _____

P Waves: _____

P-R Int: _____

QRS: _____

Intrp: _____

63

Rate: _____

Rhythm: _____

P Waves: _____

P-R Int: _____

QRS: _____

Intrp: _____

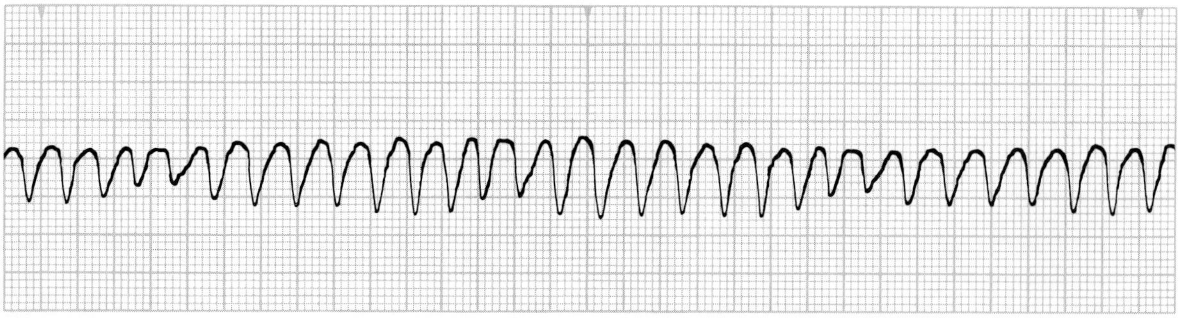

64

Rate: _____

Rhythm: _____

P Waves: _____

P-R Int: _____

QRS: _____

Intrp: _____

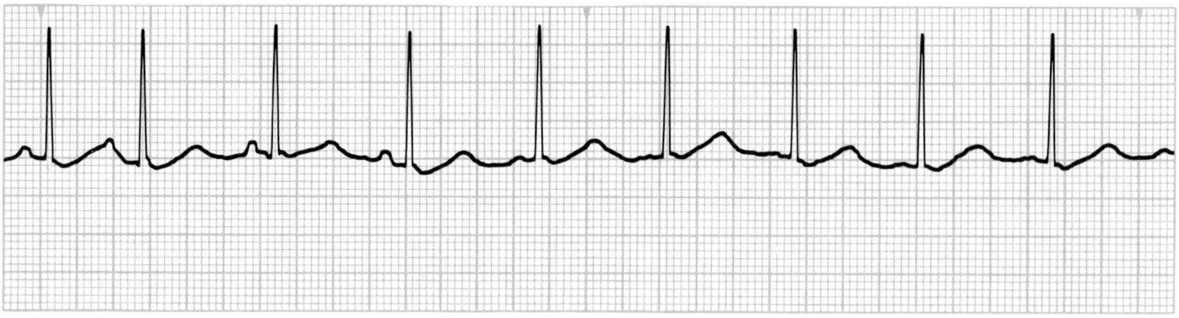

65

Rate: _____

Rhythm: _____

P Waves: _____

P-R Int: _____

QRS: _____

Intrp: _____

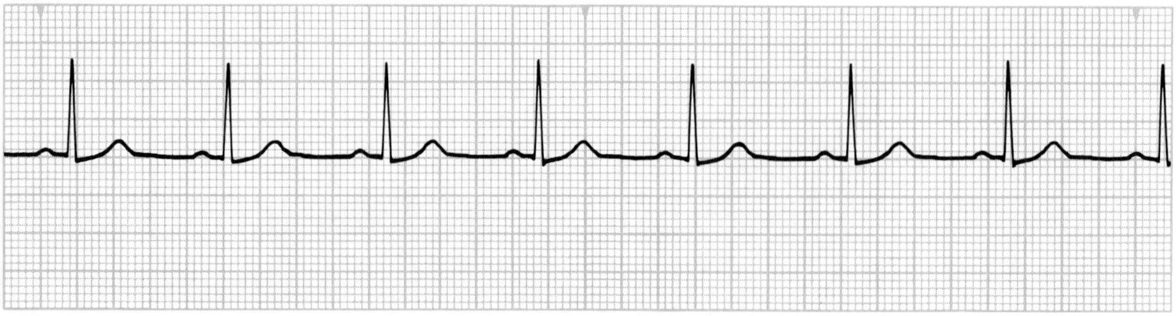

66

Rate: _____

Rhythm: _____

P Waves: _____

P-R Int: _____

QRS: _____

Intrp: _____

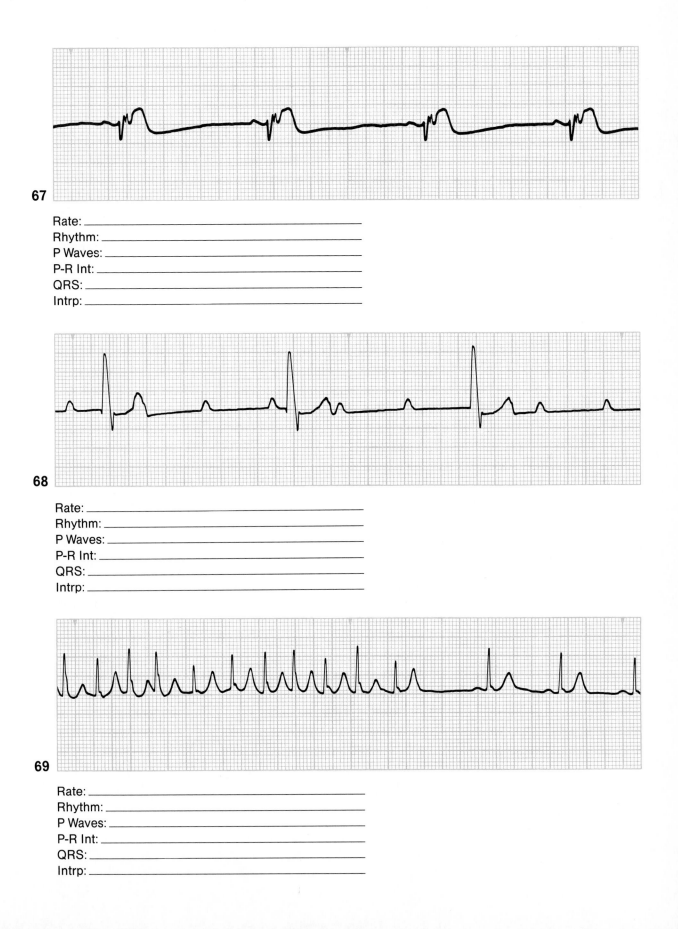

67

Rate: _____

Rhythm: _____

P Waves: _____

P-R Int: _____

QRS: _____

Intrp: _____

68

Rate: _____

Rhythm: _____

P Waves: _____

P-R Int: _____

QRS: _____

Intrp: _____

69

Rate: _____

Rhythm: _____

P Waves: _____

P-R Int: _____

QRS: _____

Intrp: _____

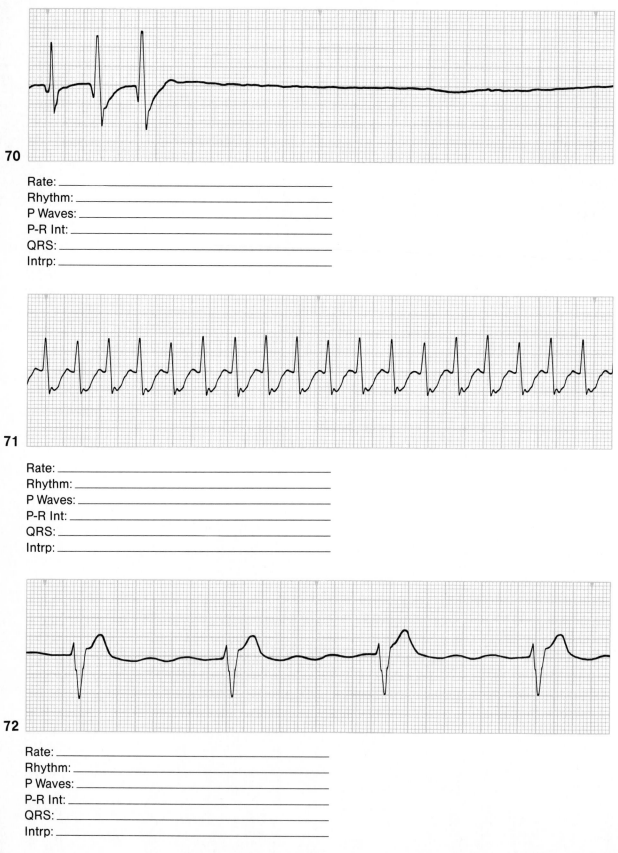

70

Rate: _____

Rhythm: _____

P Waves: _____

P-R Int: _____

QRS: _____

Intrp: _____

71

Rate: _____

Rhythm: _____

P Waves: _____

P-R Int: _____

QRS: _____

Intrp: _____

72

Rate: _____

Rhythm: _____

P Waves: _____

P-R Int: _____

QRS: _____

Intrp: _____

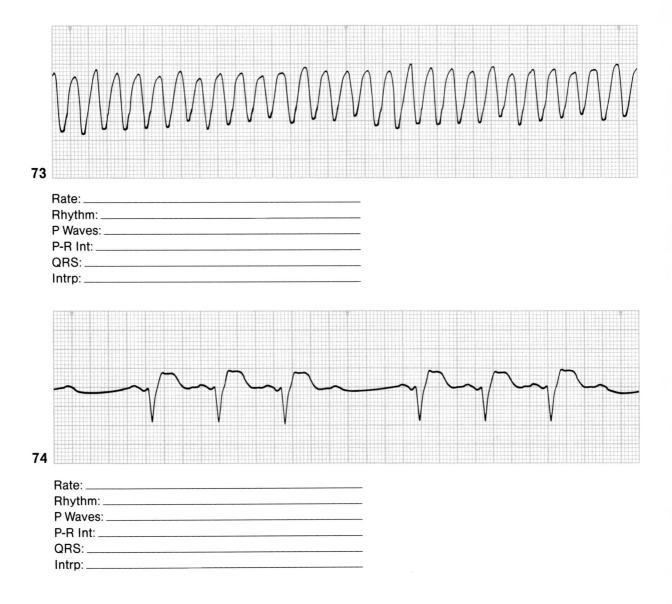

73

Rate: _____

Rhythm: _____

P Waves: _____

P-R Int: _____

QRS: _____

Intrp: _____

74

Rate: _____

Rhythm: _____

P Waves: _____

P-R Int: _____

QRS: _____

Intrp: _____

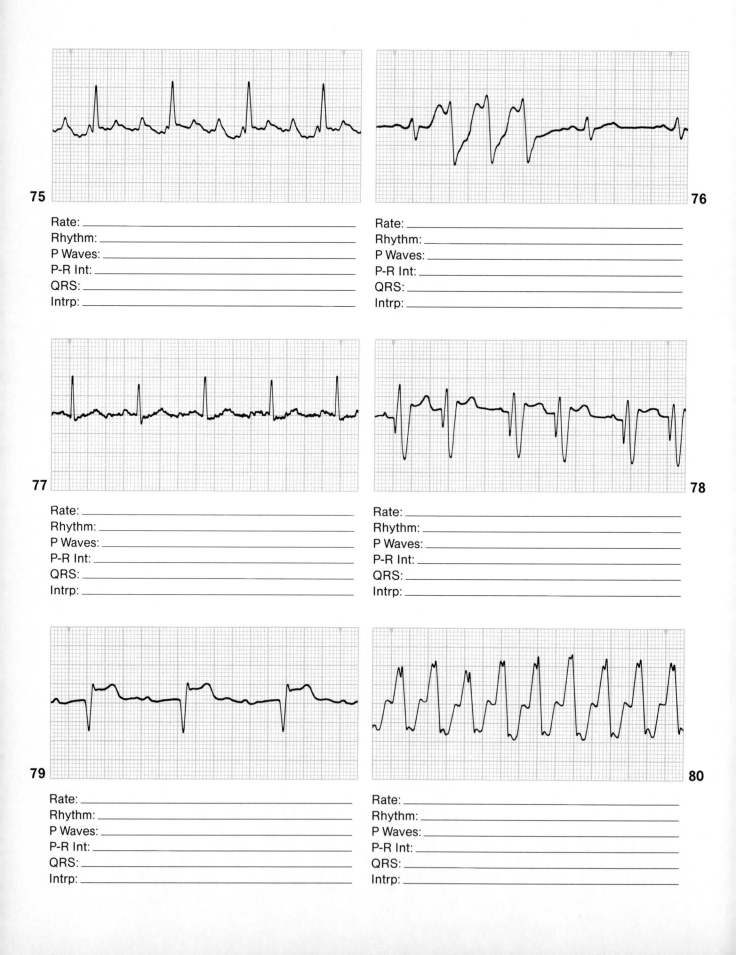

75

Rate: _____
Rhythm: _____
P Waves: _____
P-R Int: _____
QRS: _____
Intrp: _____

76

Rate: _____
Rhythm: _____
P Waves: _____
P-R Int: _____
QRS: _____
Intrp: _____

77

Rate: _____
Rhythm: _____
P Waves: _____
P-R Int: _____
QRS: _____
Intrp: _____

78

Rate: _____
Rhythm: _____
P Waves: _____
P-R Int: _____
QRS: _____
Intrp: _____

79

Rate: _____
Rhythm: _____
P Waves: _____
P-R Int: _____
QRS: _____
Intrp: _____

80

Rate: _____
Rhythm: _____
P Waves: _____
P-R Int: _____
QRS: _____
Intrp: _____

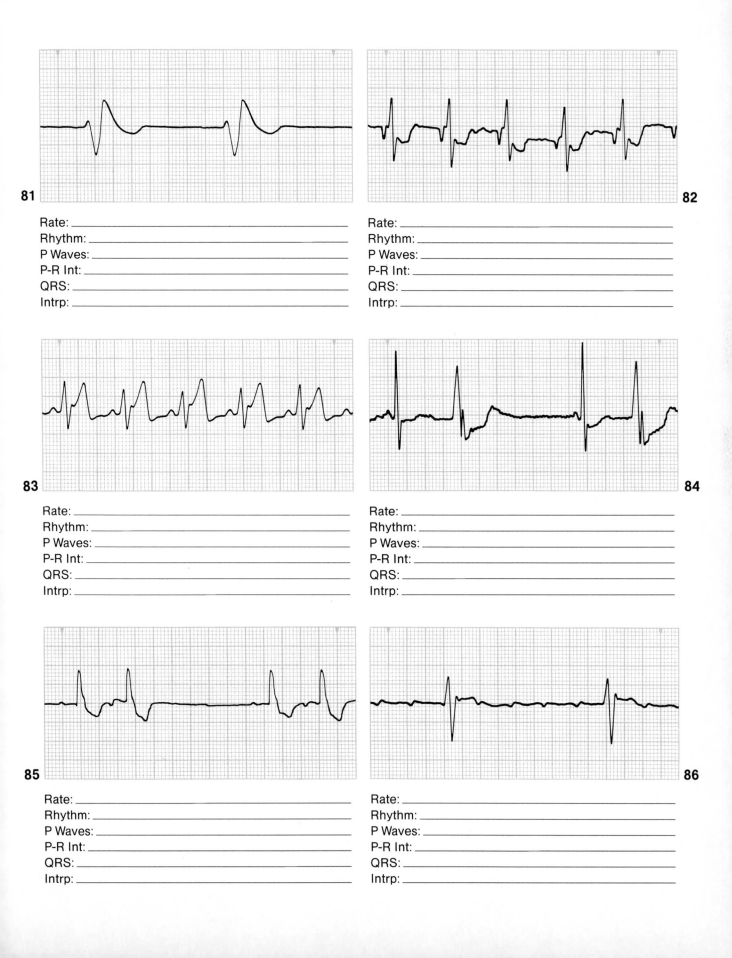

81

Rate: _____
Rhythm: _____
P Waves: _____
P-R Int: _____
QRS: _____
Intrp: _____

82

Rate: _____
Rhythm: _____
P Waves: _____
P-R Int: _____
QRS: _____
Intrp: _____

83

Rate: _____
Rhythm: _____
P Waves: _____
P-R Int: _____
QRS: _____
Intrp: _____

84

Rate: _____
Rhythm: _____
P Waves: _____
P-R Int: _____
QRS: _____
Intrp: _____

85

Rate: _____
Rhythm: _____
P Waves: _____
P-R Int: _____
QRS: _____
Intrp: _____

86

Rate: _____
Rhythm: _____
P Waves: _____
P-R Int: _____
QRS: _____
Intrp: _____

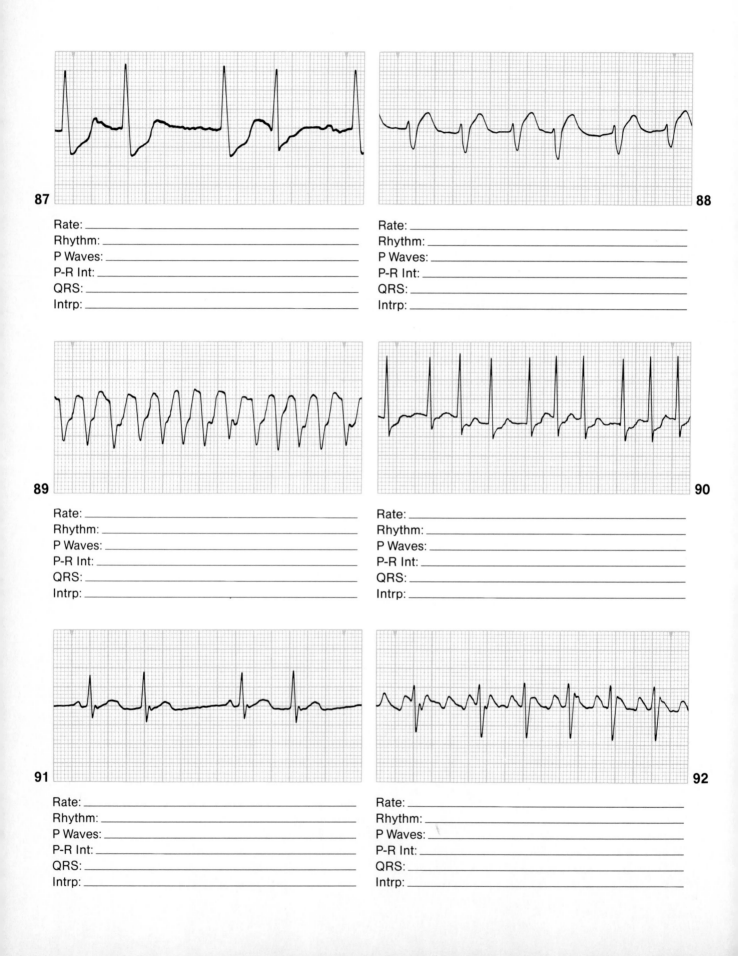

87

Rate: _____
Rhythm: _____
P Waves: _____
P-R Int: _____
QRS: _____
Intrp: _____

88

Rate: _____
Rhythm: _____
P Waves: _____
P-R Int: _____
QRS: _____
Intrp: _____

89

Rate: _____
Rhythm: _____
P Waves: _____
P-R Int: _____
QRS: _____
Intrp: _____

90

Rate: _____
Rhythm: _____
P Waves: _____
P-R Int: _____
QRS: _____
Intrp: _____

91

Rate: _____
Rhythm: _____
P Waves: _____
P-R Int: _____
QRS: _____
Intrp: _____

92

Rate: _____
Rhythm: _____
P Waves: _____
P-R Int: _____
QRS: _____
Intrp: _____

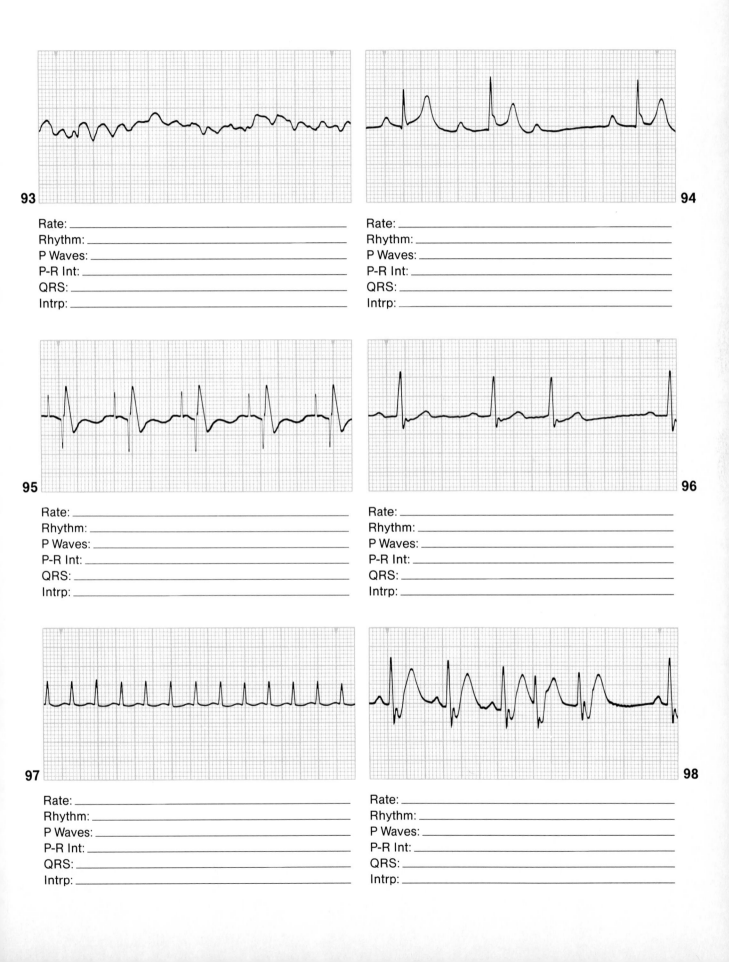

93

Rate: _____
Rhythm: _____
P Waves: _____
P-R Int: _____
QRS: _____
Intrp: _____

94

Rate: _____
Rhythm: _____
P Waves: _____
P-R Int: _____
QRS: _____
Intrp: _____

95

Rate: _____
Rhythm: _____
P Waves: _____
P-R Int: _____
QRS: _____
Intrp: _____

96

Rate: _____
Rhythm: _____
P Waves: _____
P-R Int: _____
QRS: _____
Intrp: _____

97

Rate: _____
Rhythm: _____
P Waves: _____
P-R Int: _____
QRS: _____
Intrp: _____

98

Rate: _____
Rhythm: _____
P Waves: _____
P-R Int: _____
QRS: _____
Intrp: _____

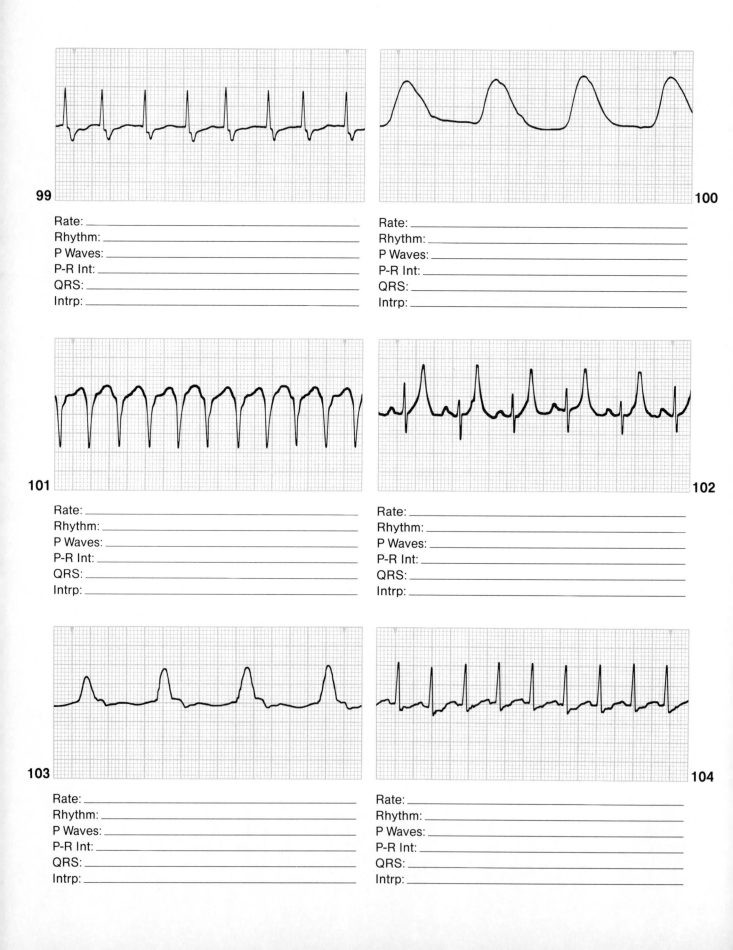

99

Rate: _____
Rhythm: _____
P Waves: _____
P-R Int: _____
QRS: _____
Intrp: _____

100

Rate: _____
Rhythm: _____
P Waves: _____
P-R Int: _____
QRS: _____
Intrp: _____

101

Rate: _____
Rhythm: _____
P Waves: _____
P-R Int: _____
QRS: _____
Intrp: _____

102

Rate: _____
Rhythm: _____
P Waves: _____
P-R Int: _____
QRS: _____
Intrp: _____

103

Rate: _____
Rhythm: _____
P Waves: _____
P-R Int: _____
QRS: _____
Intrp: _____

104

Rate: _____
Rhythm: _____
P Waves: _____
P-R Int: _____
QRS: _____
Intrp: _____

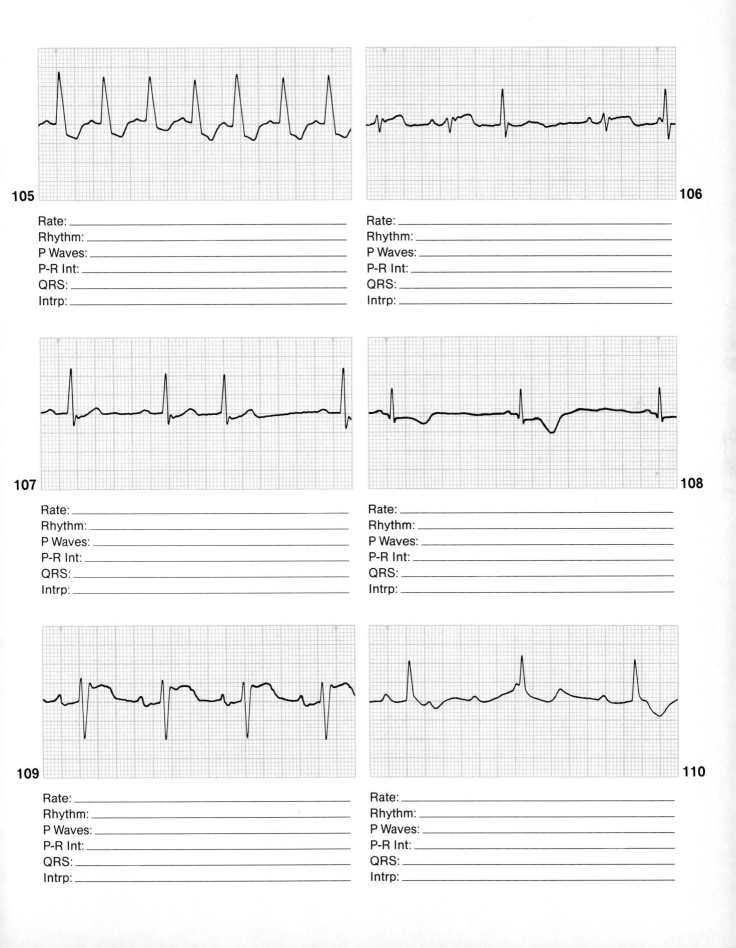

105

Rate: _____
Rhythm: _____
P Waves: _____
P-R Int: _____
QRS: _____
Intrp: _____

106

Rate: _____
Rhythm: _____
P Waves: _____
P-R Int: _____
QRS: _____
Intrp: _____

107

Rate: _____
Rhythm: _____
P Waves: _____
P-R Int: _____
QRS: _____
Intrp: _____

108

Rate: _____
Rhythm: _____
P Waves: _____
P-R Int: _____
QRS: _____
Intrp: _____

109

Rate: _____
Rhythm: _____
P Waves: _____
P-R Int: _____
QRS: _____
Intrp: _____

110

Rate: _____
Rhythm: _____
P Waves: _____
P-R Int: _____
QRS: _____
Intrp: _____

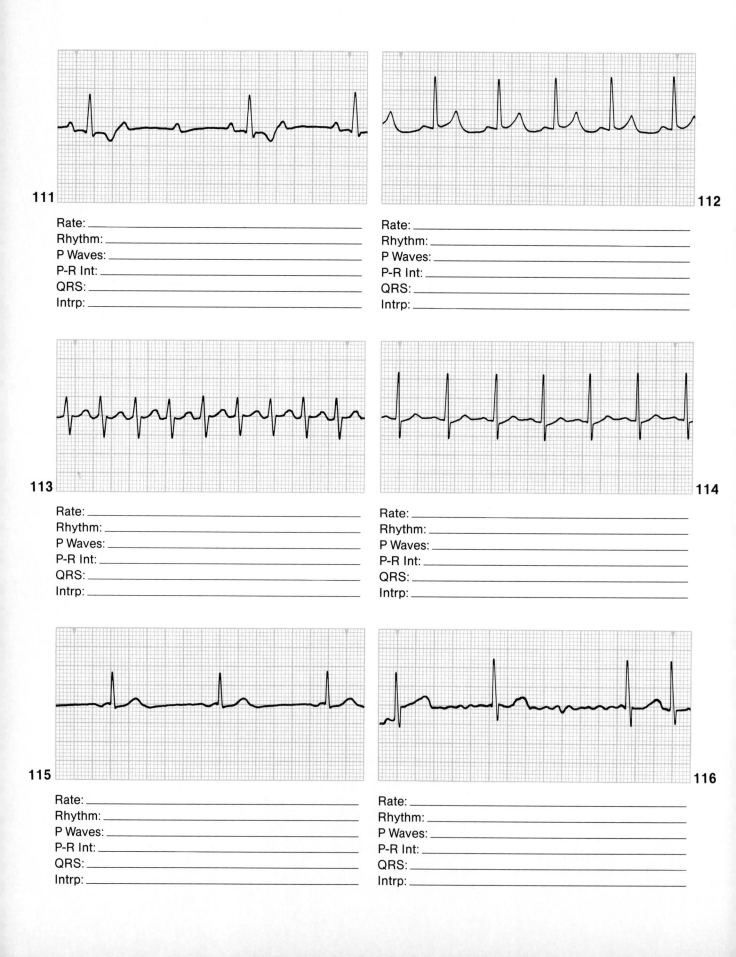

111

Rate: _____
Rhythm: _____
P Waves: _____
P-R Int: _____
QRS: _____
Intrp: _____

112

Rate: _____
Rhythm: _____
P Waves: _____
P-R Int: _____
QRS: _____
Intrp: _____

113

Rate: _____
Rhythm: _____
P Waves: _____
P-R Int: _____
QRS: _____
Intrp: _____

114

Rate: _____
Rhythm: _____
P Waves: _____
P-R Int: _____
QRS: _____
Intrp: _____

115

Rate: _____
Rhythm: _____
P Waves: _____
P-R Int: _____
QRS: _____
Intrp: _____

116

Rate: _____
Rhythm: _____
P Waves: _____
P-R Int: _____
QRS: _____
Intrp: _____

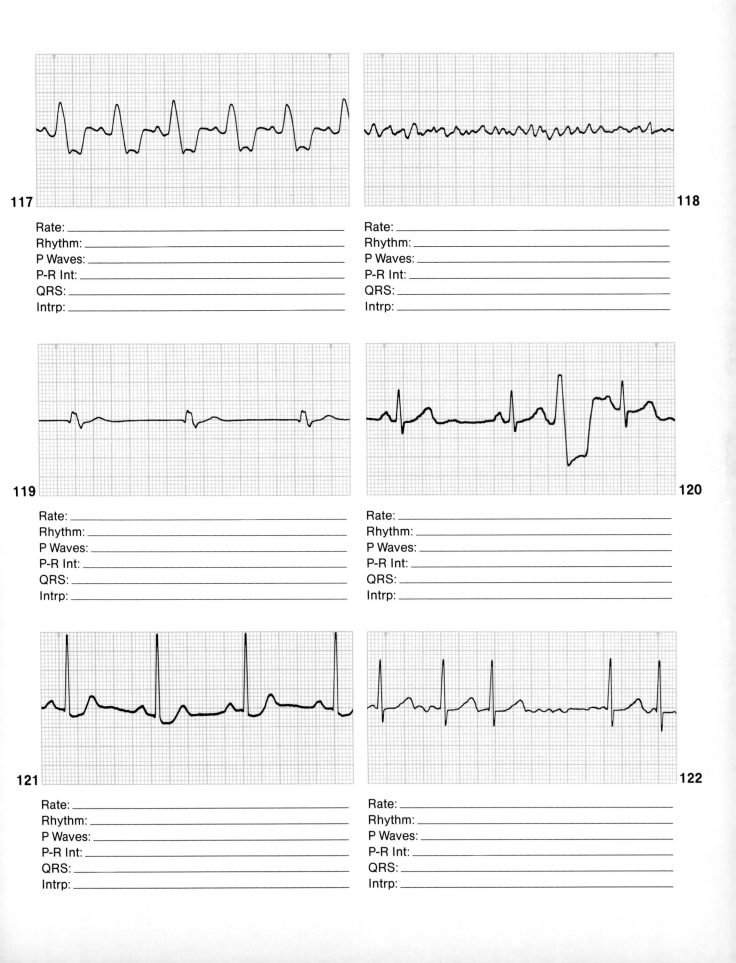

117

Rate: _____
Rhythm: _____
P Waves: _____
P-R Int: _____
QRS: _____
Intrp: _____

118

Rate: _____
Rhythm: _____
P Waves: _____
P-R Int: _____
QRS: _____
Intrp: _____

119

Rate: _____
Rhythm: _____
P Waves: _____
P-R Int: _____
QRS: _____
Intrp: _____

120

Rate: _____
Rhythm: _____
P Waves: _____
P-R Int: _____
QRS: _____
Intrp: _____

121

Rate: _____
Rhythm: _____
P Waves: _____
P-R Int: _____
QRS: _____
Intrp: _____

122

Rate: _____
Rhythm: _____
P Waves: _____
P-R Int: _____
QRS: _____
Intrp: _____

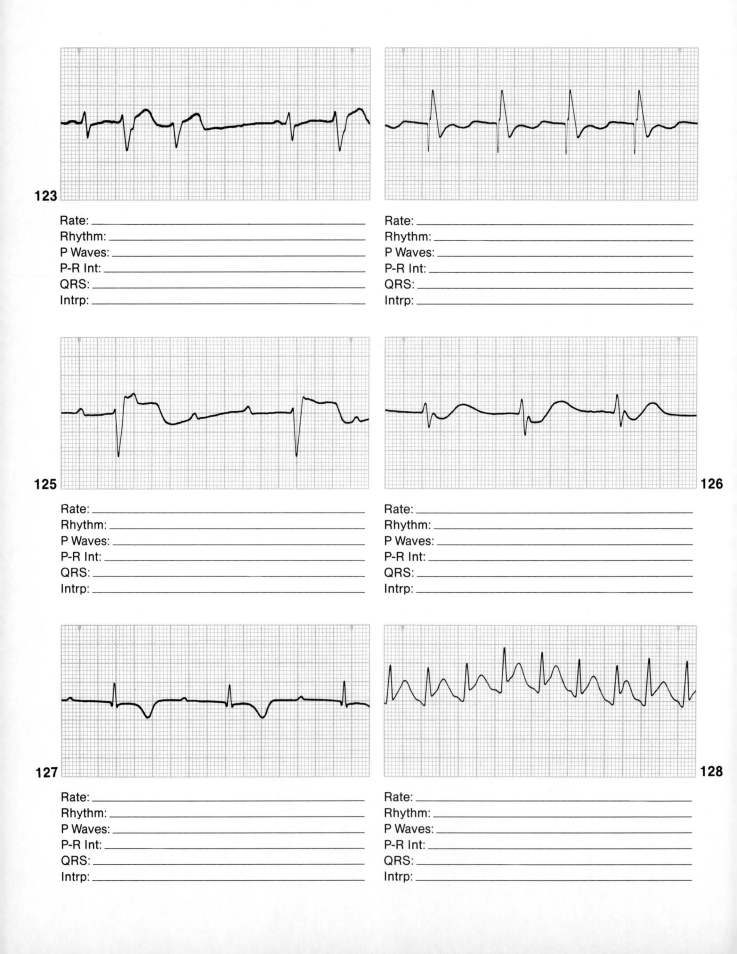

123

Rate: _____
Rhythm: _____
P Waves: _____
P-R Int: _____
QRS: _____
Intrp: _____

Rate: _____
Rhythm: _____
P Waves: _____
P-R Int: _____
QRS: _____
Intrp: _____

125

Rate: _____
Rhythm: _____
P Waves: _____
P-R Int: _____
QRS: _____
Intrp: _____

126

Rate: _____
Rhythm: _____
P Waves: _____
P-R Int: _____
QRS: _____
Intrp: _____

127

Rate: _____
Rhythm: _____
P Waves: _____
P-R Int: _____
QRS: _____
Intrp: _____

128

Rate: _____
Rhythm: _____
P Waves: _____
P-R Int: _____
QRS: _____
Intrp: _____

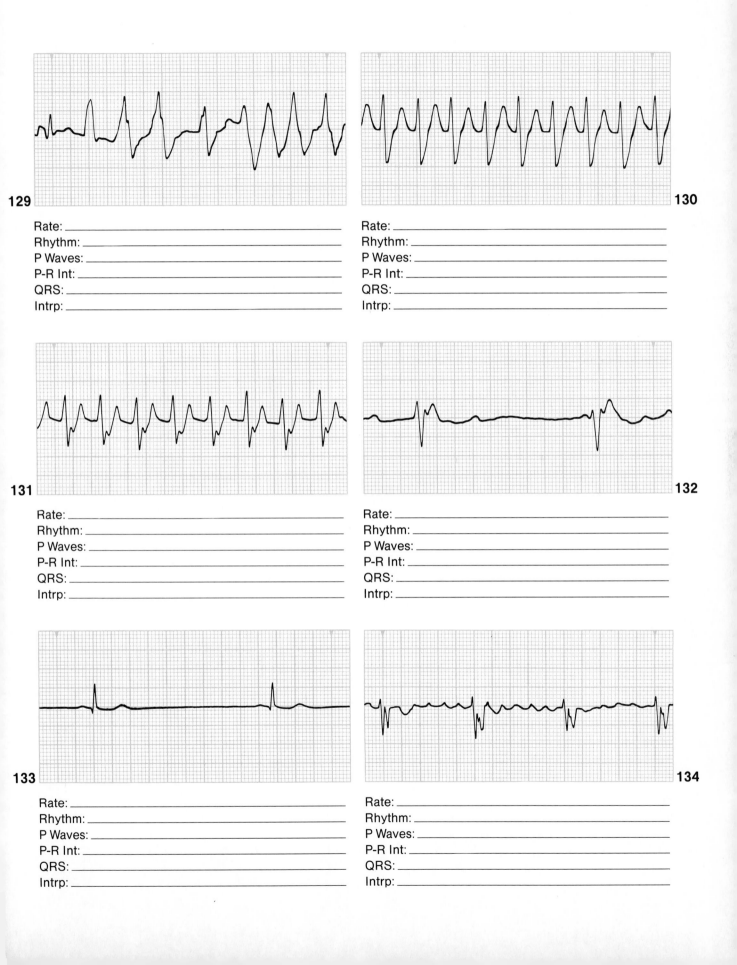

129

Rate: _____
Rhythm: _____
P Waves: _____
P-R Int: _____
QRS: _____
Intrp: _____

130

Rate: _____
Rhythm: _____
P Waves: _____
P-R Int: _____
QRS: _____
Intrp: _____

131

Rate: _____
Rhythm: _____
P Waves: _____
P-R Int: _____
QRS: _____
Intrp: _____

132

Rate: _____
Rhythm: _____
P Waves: _____
P-R Int: _____
QRS: _____
Intrp: _____

133

Rate: _____
Rhythm: _____
P Waves: _____
P-R Int: _____
QRS: _____
Intrp: _____

134

Rate: _____
Rhythm: _____
P Waves: _____
P-R Int: _____
QRS: _____
Intrp: _____

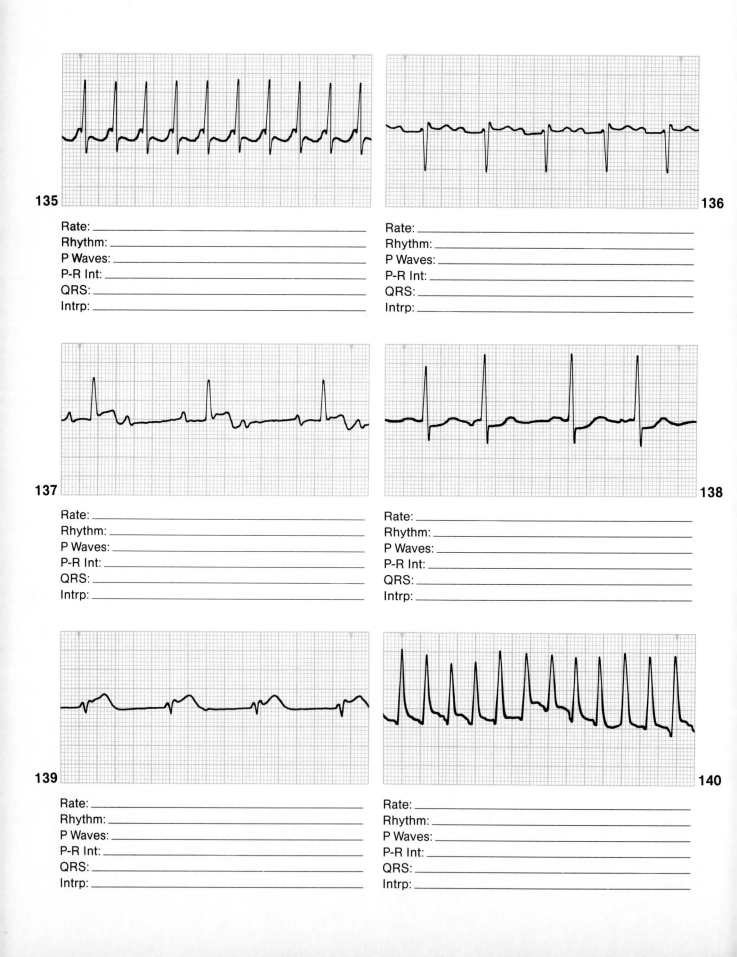

135

Rate: _____
Rhythm: _____
P Waves: _____
P-R Int: _____
QRS: _____
Intrp: _____

136

Rate: _____
Rhythm: _____
P Waves: _____
P-R Int: _____
QRS: _____
Intrp: _____

137

Rate: _____
Rhythm: _____
P Waves: _____
P-R Int: _____
QRS: _____
Intrp: _____

138

Rate: _____
Rhythm: _____
P Waves: _____
P-R Int: _____
QRS: _____
Intrp: _____

139

Rate: _____
Rhythm: _____
P Waves: _____
P-R Int: _____
QRS: _____
Intrp: _____

140

Rate: _____
Rhythm: _____
P Waves: _____
P-R Int: _____
QRS: _____
Intrp: _____

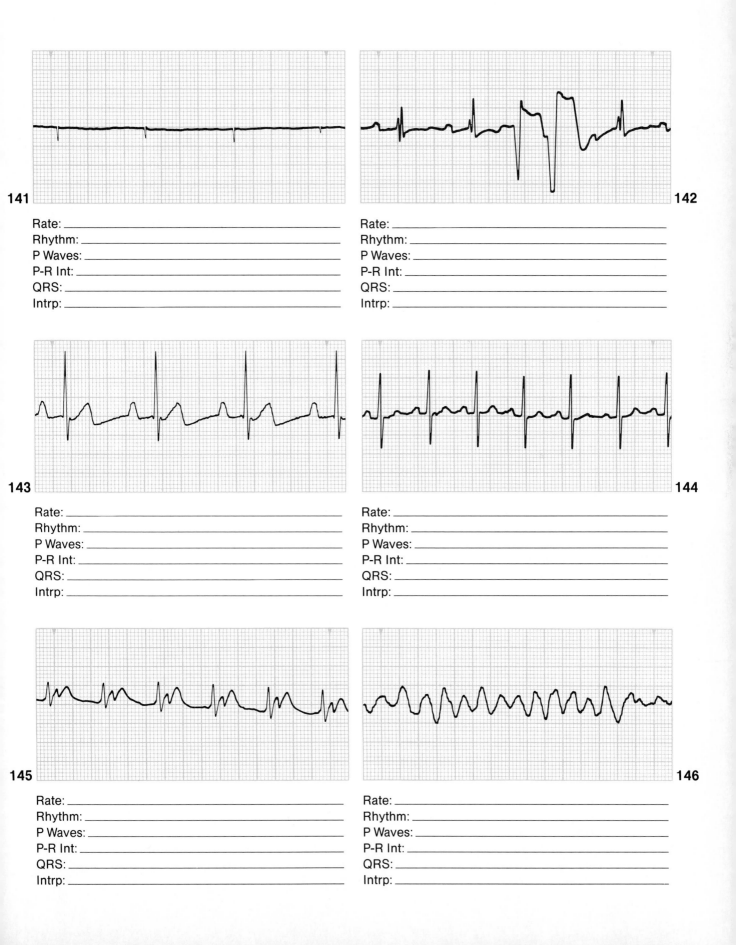

141

Rate: _____
Rhythm: _____
P Waves: _____
P-R Int: _____
QRS: _____
Intrp: _____

142

Rate: _____
Rhythm: _____
P Waves: _____
P-R Int: _____
QRS: _____
Intrp: _____

143

Rate: _____
Rhythm: _____
P Waves: _____
P-R Int: _____
QRS: _____
Intrp: _____

144

Rate: _____
Rhythm: _____
P Waves: _____
P-R Int: _____
QRS: _____
Intrp: _____

145

Rate: _____
Rhythm: _____
P Waves: _____
P-R Int: _____
QRS: _____
Intrp: _____

146

Rate: _____
Rhythm: _____
P Waves: _____
P-R Int: _____
QRS: _____
Intrp: _____

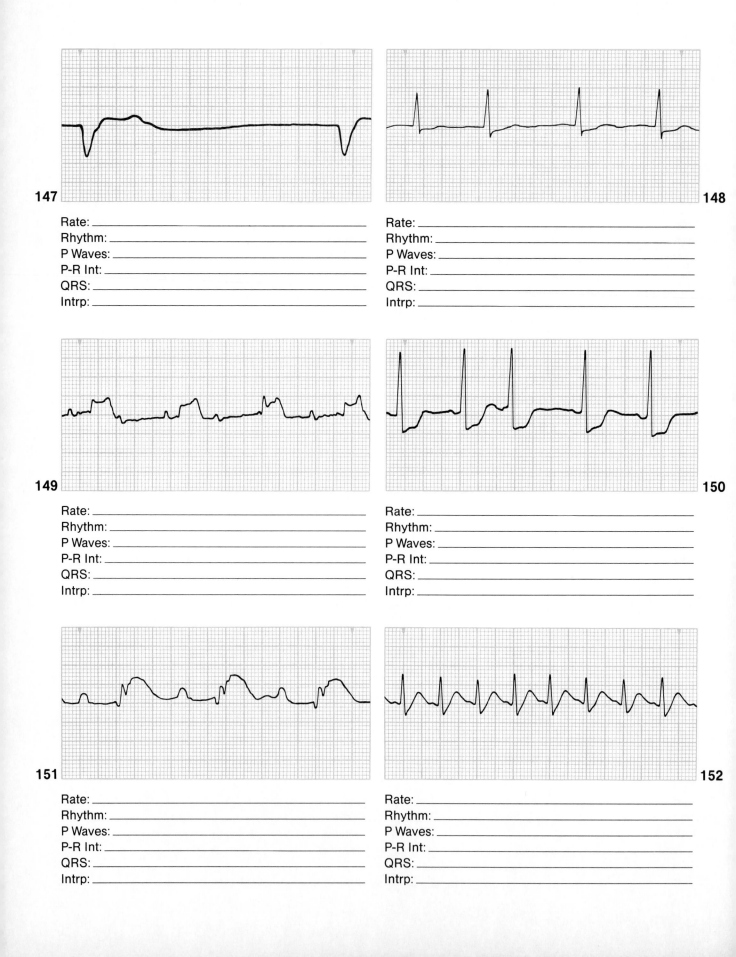

147

Rate: _____
Rhythm: _____
P Waves: _____
P-R Int: _____
QRS: _____
Intrp: _____

148

Rate: _____
Rhythm: _____
P Waves: _____
P-R Int: _____
QRS: _____
Intrp: _____

149

Rate: _____
Rhythm: _____
P Waves: _____
P-R Int: _____
QRS: _____
Intrp: _____

150

Rate: _____
Rhythm: _____
P Waves: _____
P-R Int: _____
QRS: _____
Intrp: _____

151

Rate: _____
Rhythm: _____
P Waves: _____
P-R Int: _____
QRS: _____
Intrp: _____

152

Rate: _____
Rhythm: _____
P Waves: _____
P-R Int: _____
QRS: _____
Intrp: _____

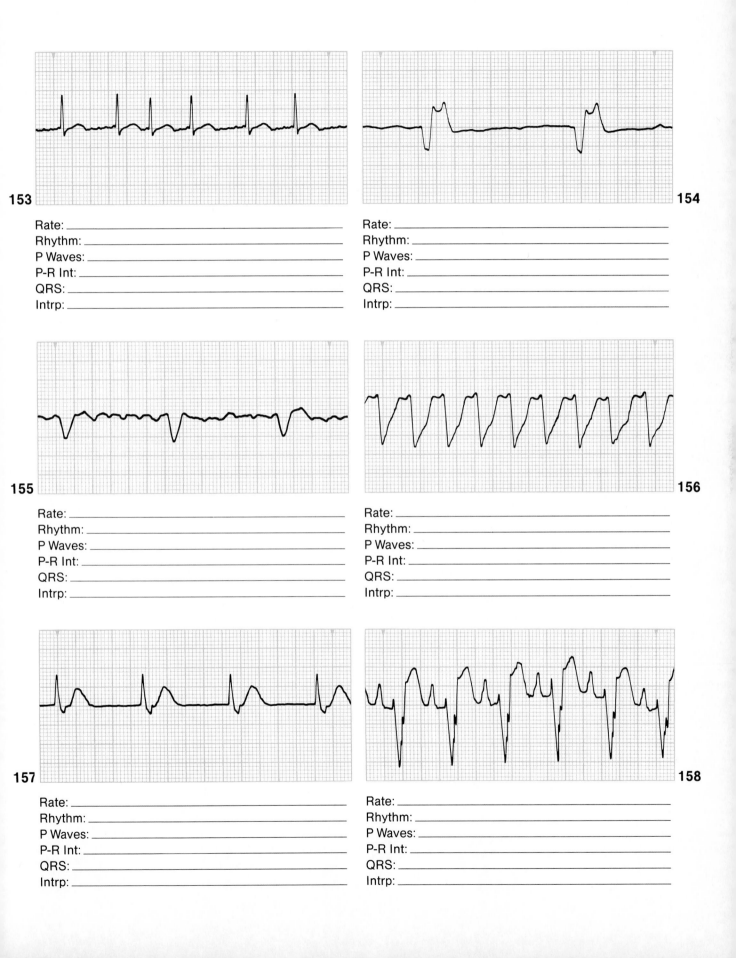

153

Rate: _____
Rhythm: _____
P Waves: _____
P-R Int: _____
QRS: _____
Intrp: _____

154

Rate: _____
Rhythm: _____
P Waves: _____
P-R Int: _____
QRS: _____
Intrp: _____

155

Rate: _____
Rhythm: _____
P Waves: _____
P-R Int: _____
QRS: _____
Intrp: _____

156

Rate: _____
Rhythm: _____
P Waves: _____
P-R Int: _____
QRS: _____
Intrp: _____

157

Rate: _____
Rhythm: _____
P Waves: _____
P-R Int: _____
QRS: _____
Intrp: _____

158

Rate: _____
Rhythm: _____
P Waves: _____
P-R Int: _____
QRS: _____
Intrp: _____

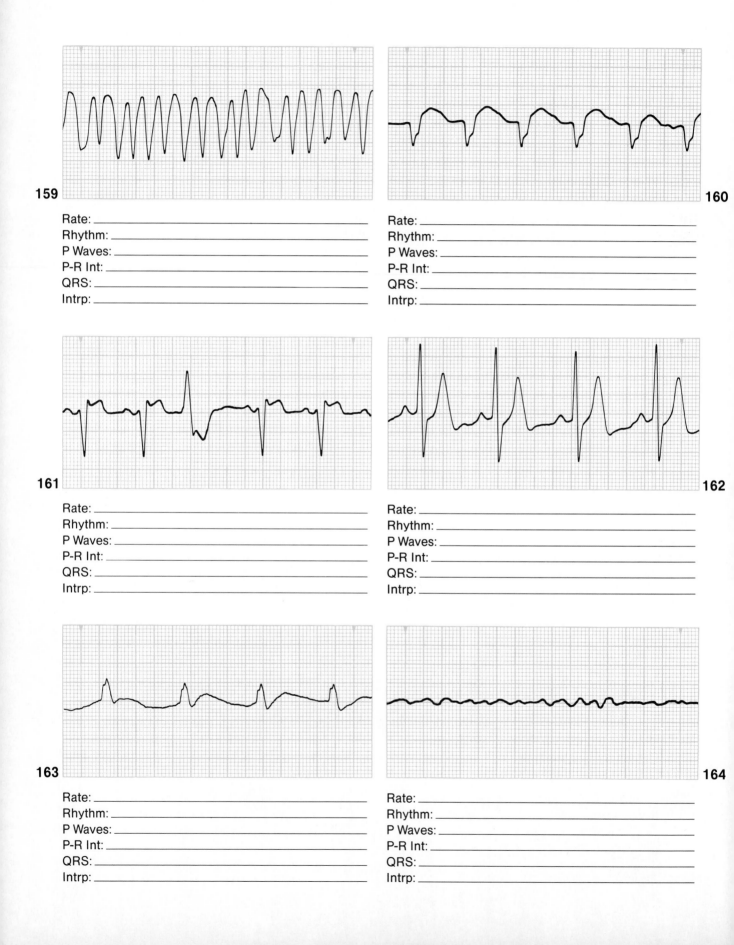

159

Rate: _____
Rhythm: _____
P Waves: _____
P-R Int: _____
QRS: _____
Intrp: _____

160

Rate: _____
Rhythm: _____
P Waves: _____
P-R Int: _____
QRS: _____
Intrp: _____

161

Rate: _____
Rhythm: _____
P Waves: _____
P-R Int: _____
QRS: _____
Intrp: _____

162

Rate: _____
Rhythm: _____
P Waves: _____
P-R Int: _____
QRS: _____
Intrp: _____

163

Rate: _____
Rhythm: _____
P Waves: _____
P-R Int: _____
QRS: _____
Intrp: _____

164

Rate: _____
Rhythm: _____
P Waves: _____
P-R Int: _____
QRS: _____
Intrp: _____

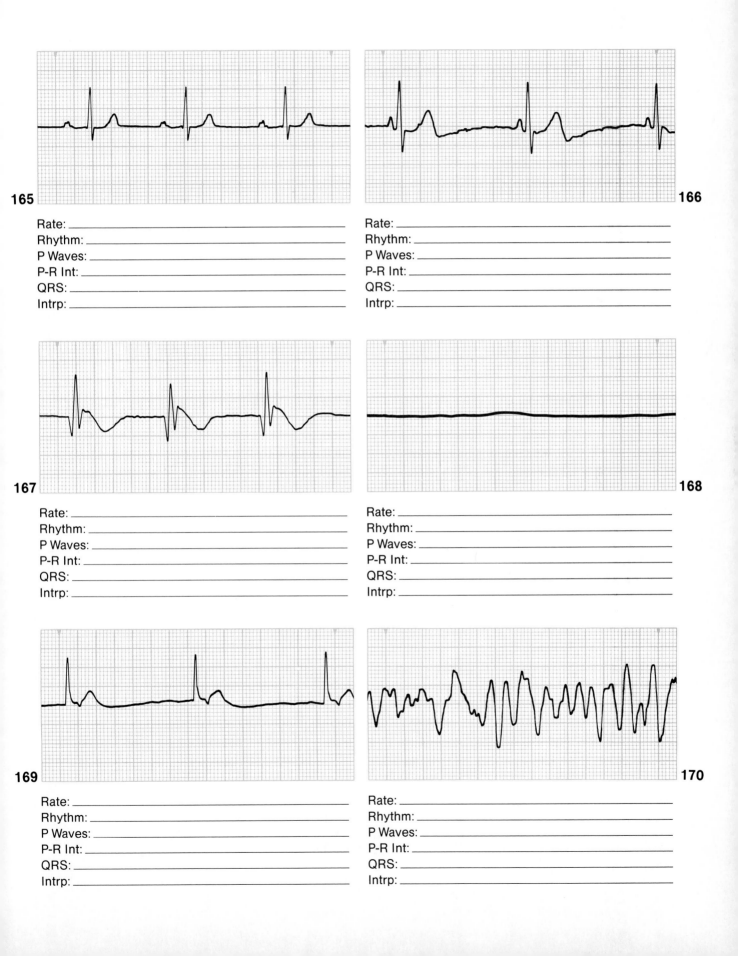

165

Rate: _____
Rhythm: _____
P Waves: _____
P-R Int: _____
QRS: _____
Intrp: _____

166

Rate: _____
Rhythm: _____
P Waves: _____
P-R Int: _____
QRS: _____
Intrp: _____

167

Rate: _____
Rhythm: _____
P Waves: _____
P-R Int: _____
QRS: _____
Intrp: _____

168

Rate: _____
Rhythm: _____
P Waves: _____
P-R Int: _____
QRS: _____
Intrp: _____

169

Rate: _____
Rhythm: _____
P Waves: _____
P-R Int: _____
QRS: _____
Intrp: _____

170

Rate: _____
Rhythm: _____
P Waves: _____
P-R Int: _____
QRS: _____
Intrp: _____

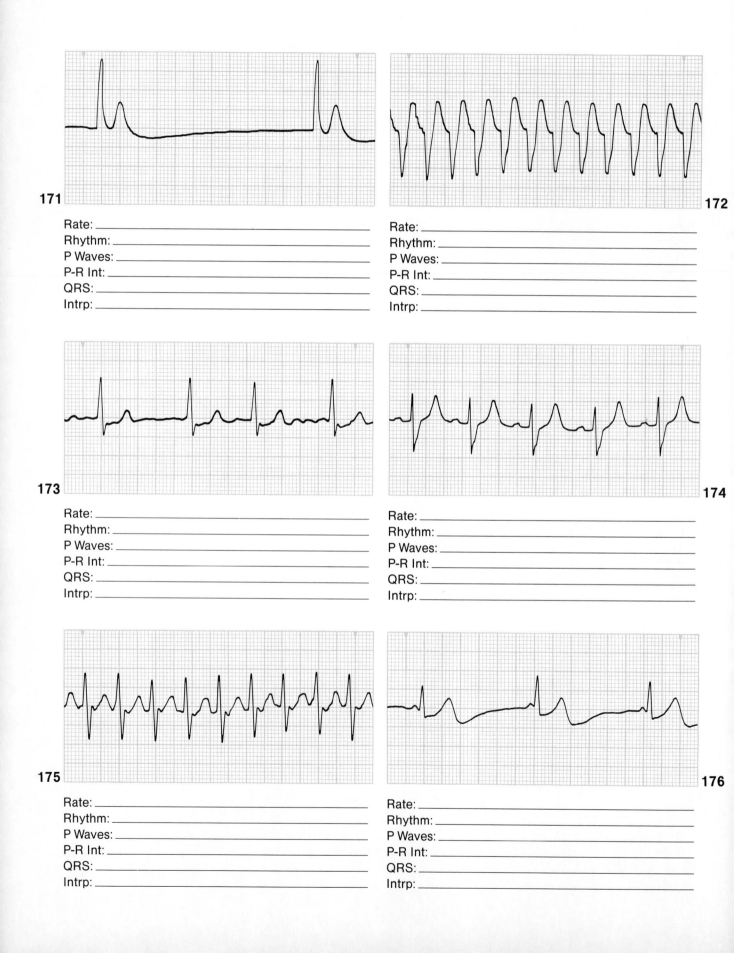

171

Rate: _____
Rhythm: _____
P Waves: _____
P-R Int: _____
QRS: _____
Intrp: _____

172

Rate: _____
Rhythm: _____
P Waves: _____
P-R Int: _____
QRS: _____
Intrp: _____

173

Rate: _____
Rhythm: _____
P Waves: _____
P-R Int: _____
QRS: _____
Intrp: _____

174

Rate: _____
Rhythm: _____
P Waves: _____
P-R Int: _____
QRS: _____
Intrp: _____

175

Rate: _____
Rhythm: _____
P Waves: _____
P-R Int: _____
QRS: _____
Intrp: _____

176

Rate: _____
Rhythm: _____
P Waves: _____
P-R Int: _____
QRS: _____
Intrp: _____

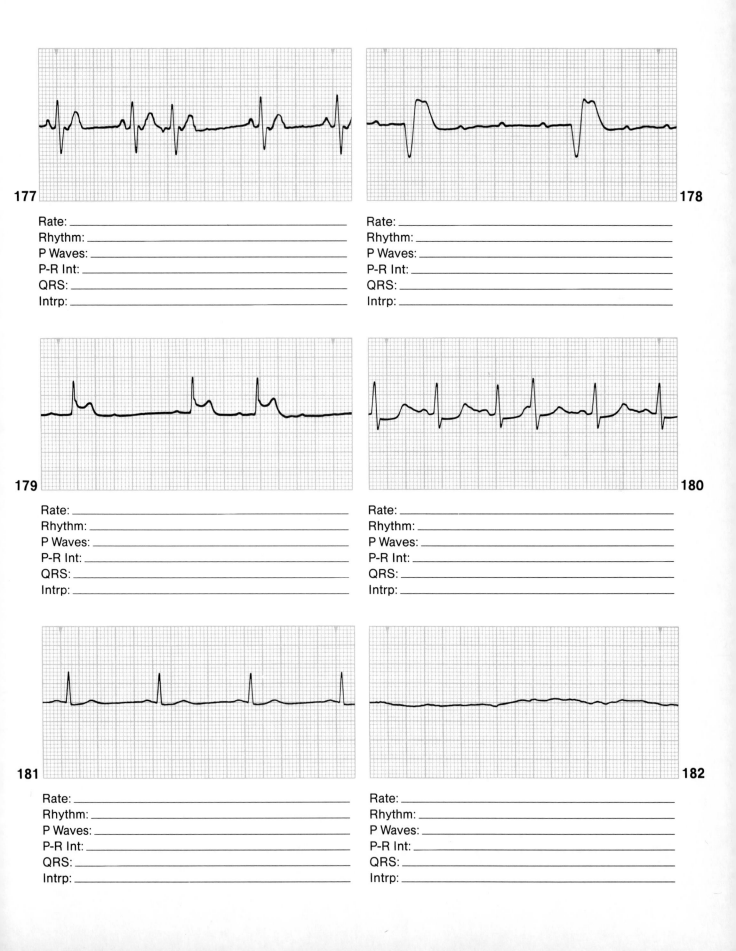

177

Rate: _____
Rhythm: _____
P Waves: _____
P-R Int: _____
QRS: _____
Intrp: _____

178

Rate: _____
Rhythm: _____
P Waves: _____
P-R Int: _____
QRS: _____
Intrp: _____

179

Rate: _____
Rhythm: _____
P Waves: _____
P-R Int: _____
QRS: _____
Intrp: _____

180

Rate: _____
Rhythm: _____
P Waves: _____
P-R Int: _____
QRS: _____
Intrp: _____

181

Rate: _____
Rhythm: _____
P Waves: _____
P-R Int: _____
QRS: _____
Intrp: _____

182

Rate: _____
Rhythm: _____
P Waves: _____
P-R Int: _____
QRS: _____
Intrp: _____

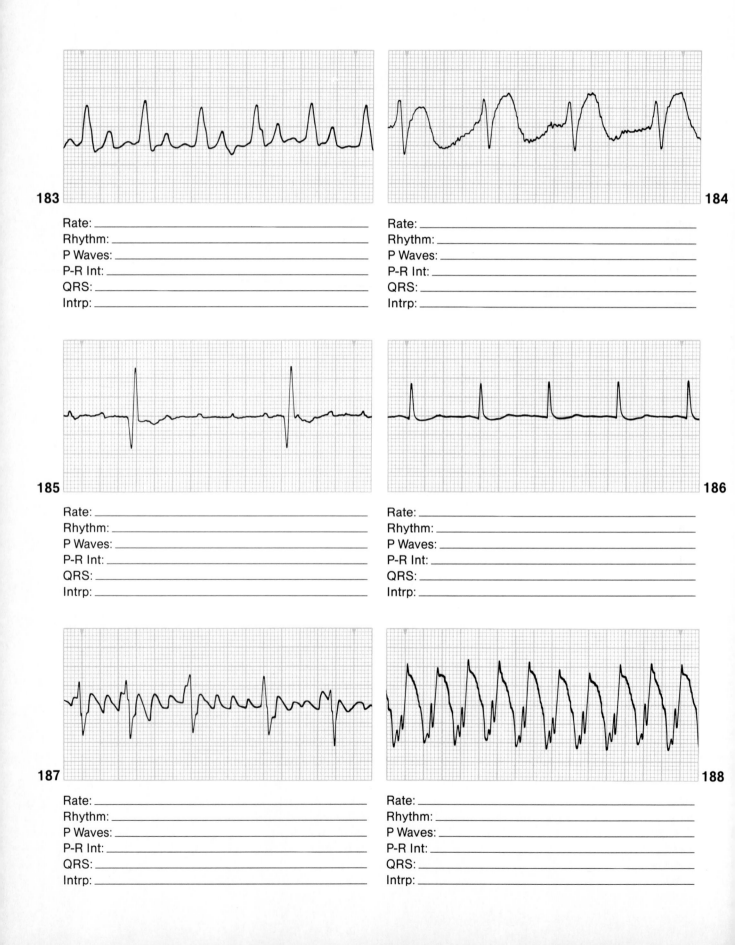

183

Rate: _____
Rhythm: _____
P Waves: _____
P-R Int: _____
QRS: _____
Intrp: _____

184

Rate: _____
Rhythm: _____
P Waves: _____
P-R Int: _____
QRS: _____
Intrp: _____

185

Rate: _____
Rhythm: _____
P Waves: _____
P-R Int: _____
QRS: _____
Intrp: _____

186

Rate: _____
Rhythm: _____
P Waves: _____
P-R Int: _____
QRS: _____
Intrp: _____

187

Rate: _____
Rhythm: _____
P Waves: _____
P-R Int: _____
QRS: _____
Intrp: _____

188

Rate: _____
Rhythm: _____
P Waves: _____
P-R Int: _____
QRS: _____
Intrp: _____

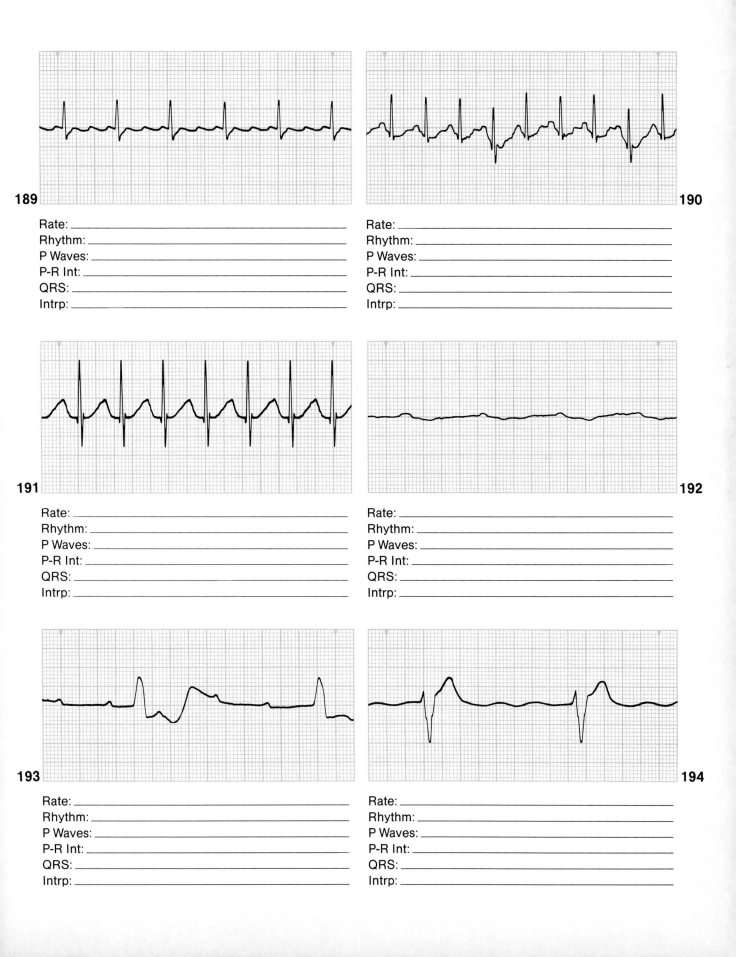

189

Rate: _____
Rhythm: _____
P Waves: _____
P-R Int: _____
QRS: _____
Intrp: _____

190

Rate: _____
Rhythm: _____
P Waves: _____
P-R Int: _____
QRS: _____
Intrp: _____

191

Rate: _____
Rhythm: _____
P Waves: _____
P-R Int: _____
QRS: _____
Intrp: _____

192

Rate: _____
Rhythm: _____
P Waves: _____
P-R Int: _____
QRS: _____
Intrp: _____

193

Rate: _____
Rhythm: _____
P Waves: _____
P-R Int: _____
QRS: _____
Intrp: _____

194

Rate: _____
Rhythm: _____
P Waves: _____
P-R Int: _____
QRS: _____
Intrp: _____

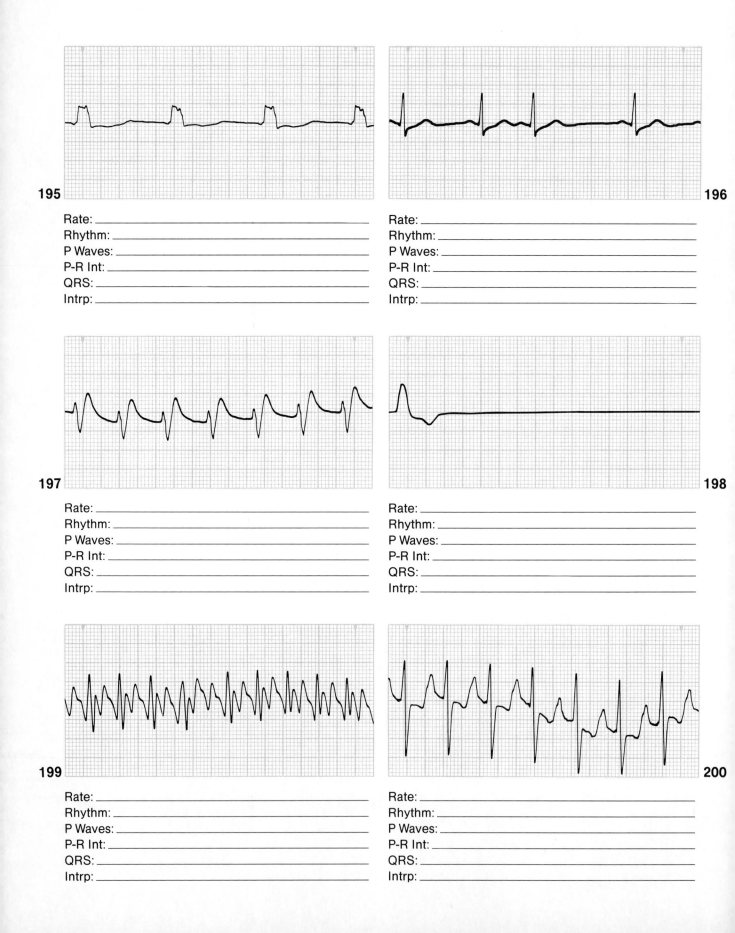

195

Rate: _____

Rhythm: _____

P Waves: _____

P-R Int: _____

QRS: _____

Intrp: _____

196

Rate: _____

Rhythm: _____

P Waves: _____

P-R Int: _____

QRS: _____

Intrp: _____

197

Rate: _____

Rhythm: _____

P Waves: _____

P-R Int: _____

QRS: _____

Intrp: _____

198

Rate: _____

Rhythm: _____

P Waves: _____

P-R Int: _____

QRS: _____

Intrp: _____

199

Rate: _____

Rhythm: _____

P Waves: _____

P-R Int: _____

QRS: _____

Intrp: _____

200

Rate: _____

Rhythm: _____

P Waves: _____

P-R Int: _____

QRS: _____

Intrp: _____

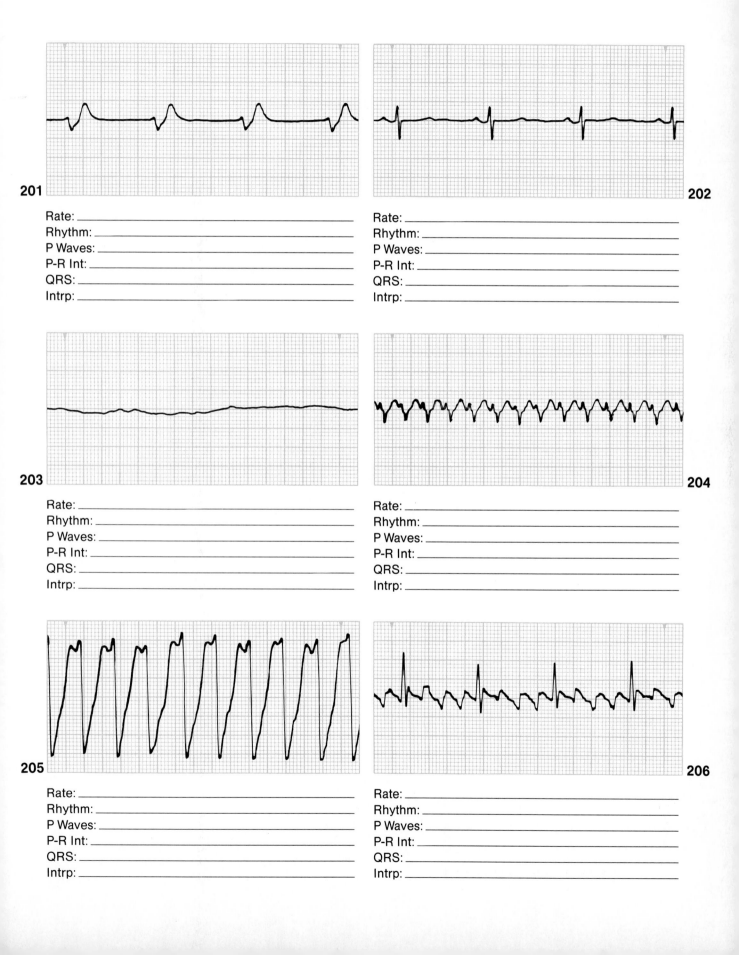

201

Rate: _____
Rhythm: _____
P Waves: _____
P-R Int: _____
QRS: _____
Intrp: _____

202

Rate: _____
Rhythm: _____
P Waves: _____
P-R Int: _____
QRS: _____
Intrp: _____

203

Rate: _____
Rhythm: _____
P Waves: _____
P-R Int: _____
QRS: _____
Intrp: _____

204

Rate: _____
Rhythm: _____
P Waves: _____
P-R Int: _____
QRS: _____
Intrp: _____

205

Rate: _____
Rhythm: _____
P Waves: _____
P-R Int: _____
QRS: _____
Intrp: _____

206

Rate: _____
Rhythm: _____
P Waves: _____
P-R Int: _____
QRS: _____
Intrp: _____

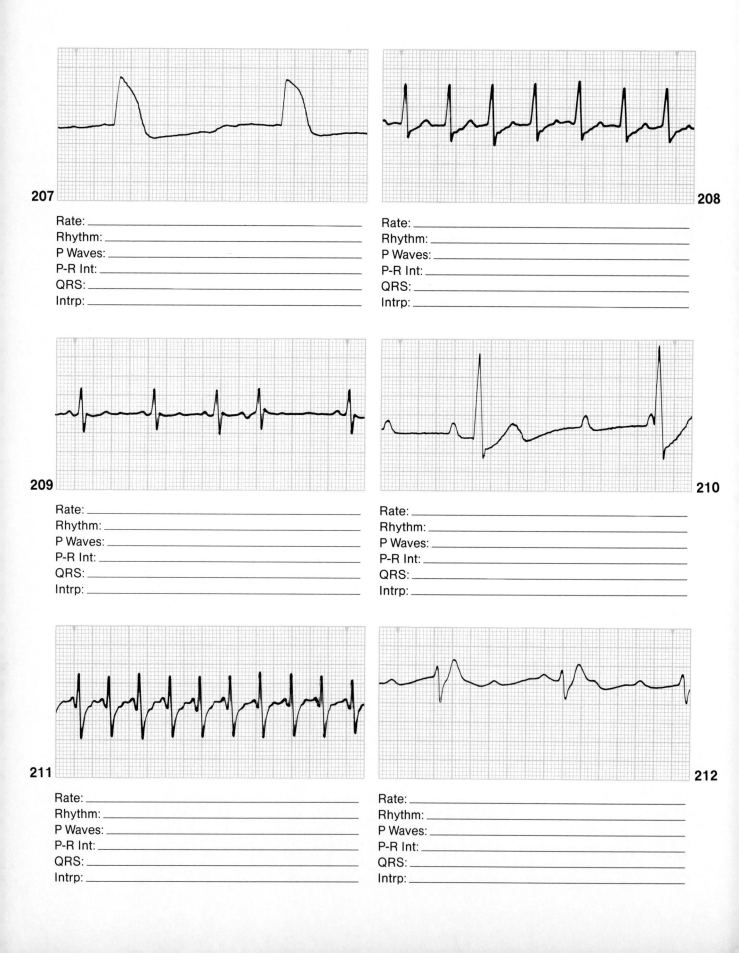

207

Rate: _____

Rhythm: _____

P Waves: _____

P-R Int: _____

QRS: _____

Intrp: _____

208

Rate: _____

Rhythm: _____

P Waves: _____

P-R Int: _____

QRS: _____

Intrp: _____

209

Rate: _____

Rhythm: _____

P Waves: _____

P-R Int: _____

QRS: _____

Intrp: _____

210

Rate: _____

Rhythm: _____

P Waves: _____

P-R Int: _____

QRS: _____

Intrp: _____

211

Rate: _____

Rhythm: _____

P Waves: _____

P-R Int: _____

QRS: _____

Intrp: _____

212

Rate: _____

Rhythm: _____

P Waves: _____

P-R Int: _____

QRS: _____

Intrp: _____

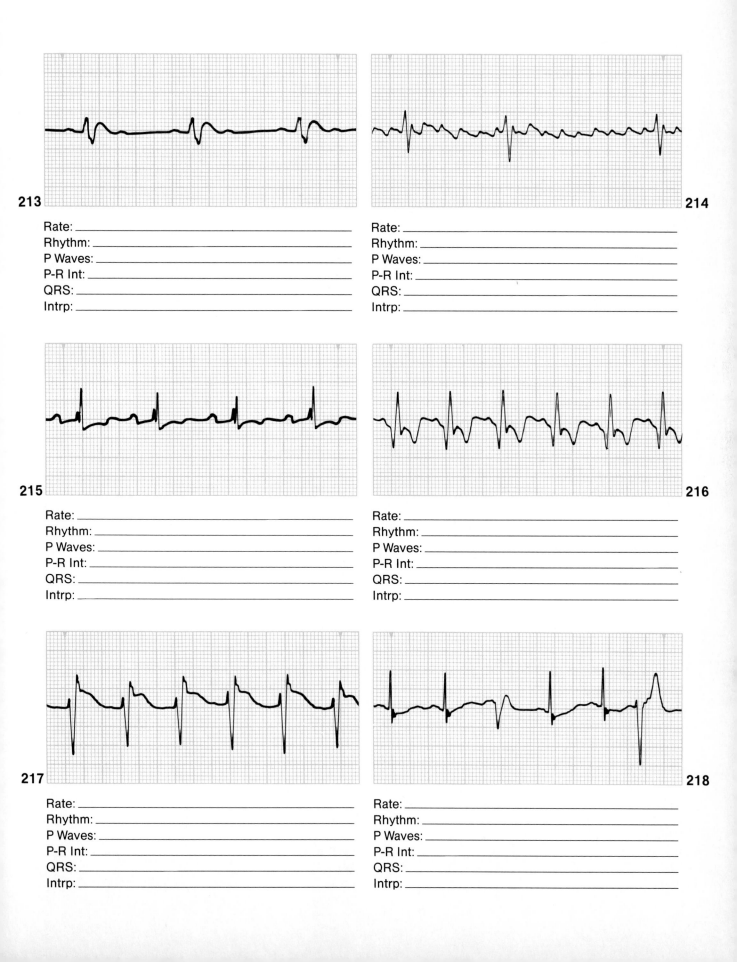

213

Rate: _____
Rhythm: _____
P Waves: _____
P-R Int: _____
QRS: _____
Intrp: _____

214

Rate: _____
Rhythm: _____
P Waves: _____
P-R Int: _____
QRS: _____
Intrp: _____

215

Rate: _____
Rhythm: _____
P Waves: _____
P-R Int: _____
QRS: _____
Intrp: _____

216

Rate: _____
Rhythm: _____
P Waves: _____
P-R Int: _____
QRS: _____
Intrp: _____

217

Rate: _____
Rhythm: _____
P Waves: _____
P-R Int: _____
QRS: _____
Intrp: _____

218

Rate: _____
Rhythm: _____
P Waves: _____
P-R Int: _____
QRS: _____
Intrp: _____

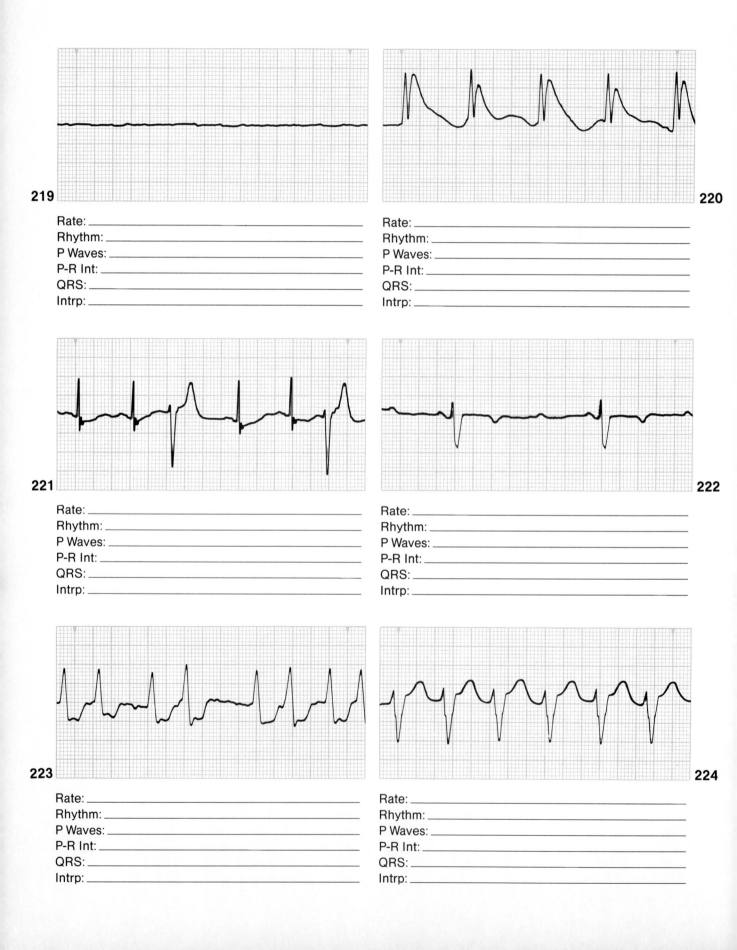

219

Rate: _____
Rhythm: _____
P Waves: _____
P-R Int: _____
QRS: _____
Intrp: _____

220

Rate: _____
Rhythm: _____
P Waves: _____
P-R Int: _____
QRS: _____
Intrp: _____

221

Rate: _____
Rhythm: _____
P Waves: _____
P-R Int: _____
QRS: _____
Intrp: _____

222

Rate: _____
Rhythm: _____
P Waves: _____
P-R Int: _____
QRS: _____
Intrp: _____

223

Rate: _____
Rhythm: _____
P Waves: _____
P-R Int: _____
QRS: _____
Intrp: _____

224

Rate: _____
Rhythm: _____
P Waves: _____
P-R Int: _____
QRS: _____
Intrp: _____

Answer Keys

1. Rate: 126 beats/minute.*
   Rhythm: Irregular.
   P Waves: None; fine atrial fibrillation waves are present.
   P-R Int: None.
   QRS: 0.10 second.
   Intrp: Atrial fibrillation (fine).

2. Rate: 33 beats/minute.
   Rhythm: Irregular.
   P Waves: Present; the first, second, third, and fifth P waves are followed by QRS complexes.
   P-R Int: 0.22 to 0.36 second. The P-R intervals progressively increase until a QRS complex fails to follow the P wave.
   QRS: 0.10 second.
   Intrp: Sinus rhythm with second-degree, Type I AV block (Wenckebach).

3. Rate: 41 beats/minute.
   Rhythm: Irregular.
   P Waves: Present; precede each QRS complex.
   P-R Int: 0.16 second.
   QRS: 0.08 second.
   Intrp: Sinus bradycardia with sinus arrhythmia.

4. Rate: 170 beats/minute.
   Rhythm: Regular.
   P Waves: Present; precede each QRS complex.
   P-R Int: 0.12 second.
   QRS: 0.12 second.
   Intrp: Atrial tachycardia with bundle branch block.

5. Rate: 62 beats/minute.
   Rhythm: Irregular.
   P Waves: Present; precede the second, fourth, fifth, sixth, and seventh QRS complexes. The P waves are abnormal (0.16 second in duration and notched).
   P-R Int: 0.26 second.
   QRS: 0.12 second (all QRS complexes except the third QRS complex); 0.14 second (third QRS complex).
   Intrp: Sinus rhythm with first-degree AV block, bundle branch block, and an isolated premature ventricular contraction.

6. Rate: 107 beats/minute.
   Rhythm: Irregular.
   P Waves: Present; precede all QRS complexes except the fifth, eighth, ninth, and tenth QRS complexes.
   P-R Int: 0.16 second.
   QRS: 0.09 to 0.10 second.
   Intrp: Normal sinus rhythm with premature junctional contractions (fifth, eighth, ninth, and tenth QRS complexes) occurring singly and in group beats; the latter may be considered a short episode of paroxysmal junctional tachycardia.

7. Rate: 182 beats/minute.
   Rhythm: Regular.
   P Waves: Present; precede each QRS complex.
   P-R Int: 0.08 second.
   QRS: 0.09 second.
   Intrp: Atrial tachycardia.

8. Rate: Unmeasurable.
   Rhythm: Irregular.
   P Waves: None; coarse ventricular fibrillation waves are present.
   P-R Int: None.
   QRS: None.
   Intrp: Ventricular fibrillation (coarse).

9. Rate: 89 beats/minute.
   Rhythm: Irregular.
   P Waves: Present; precede all except the third and sixth QRS complexes. The shape and direction of the P waves vary from positive to negative.
   P-R Int: 0.14 second.
   QRS: 0.10 second (all QRS complexes except the third and sixth QRS complexes); 0.12 second (third and sixth QRS complexes).
   Intrp: Wandering atrial pacemaker with unifocal premature ventricular contractions. Trigeminy is present in the first part of the tracing.

10. Rate: 61 beats/minute.
    Rhythm: Irregular.
    P Waves: Present; precede each QRS complex.
    P-R Int: 0.12 second.
    QRS: 0.14 second.
    Intrp: Sinus arrhythmia with bundle branch block.

11. Rate: 89 beats/minute.
    Rhythm: Irregular.
    P Waves: Present; precede all QRS complexes except the second and eighth QRS complexes.
    P-R Int: 0.18 second.
    QRS: 0.08 second (all QRS complexes except the second and eighth QRS complexes); 0.12 second (second and eighth QRS complexes).
    Intrp: Normal sinus rhythm with isolated unifocal premature ventricular contractions.

12. Rate: 145 beats/minute.
    Rhythm: Regular.
    P Waves: Present; precede each QRS complex.
    P-R Int: 0.12 second.
    QRS: 0.08 second.
    Intrp: Sinus tachycardia.

13. Rate: 87 beats/minute.
    Rhythm: Irregular.
    P Waves: Present; precede each QRS complex.
    P-R Int: 0.18 second.
    QRS: 0.05 second.
    Intrp: Sinus arrhythmia.

14. Rate: 164 beats/minute.
    Rhythm: Regular.
    P Waves: None.
    P-R Int: None.
    QRS: 0.12 second.
    Intrp: Ventricular tachycardia.

15. Rate: 74 beats/minute.
    Rhythm: Regular.
    P Waves: Present; precede each QRS complex; shape and direction vary from positive to negative.
    P-R Int: 0.08 to 0.12 second.
    QRS: 0.08 second.
    Intrp: Wandering atrial pacemaker.

16. Rate: 70 beats/minute (atrial rate: 52 beats/minute).
    Rhythm: Regular.
    P Waves: Present, but have no set relation to the QRS complexes.
    P-R Int: None.
    QRS: 0.14 second.
    Intrp: Accelerated idioventricular rhythm with AV dissociation.

    *The heart rates were calculated using R-R interval method 3.

17. Rate: 83 beats/minute.
     Rhythm: Regular.
     P Waves: Present; precede each QRS complex.
     P-R Int: 0.16 second.
     QRS: 0.06 second.
     Intrp: Normal sinus rhythm.

18. Rate: 229 beats/minute.
     Rhythm: Regular.
     P Waves: None.
     P-R Int: None.
     QRS: 0.12 second.
     Intrp: Ventricular tachycardia.

19. Rate: 26 beats/minute.
     Rhythm: Regular.
     P Waves: Present; the first, third, and fifth P waves are
              followed by QRS complexes. AV conduction
              ratio is 2:1.
     P-R Int: 0.19 second.
     QRS: 0.10 second.
     Intrp: Sinus rhythm with second-degree, 2:1 AV
              block.

20. Rate: 84 beats/minute.
     Rhythm: Regular.
     P Waves: None; atrial flutter waves are present.
     P-R Int: None.
     QRS: 0.08 second.
     Intrp: Atrial flutter.

21. Rate: 30 beats/minute.
     Rhythm: Regular.
     P Waves: Present; precede each QRS complex.
     P-R Int: 0.17 to 0.18 second.
     QRS: 0.12 second.
     Intrp: Sinus bradycardia with bundle branch block.

22. Rate: 98 beats/minute.
     Rhythm: Regular.
     P Waves: Present; precede each QRS complex.
     P-R Int: About 0.16 second.
     QRS: About 0.19 second.
     Intrp: Normal sinus rhythm with bundle branch
              block.

23. Rate: 62 beats/minute.
     Rhythm: Irregular.
     P Waves: Present; precede the first, second, third, and
              fifth QRS complexes.
     P-R Int: 0.18 second.
     QRS: 0.12 second.
     Intrp: Normal sinus rhythm with bundle branch block
              and premature junctional contractions.

24. Rate: 82 beats/minute.
     Rhythm: Regular.
     P Waves: Present; precede each QRS complex. The P
              waves are abnormally wide.
     P-R Int: 0.16 second.
     QRS: 0.16 second.
     Intrp: Normal sinus rhythm with bundle branch
              block.

25. Rate: 129 beats/minute.
     Rhythm: Irregular.
     P Waves: None; fine atrial fibrillation waves are present.
     P-R Int: None.
     QRS: 0.08 second.
     Intrp: Atrial fibrillation (fine).

26. Rate: 31 beats/minute.
     Rhythm: Irregular.
     P Waves: Present; a QRS complex follows the first, fifth,
              and tenth P waves. AV conduction ratios are
              4:1 and 5:1.
     P-R Int: 0.34 second.
     QRS: 0.16 second.
     Intrp: Sinus rhythm with second-degree, high-degree
              AV block and bundle branch block.

27. Rate: 75 beats/minute.
     Rhythm: Regular.
     P Waves: Present; negative P waves precede each QRS
              complex.
     P-R Int: 0.08 second.
     QRS: 0.08 second.
     Intrp: Accelerated junctional rhythm.

28. Rate: 62 beats/minute.
     Rhythm: Irregular. The R-R intervals between the third
              and fourth QRS complexes and the fifth and
              sixth QRS complexes are twice the R-R interval
              of the underlying sinus rhythm.
     P Waves: Present; precede each QRS complex.
     P-R Int: 0.18 second.
     QRS: 0.16 second.
     Intrp: Sinus rhythm with sinoatrial (SA) exit block
              and bundle branch block.

29. Rate: 37 beats/minute.
     Rhythm: Regular.
     P Waves: None; atrial fibrillation waves are present.
     P-R Int: None.
     QRS: About 0.24 second.
     Intrp: Atrial fibrillation (fine) with third-degree AV
              block, bundle branch block, and ventricular
              escape rhythm. AV dissociation is present.

30. Rate: 60 beats/minute.
     Rhythm: Regular.
     P Waves: Present; precede each QRS complex.
     P-R Int: 0.16 second.
     QRS: 0.16 second.
     Intrp: Normal sinus rhythm with bundle branch block.

31. Rate: 135 beats/minute.
     Rhythm: Regular.
     P Waves: None.
     P-R Int: None.
     QRS: 0.26 second.
     Intrp: Ventricular tachycardia.

32. Rate: 163 beats/minute.
     Rhythm: Regular.
     P Waves: None.
     P-R Int: None.
     QRS: 0.10 second.
     Intrp: Junctional tachycardia.

33. Rate: 41 beats/minute.
     Rhythm: Irregular.
     P Waves: Present; precede the first, second, fourth, and
              fifth QRS complexes. The R-R interval between
              the second and fourth QRS complexes is four
              times the R-R interval of the underlying sinus
              rhythm.
     P-R Int: 0.14 second.
     QRS: 0.12 second.
     Intrp: Sinus rhythm with sinoatrial (SA) exit block,
              first-degree AV block, bundle branch block, and
              an isolated junctional escape beat (third QRS
              complex).

34.   Rate: 17 beats/minute.
     Rhythm: Undeterminable.
     P Waves: None.
     P-R Int: None.
     QRS: 0.14 second.
     Intrp: Ventricular escape rhythm.

35.   Rate: 70 beats/minute.
     Rhythm: Regular.
     P Waves: Present; precede each QRS complex.
     P-R Int: 0.16 second.
     QRS: 0.06 second.
     Intrp: Normal sinus rhythm

36.   Rate: 64 beats/minute.
     Rhythm: Irregular.
     P Waves: Present; precede the first and second QRS complexes. Pacemaker spikes precede the rest of the QRS complexes.
     P-R Int: 0.26 second.
     QRS: 0.08 second (first and second QRS complexes); 0.16 second (third, fourth, fifth, sixth, and seventh QRS complexes).
     Intrp: Sinus rhythm with first-degree AV block followed by ventricular asystole and a ventricular demand pacemaker rhythm.

37.   Rate: 72 beats/minute.
     Rhythm: Irregular.
     P Waves: Present; precede each QRS complex.
     P-R Int: 0.16 second.
     QRS: 0.08 second.
     Intrp: Sinus arrhythmia.

38.   Rate: 75 beats/minute.
     Rhythm: Irregular.
     P Waves: Present; all but the first and sixth P waves are followed by QRS complexes. AV conduction ratio is 3:4.
     P-R Int: 0.12 to 0.13 second.
     QRS: 0.14 second.
     Intrp: Sinus rhythm with second-degree, type II AV block and bundle branch block.

39.   Rate: 101 beats/minute.
     Rhythm: Irregular.
     P Waves: Present; precede each QRS complex. The shape and direction of the P waves vary from positive to negative.
     P-R Int: 0.12 to 0.18 second.
     QRS: 0.06 second.
     Intrp: Wandering atrial pacemaker.

40.   Rate: 37 beats/minute.
     Rhythm: Regular.
     P Waves: Present; precede each QRS complex.
     P-R Int: 0.34 second.
     QRS: 0.08 second.
     Intrp: Sinus bradycardia with first-degree AV block.

41.   Rate: 42 beats/minute.
     Rhythm: Irregular.
     P Waves: Present; precede each QRS complex. The fourth P wave is negative; the rest are positive.
     P-R Int: 0.18 to 0.20 second.
     QRS: 0.12 second.
     Intrp: Sinus bradycardia with bundle branch block and an isolated premature atrial contraction.

42.   Rate: 66 beats/minute.
     Rhythm: Irregular.
     P Waves: Present; all the P waves except the fourth and eighth P waves are followed by QRS complexes.
     P-R Int: 0.22 to 0.36 second. The P-R intervals progressively increase until a QRS complex fails to follow the P wave.
     QRS: 0.14 second.
     Intrp: Sinus rhythm with second-degree, type I AV block (Wenckebach) and bundle branch block.

43.   Rate: 74 beats/minute.
     Rhythm: Regular.
     P Waves: None.
     P-R Int: None.
     QRS: 0.12 second.
     Intrp: Pacemaker rhythm (ventricular pacemaker).

44.   Rate: 88 beats/minute.
     Rhythm: Regular.
     P Waves: Present; precede each QRS complex.
     P-R Int: 0.12 second.
     QRS: 0.14 second.
     Intrp: Normal sinus rhythm with bundle branch block.

45.   Rate: 61 beats/minute.
     Rhythm: Irregular.
     P Waves: Present; precede all but the fourth QRS complex.
     P-R Int: 0.12 second.
     QRS: 0.08 second.
     Intrp: Sinus rhythm with sinus arrest.

46.   Rate: 71 beats/minute.
     Rhythm: Regular.
     P Waves: Present; precede each QRS complex.
     P-R Int: 0.18 second.
     QRS: 0.08 second.
     Intrp: Normal sinus rhythm.

47.   Rate: 66 beats/minute.
     Rhythm: Irregular.
     P Waves: Present; all but the fourth and eighth P waves are followed by QRS complexes.
     P-R Int: 0.22 to 0.40 second. The P-R intervals progressively increase until a QRS complex fails to follow the P wave.
     QRS: About 0.15 second.
     Intrp: Sinus rhythm with second-degree, type I AV block (Wenckebach) and bundle branch block.

48.   Rate: 102 beats/minute.
     Rhythm: Irregular.
     P Waves: None; fine atrial fibrillation waves are present.
     P-R Int: None.
     QRS: 0.09 to 0.10 second (first, fifth, seventh, eighth, ninth, and tenth QRS complexes); 0.12 to 0.16 second (second, third, fourth, sixth, and tenth QRS complexes). The shape and direction of the second, third, and fourth QRS complexes differ from each other. The second QRS complex is similar to the sixth QRS complex; the fourth QRS complex is similar to the tenth QRS complex.
     Intrp: Atrial fibrillation (fine) with third-degree AV block, accelerated junctional rhythm, multifocal (multiform) premature ventricular contractions (group beats), and a short burst of ventricular tachycardia. AV dissociation is present.

49.
Rate: 63 beats/minute.
Rhythm: Irregular.
P Waves: None; coarse atrial fibrillation waves are present.
P-R Int: None.
QRS: 0.13 second.
Intrp: Atrial fibrillation (coarse) with bundle branch block.

50.
Rate: 57 beats/minute.
Rhythm: Irregular. The R-R interval between the fourth and fifth QRS complexes is less than twice the R-R interval of the underlying sinus rhythm.
P Waves: Present; precede all but the fifth QRS complex.
P-R Int: 0.12 second.
QRS: 0.11 second.
Intrp: Sinus rhythm with sinus arrest and incomplete bundle branch block.

51.
Rate: 52 beats/minute.
Rhythm: Regular.
P Waves: Present; precede each QRS complex.
P-R Int: 0.20 second.
QRS: 0.06 second.
Intrp: Normal sinus rhythm.

52.
Rate: 183 beats/minute.
Rhythm: Regular.
P Waves: None.
P-R Int: None.
QRS: 0.12 second.
Intrp: Ventricular tachycardia.

53.
Rate: 65 beats/minute.
Rhythm: Irregular.
P Waves: Present; precede each QRS complex.
P-R Int: 0.16 second.
QRS: 0.08 second.
Intrp: Sinus arrhythmia.

54.
Rate: 27 beats/minute.
Rhythm: Regular.
P Waves: None.
P-R Int: None.
QRS: 0.12 second.
Intrp: Junctional escape rhythm with bundle branch block.

55.
Rate: 40 beats/minute.
Rhythm: Regular.
P Waves: None.
P-R Int: None.
QRS: 0.16 second.
Intrp: Ventricular escape rhythm.

56.
Rate: 59 beats/minute.
Rhythm: Irregular.
P Waves: Present; the second, third, fifth, sixth, eighth, and tenth P waves are followed by QRS complexes. AV conduction ratios are 3:1 and 2:1.
P-R Int: About 0.16 second.
QRS: About 0.16 second.
Intrp: Sinus rhythm with second-degree, 2:1 and high-degree AV block and bundle branch block.

57.
Rate: 58 beats/minute.
Rhythm: Regular.
P Waves: Present; negative P waves follow each QRS complex.
P-R Int: None.
QRS: 0.11 second.
Intrp: Accelerated junctional rhythm with incomplete bundle branch block.

58.
Rate: 53 beats/minute.
Rhythm: Irregular.
P Waves: Present; the first, second, fourth, fifth, and sixth P waves are followed by QRS complexes.
P-R Int: 0.22 to 0.46 second. The P-R intervals progressively increase until a QRS complex fails to follow the P wave.
QRS: 0.08 second.
Intrp: Sinus rhythm with second-degree, type I AV block (Wenckebach).

59.
Rate: 80 beats/minute.
Rhythm: Irregular.
P Waves: Present; precede the first, second, third, sixth, eighth, and ninth QRS complexes. The third P wave is negative; the fifth wave is buried in the preceding T wave. Pacemaker spikes precede the third, fourth, fifth, and seventh QRS complexes.
P-R Int: 0.12 to 0.18 second.
QRS: 0.07 second (first, second, sixth, eighth, and ninth QRS complexes); 0.16 second (fourth, fifth, and seventh QRS complexes). The third QRS complex is a fusion beat—a combination of the normally conducted QRS complex and the pacemaker induced ventricular QRS complex.
Intrp: Sinus rhythm with episodes of ventricular demand pacemaker rhythm.

60.
Rate: 134 beats/minute.
Rhythm: Regular.
P Waves: None.
P-R Int: None.
QRS: About 0.32 to 0.36 second.
Intrp: Ventricular tachycardia.

61.
Rate: 70 beats/minute.
Rhythm: Regular.
P Waves: Present; precede each QRS complex.
P-R Int: 0.15 second.
QRS: 0.06 second.
Intrp: Normal sinus rhythm.

62.
Rate: 52 beats/minute.
Rhythm: Irregular.
P Waves: Present; the second, third, fifth, and sixth P waves are followed by QRS complexes. The AV conduction ratio is 3:2.
P-R Int: 0.24 to 0.26 second.
QRS: 0.16 second.
Intrp: Sinus rhythm with second-degree, type II AV block and bundle branch block.

63.
Rate: 64 beats/minute.
Rhythm: Irregular.
P Waves: Present; the first, second, fourth, fifth, and sixth P waves are followed by QRS complexes.
P-R Int: 0.24 to 0.36 second. The P-R intervals progressively increase until a QRS complex fails to follow the P wave.
QRS: 0.12 second.
Intrp: Sinus rhythm with second-degree, type I AV block (Wenckebach) and bundle branch block.

64.
Rate: 284 beats/minute.
Rhythm: Regular.
P Waves: None.
P-R Int: None.
QRS: About 0.12 second.
Intrp: Ventricular tachycardia.

65. Rate: 87 beats/minute.
     Rhythm: Irregular.
     P Waves: Present; precede each QRS complex.
     P-R Int: 0.12 to 0.16 second.
     QRS: 0.04 second.
     Intrp: Wandering atrial pacemaker.

66. Rate: 70 beats/minute.
     Rhythm: Regular.
     P Waves: Present; precede each QRS complex.
     P-R Int: 0.16 second.
     QRS: 0.05 second.
     Intrp: Normal sinus rhythm.

67. Rate: 37 beats/minute.
     Rhythm: Regular.
     P Waves: Present; precede each QRS complex.
     P-R Int: 0.18 second.
     QRS: 0.12 second.
     Intrp: Sinus bradycardia with bundle branch block.

68. Rate: 30 beats/minute (atrial rate: 82 beats/minute).
     Rhythm: Regular.
     P Waves: Present, but have no set relation to the QRS complexes.
     P-R Int: None.
     QRS: 0.14 second.
     Intrp: Third-degree AV block with wide QRS complexes.

69. Rate: 125 beats/minute (average); 165 beats/minute (first part); 79 beats/minute (second part).
     Rhythm: Irregular.
     P Waves: Present; precede each QRS complex. In the first part, the P waves are superimposed on the preceding T waves.
     P-R Int: 0.16 second.
     QRS: About 0.04 second.
     Intrp: Paroxysmal atrial tachycardia with reversion to normal sinus rhythm.

70. Rate: 120 beats/minute (three beats).
     Rhythm: Regular (three beats).
     P Waves: None.
     P-R Int: None.
     QRS: 0.14 second.
     Intrp: Supraventricular tachycardia with wide QRS complexes or ventricular tachycardia followed by ventricular asystole.

71. Rate: 174 beats/minute.
     Rhythm: Regular.
     P Waves: None.
     P-R Int: None.
     QRS: 0.10 second.
     Intrp: Supraventricular tachycardia.

72. Rate: 36 beats/minute.
     Rhythm: Regular.
     P Waves: None.
     P-R Int: None.
     QRS: 0.18 second.
     Intrp: Junctional escape rhythm with bundle branch block or ventricular escape rhythm.

73. Rate: 263 beats/minute.
     Rhythm: Regular.
     P Waves: None.
     P-R Int: None.
     QRS: About 0.12 second.
     Intrp: Ventricular tachycardia.

74. Rate: 69 beats/minute.
     Rhythm: Irregular.
     P Waves: Present; the second, third, fourth, sixth, seventh, and eighth P waves are followed by QRS complexes. AV conduction ratio is 4:3.
     P-R Int: 0.30 second.
     QRS: 0.12 second.
     Intrp: Sinus rhythm with second-degree, type II AV block and bundle branch block.

75. Rate: 72 beats/minute.
     Rhythm: Regular.
     P Waves: Ectopic atrial P waves are present. A QRS complex follows every third P' wave.
     P-R Int: Unmeasurable.
     QRS: 0.08 second.
     Intrp: Atrial tachycardia with AV block.

76. Rate: 104 beats/minute.
     Rhythm: Irregular.
     P Waves: Present; precede the first, fifth, and sixth QRS complex.
     P-R Int: 0.18 second.
     QRS: 0.12 second (first, fifth, and sixth complexes); About 0.16 second (second, third, and fourth QRS complex).
     Intrp: Sinus rhythm with bundle branch block and unifocal premature ventricular contractions occurring in a burst of three (ventricular tachycardia); R-on-T phenomenon.

77. Rate: 82 beats/minute.
     Rhythm: Regular.
     P Waves: Present; precede each QRS complex.
     P-R Int: About 0.16 second.
     QRS: 0.08 second.
     Intrp: Normal sinus rhythm.

78. Rate: 100 beats/minute.
     Rhythm: Irregular.
     P Waves: Present; precede each QRS complex.
     P-R Int: 0.12 to 0.14 second.
     QRS: 0.16 second.
     Intrp: Sinus rhythm with bundle branch block and premature atrial contractions (atrial bigeminy).

79. Rate: 56 beats/minute.
     Rhythm: Regular.
     P Waves: Present; precede each QRS complex.
     P-R Int: 0.36 to 0.42 second. The P-R intervals progressively increase.
     QRS: About 0.12 second.
     Intrp: Sinus rhythm with second-degree AV block (type undeterminable, probably type I AV block [Wenckebach]) and bundle branch block.

80. Rate: 181 beats/minute.
     Rhythm: Regular.
     P Waves: None.
     P-R Int: None.
     QRS: About 0.18 second.
     Intrp: Supraventricular tachycardia with wide QRS complexes or ventricular tachycardia.

81. Rate: 40 beats/minute.
     Rhythm: Undeterminable.
     P Waves: None.
     P-R Int: None.
     QRS: 0.16 second.
     Intrp: Ventricular escape rhythm.

82. Rate: 94 beats/minute.
    Rhythm: Regular.
    P Waves: Present; negative P waves precede each QRS complex.
    P-R Int: 0.08 second.
    QRS: 0.10 second.
    Intrp: Accelerated junctional rhythm.

83. Rate: 94 beats/minute.
    Rhythm: Regular.
    P Waves: Present; precede each QRS complex.
    P-R Int: 0.12 second.
    QRS: 0.12 second.
    Intrp: Normal sinus rhythm with bundle branch block.

84. Rate: 68 beats/minute.
    Rhythm: Irregular.
    P Waves: Present; precede the first and third QRS complexes.
    P-R Int: About 0.08 second.
    QRS: 0.08 second (first and third QRS complex); 0.18 second (second and fourth QRS complex).
    Intrp: Atrial rhythm with premature ventricular contractions (ventricular bigeminy).

85. Rate: 68 beats/minute.
    Rhythm: Irregular.
    P Waves: Present; precede each QRS complex. The first and third P waves are positive; the second and fourth P waves are negative.
    P-R Int: 0.20 second.
    QRS: 0.12 second.
    Intrp: Sinus rhythm with first-degree AV block, bundle branch block, and premature atrial contractions (atrial bigeminy).

86. Rate: 34 beats/minute (atrial rate: 163 beats/minute).
    Rhythm: Undeterminable.
    P Waves: Present, but the negative P waves have no set relation to the QRS complexes.
    P-R Int: None.
    QRS: 0.16 second.
    Intrp: Third-degree AV block with wide QRS complexes.

87. Rate: 75 beats/minute.
    Rhythm: Irregular.
    P Waves: None; fine atrial fibrillation waves are present.
    P-R Int: None.
    QRS: 0.16 second.
    Intrp: Atrial fibrillation (fine).

88. Rate: 107 beats/minute.
    Rhythm: Irregular.
    P Waves: Present; precede each QRS complex.
    P-R Int: 0.14 second.
    QRS: 0.12 second.
    Intrp: Sinus tachycardia with first-degree AV block, bundle branch block, and an isolated premature junctional contraction (fourth QRS complex).

89. Rate: 230 beats/minute.
    Rhythm: Slightly Irregular.
    P Waves: None.
    P-R Int: None.
    QRS: 0.12 second.
    Intrp: Ventricular tachycardia.

90. Rate: 170 beats/minute.
    Rhythm: Irregular.
    P Waves: None; fine atrial fibrillation waves are present.
    P-R Int: None.
    QRS: 0.08 second.
    Intrp: Atrial fibrillation (fine).

91. Rate: 80 second beats/minute.
    Rhythm: Irregular.
    P Waves: Present; precede the first and third QRS complexes.
    P-R Int: 0.14 second.
    QRS: 0.12 second.
    Intrp: Sinus rhythm with bundle branch block and premature junctional contractions (bigeminy).

92. Rate: 115 beats/minute.
    Rhythm: Irregular.
    P Waves: None; atrial flutter waves are present.
    P-R Int: None.
    QRS: 0.12 second.
    Intrp: Atrial flutter.

93. Rate: Unmeasurable.
    Rhythm: Irregular.
    P Waves: None; coarse ventricular fibrillation waves are present.
    P-R Int: None.
    QRS: None.
    Intrp: Ventricular fibrillation (coarse).

94. Rate: 46 beats/minute.
    Rhythm: Irregular.
    P Waves: Present; the first, second, and fourth P waves are followed by QRS complexes.
    P-R Int: 0.20 to 0.32 second. The P-R intervals progressively increase until a QRS complex fails to follow the P wave.
    QRS: 0.10 second.
    Intrp: Sinus rhythm with second-degree, type I AV block (Wenckebach).

95. Rate: 82 beats/minute.
    Rhythm: Regular.
    P Waves: None; atrial and ventricular pacemaker spikes are present.
    P-R Int: None.
    QRS: 0.16 second.
    Intrp: Pacemaker rhythm (AV sequential pacemaker).

96. Rate: 61 beats/minute.
    Rhythm: Irregular.
    P Waves: Present; precede the first, second, and fourth QRS complexes.
    P-R Int: 0.22 second.
    QRS: 0.11 second.
    Intrp: Normal sinus rhythm with incomplete bundle branch block and an isolated premature junctional contraction (third QRS complex).

97. Rate: 224 beats/minute.
    Rhythm: Regular.
    P Waves: None.
    P-R Int: None.
    QRS: 0.06 second.
    Intrp: Supraventricular tachycardia.

98. Rate: 98 beats/minute.
    Rhythm: Irregular.
    P Waves: Present; precede the first, second, third, and sixth QRS complexes.
    P-R Int: 0.16 second.
    QRS: 0.16 to 0.18 second.
    Intrp: Normal sinus rhythm with bundle branch block and premature junctional contractions (group beats).

99. Rate: 136 beats/minute.
Rhythm: Regular.
P Waves: Present; negative P waves follow each QRS complex.
P-R Int: None.
QRS: 0.06 second.
Intrp: Junctional tachycardia.

100. Rate: 63 beats/minute.
Rhythm: None.
P Waves: None; positive wide artifacts are present.
P-R Int: None.
QRS: None.
Intrp: Ventricular asystole with artifacts (chest compressions).

101. Rate: 184 beats/minute.
Rhythm: Regular.
P Waves: None.
P-R Int: None.
QRS: 0.10 second.
Intrp: Supraventricular tachycardia.

102. Rate: 102 beats/minute.
Rhythm: Regular.
P Waves: Present; precede each QRS complex.
P-R Int: 0.16 second.
QRS: 0.06 second.
Intrp: Sinus tachycardia. Abnormally tall T waves characteristic of hyperkalemia are present.

103. Rate: 68 beats/minute.
Rhythm: Regular.
P Waves: None.
P-R Int: None.
QRS: 0.18 to 0.24 second.
Intrp: Accelerated idioventricular rhythm.

104. Rate: 164 beats/minute.
Rhythm: Regular.
P Waves: Present; precede each QRS complex.
P-R Int: 0.12 second.
QRS: 0.08 second.
Intrp: Atrial tachycardia.

105. Rate: 123 beats/minute.
Rhythm: Regular.
P Waves: Present; precede each QRS complex.
P-R Int: 0.14 second.
QRS: 0.12 second.
Intrp: Sinus tachycardia with bundle branch block.

106. Rate: 76 beats/minute.
Rhythm: Irregular.
P Waves: Present; precede the second and fourth QRS complex. The fifth QRS complex is superimposed on a P wave.
P-R Int: 0.16 second.
QRS: 0.08 second (third and fifth QRS complexes); 0.12 second (first, second, and fourth QRS complexes).
Intrp: Normal sinus rhythm with bundle branch block and premature junctional contractions.

107. Rate: 61 beats/minute.
Rhythm: Irregular.
P Waves: Present; precede the first, second, and fourth QRS complexes.
P-R Int: 0.24 second.
QRS: 0.10 second.
Intrp: Sinus rhythm with first-degree AV block and an isolated premature junctional contraction.

108. Rate: 41 beats/minute.
Rhythm: Regular.
P Waves: Present; precede each QRS complex.
P-R Int: About 0.14 second.
QRS: 0.08 second.
Intrp: Sinus bradycardia.

109. Rate: 69 beats/minute.
Rhythm: Regular.
P Waves: Present; precede each QRS complex.
P-R Int: 0.22 to 0.26 second.
QRS: 0.16 second.
Intrp: Sinus rhythm with first-degree AV block and bundle branch block.

110. Rate: 48 beats/minute (atrial rate: 125 beats/minute).
Rhythm: Regular.
P Waves: Present, but have no set relation to the QRS complexes.
P-R Int: None.
QRS: 0.10 second.
Intrp: Third-degree AV block.

111. Rate: 41 beats/minute.
Rhythm: Irregular.
P Waves: Present; the first, fourth, and sixth P waves are followed by QRS complexes. AV conduction ratios are 2:1 and 3:1.
P-R Int: 0.20 second.
QRS: 0.12 second.
Intrp: Sinus rhythm with second-degree, 2:1 and high-degree AV block.

112. Rate: 92 beats/minute.
Rhythm: Regular.
P Waves: Present; precede each QRS complex.
P-R Int: 0.14 second.
QRS: About 0.06 second.
Intrp: Normal sinus rhythm.

113. Rate: 161 beats/minute.
Rhythm: Regular.
P Waves: None.
P-R Int: None.
QRS: 0.09 second.
Intrp: Supraventricular tachycardia.

114. Rate: 115 beats/minute.
Rhythm: Regular.
P Waves: Present; precede each QRS complex.
P-R Int: 0.20 second.
QRS: 0.06 second.
Intrp: Sinus tachycardia.

115. Rate: 50 beats/minute.
Rhythm: Regular.
P Waves: Present; precede each QRS complex.
P-R Int: 0.16 second.
QRS: 0.05 second.
Intrp: Junctional escape rhythm with first-degree AV block.

116. Rate: 60 beats/minute.
Rhythm: Irregular.
P Waves: None; fine atrial fibrillation waves are present.
P-R Int: None.
QRS: 0.07 second.
Intrp: Atrial fibrillation (fine).

117. Rate: 97 beats/minute.
Rhythm: Regular.
P Waves: Present; precede each QRS complex.
P-R Int: 0.16 second.
QRS: 0.16 second.
Intrp: Normal sinus rhythm with bundle branch block.

118. Rate: Unmeasurable.
Rhythm: Irregular.
P Waves: None; coarse ventricular fibrillation waves present.
P-R Int: None.
QRS: None.
Intrp: Ventricular fibrillation (coarse).

119. Rate: 48 beats/minute.
Rhythm: Regular.
P Waves: Present; follow each QRS complex.
P-R Int: None.
QRS: 0.11 to 0.12 second.
Intrp: Junctional escape rhythm with bundle branch block.

120. Rate: 73 beats/minute.
Rhythm: Irregular.
P Waves: Present; precede the first, second, and fourth QRS complexes.
P-R Int: 0.18 second.
QRS: 0.08 second (first, second, and fourth QRS complexes); 0.16 second (third QRS complex).
Intrp: Normal sinus rhythm with an isolated premature ventricular complex (interpolated).

121. Rate: 62 beats/minute.
Rhythm: Regular.
P Waves: Present; precede each QRS complex.
P-R Int: 0.20 second.
QRS: 0.10 second.
Intrp: Normal sinus rhythm.

122. Rate: 78 beats/minute.
Rhythm: Irregular.
P Waves: None; fine atrial fibrillation waves are present.
P-R Int: None.
QRS: 0.08 second.
Intrp: Atrial fibrillation (fine).

123. Rate: 87 beats/minute.
Rhythm: Irregular.
P Waves: Present; precede the first and fourth QRS complexes.
P-R Int: 0.16 second.
QRS: 0.09 second (first and fourth QRS complexes); 0.16 second (second, third, and fifth QRS complexes).
Intrp: Normal sinus rhythm with multiform premature ventricular contractions (group beats).

124. Rate: 80 beats/minute.
Rhythm: Regular.
P Waves: None; ventricular pacemaker spikes are present.
P-R Int: None.
QRS: 0.12 second.
Intrp: Pacemaker rhythm (ventricular pacemaker).

125. Rate: 31 beats/minute (atrial rate: 97 beats/minute).
Rhythm: Undeterminable.
P Waves: Present, but have no set relation to the QRS complexes.
P-R Int: None.
QRS: 0.12 to 0.14 second.
Intrp: Third-degree AV block with wide QRS complexes.

126. Rate: 57 beats/minute.
Rhythm: Regular.
P Waves: None.
P-R Int: None.
QRS: 0.11 to 0.13 second.
Intrp: Junctional escape rhythm with bundle branch block.

127. Rate: 47 beats/minute.
Rhythm: Regular.
P Waves: Present; precede each QRS complex.
P-R Int: 0.48 second.
QRS: 0.08 second.
Intrp: Sinus bradycardia with first-degree AV block.

128. Rate: 149 beats/minute.
Rhythm: Regular.
P Waves: Present; precede each QRS complex.
P-R Int: Unmeasurable.
QRS: 0.08 second.
Intrp: Atrial tachycardia.

129. Rate: 160 beats/minute.
Rhythm: Irregular.
P Waves: Undeterminable.
P-R Int: Undeterminable.
QRS: 0.12 second. (first QRS complex); 0.16 second (rest of the QRS complexes).
Intrp: A wide QRS complex followed by multiform ventricular tachycardia.

130. Rate: 160 beats/minute.
Rhythm: Regular.
P Waves: None.
P-R Int: None.
QRS: 0.14 second.
Intrp: Supraventricular tachycardia with wide QRS complexes or ventricular tachycardia.

131. Rate: 150 beats/minute.
Rhythm: Regular.
P Waves: Present; follow each QRS complex.
P-R Int: None.
QRS: 0.10 second.
Intrp: Junctional tachycardia.

132. Rate: 31 beats/minute (atrial rate: unmeasurable).
Rhythm: Undeterminable.
P Waves: Present, but have no set relation to the QRS complexes.
P-R Int: None.
QRS: About 0.15 second.
Intrp: Third-degree AV block with wide QRS complexes.

133. Rate: 31 beats/minute.
Rhythm: Undeterminable.
P Waves: Present; precede each QRS complex.
P-R Int: 0.14 second.
QRS: 0.08 second.
Intrp: Sinus bradycardia.

134. Rate: 59 beats/minute.
Rhythm: Regular.
P Waves: None; atrial flutter waves are present.
P-R Int: None.
QRS: 0.12 to 0.14 second.
Intrp: Atrial flutter with bundle branch block.

135. Rate: 178 beats/minute.
Rhythm: Regular.
P Waves: None.
P-R Int: None.
QRS: 0.08 second.
Intrp: Supraventricular tachycardia.

136. Rate: 91 beats/minute.
Rhythm: Regular.
P Waves: Present; precede each QRS complex.
P-R Int: 0.28 second.
QRS: 0.12 second.
Intrp: Sinus rhythm with first-degree AV block and bundle branch block.

137. Rate: 47 beats/minute.
Rhythm: Regular.
P Waves: Present; the first, third, and fifth P waves are followed by QRS complexes.
P-R Int: 0.28 second.
QRS: 0.12 second.
Intrp: Sinus rhythm with second-degree, 2:1 AV block and bundle branch block.

138. Rate: 78 beats/minute.
Rhythm: Irregular.
P Waves: Present; precede each QRS complex. The second and fourth P waves are abnormal, each in a different way.
P-R Int: 0.20 second (first and third P-R intervals); 0.11 to 0.12 second (second and fourth P-R intervals).
QRS: 0.08 to 0.09 second.
Intrp: Sinus rhythm with multifocal premature atrial contractions.

139. Rate: 64 beats/minute.
Rhythm: Regular.
P Waves: None.
P-R Int: None.
QRS: About 0.10 second.
Intrp: Accelerated junctional rhythm.

140. Rate: 222 beats/minute.
Rhythm: Regular.
P Waves: None.
P-R Int: None.
QRS: 0.12 second.
Intrp: Supraventricular tachycardia with wide QRS complexes or ventricular tachycardia.

141. Rate: None (pacemaker spikes: 63 beats/minute).
Rhythm: Regular.
P Waves: None; pacemaker spikes are present.
P-R Int: None.
QRS: None.
Intrp: Ventricular asystole with pacemaker spikes without capture.

142. Rate: 99 beats/minute.
Rhythm: Irregular.
P Waves: Present; precede the first, second, and fifth QRS complexes.
P-R Int: 0.28 second.
QRS: 0.10 second (first, second, and fifth QRS complexes); 0.12 to 0.16 second (third and fourth QRS complexes).
Intrp: Sinus rhythm with first-degree AV block and multiform premature ventricular contractions (group beats).

143. Rate: 61 beats/minute.
Rhythm: Regular.
P Waves: Present; precede each QRS complex. P waves are abnormally tall (P pulmonale).
P-R Int: 0.26 second.
QRS: 0.10 to 0.12 second.
Intrp: Sinus rhythm with first-degree AV block and bundle branch block.

144. Rate: 114 beats/minute.
Rhythm: Regular.
P Waves: Present; precede each QRS complex.
P-R Int: 0.16 second.
QRS: 0.08 second.
Intrp: Sinus tachycardia.

145. Rate: 100 beats/minute.
Rhythm: Regular.
P Waves: Present; negative P waves follow each QRS complex.
P-R Int: None.
QRS: 0.10 second.
Intrp: Junctional tachycardia.

146. Rate: Unmeasurable.
Rhythm: Irregular.
P Waves: None; coarse ventricular fibrillation waves are present.
P-R Int: None.
QRS: None.
Intrp: Ventricular fibrillation (coarse).

147. Rate: 21 beats/minute.
Rhythm: Undeterminable.
P Waves: None.
P-R Int: None.
QRS: 0.16 second.
Intrp: Ventricular escape rhythm.

148. Rate: 68 beats/minute.
Rhythm: Irregular.
P Waves: None; fine atrial fibrillation waves are present.
P-R Int: None.
QRS: 0.10 second.
Intrp: Atrial fibrillation (fine).

149. Rate: 65 beats/minute (atrial rate: 113 beats/minute).
Rhythm: Regular.
P Waves: Present, but have no set relation to the QRS complexes.
P-R Int: None.
QRS: About 0.10 second.
Intrp: Third-degree AV block.

150. Rate: 88 beats/minute.
Rhythm: Irregular.
P Waves: None; fine atrial fibrillation waves are present.
P-R Int: None.
QRS: About 0.08 second.
Intrp: Atrial fibrillation (fine).

151. Rate: 55 beats/minute.
Rhythm: Regular.
P Waves: Present; abnormally wide positive P waves precede each QRS complex.
P-R Int: About 0.40 second.
QRS: About 0.10 second.
Intrp: Sinus rhythm with first-degree AV block.

152. Rate: 148 beats/minute.
Rhythm: Regular.
P Waves: Present; precede each QRS complex.
P-R Int: Undeterminable; P waves are buried in the preceding QRS complexes.
QRS: 0.10 second.
Intrp: Atrial tachycardia.

153. Rate: 118 beats/minute.
Rhythm: Irregular.
P Waves: None; fine atrial fibrillation waves are present.
P-R Int: None.
QRS: 0.10 second.
Intrp: Atrial fibrillation (fine).

154. Rate: 36 beats/minute.
Rhythm: Undeterminable.
P Waves: None.
P-R Int: None.
QRS: About 0.16 second.
Intrp: Ventricular escape rhythm.

155. Rate: 50 beats/minute.
Rhythm: Regular.
P Waves: None; atrial flutter waves are present.
P-R Int: None.
QRS: 0.16 second.
Intrp: Atrial flutter with bundle branch block.

156. Rate: 163 beats/minute.
Rhythm: Regular.
P Waves: None.
P-R Int: None.
QRS: 0.16 second.
Intrp: Ventricular tachycardia.

157. Rate: 63 beats/minute.
Rhythm: Regular.
P Waves: Present; negative P waves follow each QRS complex.
P-R Int: None.
QRS: 0.06 second.
Intrp: Accelerated junctional rhythm.

158. Rate: 103 beats/minute.
Rhythm: Regular.
P Waves: Present; P waves precede each QRS complex. The P waves are abnormally tall (P pulmonale).
P-R Int: 0.19 second.
QRS: 0.14 second.
Intrp: Sinus tachycardia with bundle branch block.

159. Rate: 312 beats/minute.
Rhythm: Slightly irregular.
P Waves: None.
P-R Int: None.
QRS: 0.12 to 0.14 second.
Intrp: Ventricular tachycardia (multiform).

160. Rate: 101 beats/minute.
Rhythm: Regular.
P Waves: None.
P-R Int: None.
QRS: 0.14 second.
Intrp: Accelerated junctional rhythm with wide QRS complexes or accelerated idioventricular rhythm.

161. Rate: 92 beats/minute.
Rhythm: Irregular.
P Waves: Present; precede the first, second, fourth, and fifth QRS complexes.
P-R Int: 0.14 second.
QRS: 0.16 second.
Intrp: Normal sinus rhythm with bundle branch block and an isolated premature ventricular contraction (interpolated).

162. Rate: 70 beats/minute.
Rhythm: Regular.
P Waves: Present; precede each QRS complex.
P-R Int: 0.16 to 0.18 second.
QRS: 0.12 second.
Intrp: Normal sinus rhythm with bundle branch block.

163. Rate: 72 beats/minute.
Rhythm: Regular.
P Waves: None.
P-R Int: None.
QRS: 0.12 to 0.16 second.
Intrp: Accelerated idioventricular rhythm.

164. Rate: Unmeasurable.
Rhythm: Irregular.
P Waves: None; fine ventricular waves are present.
P-R Int: None.
QRS: None.
Intrp: Ventricular fibrillation (fine).

165. Rate: 57 beats/minute.
Rhythm: Regular.
P Waves: Present; precede each QRS complex.
P-R Int: 0.24 second.
QRS: 0.08 second.
Intrp: Sinus bradycardia with first-degree AV block.

166. Rate: 43 beats/minute.
Rhythm: Regular.
P Waves: Present; positive P waves precede each QRS complex.
P-R Int: 0.10 second.
QRS: 0.09 second.
Intrp: Bradycardia, probably atrial in origin.

167. Rate: 57 beats/minute.
Rhythm: Regular.
P Waves: None.
P-R Int: None.
QRS: About 0.16 second.
Intrp: Accelerated idioventricular rhythm.

168. Rate: None.
Rhythm: None.
P Waves: None.
P-R Int: None.
QRS: None.
Intrp: Ventricular asystole.

169. Rate: 43 beats/minute.
Rhythm: Regular.
P Waves: Present; negative P waves follow each QRS complex.
P-R Int: None.
QRS: 0.09 second.
Intrp: Junctional escape rhythm.

170. Rate: Unmeasurable.
Rhythm: Irregular.
P Waves: None; coarse ventricular fibrillation waves are present.
P-R Int: None.
QRS: None.
Intrp: Ventricular fibrillation (coarse).

171. Rate: 25 beats/minute.
Rhythm: Undeterminable.
P Waves: None.
P-R Int: None.
QRS: 0.12 second.
Intrp: Junctional escape rhythm with bundle branch block.

172. Rate: 213 beats/minute.
Rhythm: Regular.
P Waves: None.
P-R Int: None.
QRS: 0.12 second.
Intrp: Supraventricular tachycardia with wide QRS complexes or ventricular tachycardia.

173. Rate: 70 beats/minute.
    Rhythm: Irregular.
    P Waves: None; fine atrial fibrillation waves are present.
    P-R Int: None.
    QRS: 0.10 second.
    Intrp: Atrial fibrillation (fine).

174. Rate: 89 beats/minute.
    Rhythm: Regular.
    P Waves: Present; precede each QRS complex.
    P-R Int: About 0.18 second.
    QRS: 0.12 second.
    Intrp: Normal sinus rhythm with bundle branch block.

175. Rate: 165 beats/minute.
    Rhythm: Regular.
    P Waves: None.
    P-R Int: None.
    QRS: 0.10 second.
    Intrp: Supraventricular tachycardia.

176. Rate: 48 beats/minute.
    Rhythm: Regular.
    P Waves: Present; appear to precede each QRS complex.
    P-R Int: 0.08 second.
    QRS: 0.08 second.
    Intrp: Bradycardia, probably atrial in origin. (A third-degree AV block cannot be ruled out.)

177. Rate: 79 beats/minute.
    Rhythm: Irregular.
    P Waves: Present; positive P waves precede the first, second, fourth, and fifth QRS complexes. A negative P wave precedes the third QRS complex.
    P-R Int: 0.12 second (first, second, fourth, and fifth QRS complexes); 0.09 second (third QRS complex).
    QRS: 0.10 second.
    Intrp: Normal sinus rhythm with an isolated premature junctional contraction.

178. Rate: 33 beats/minute (atrial rate: 39 beats/minute).
    Rhythm: Undeterminable.
    P Waves: Present, but have no set relation to the QRS complexes.
    P-R Int: None.
    QRS: 0.12 second.
    Intrp: Third-degree AV block with wide QRS complexes.

179. Rate: 59 beats/minute.
    Rhythm: Irregular.
    P Waves: Present; the first, third, and fourth P waves are followed by QRS complexes.
    P-R Int: 0.20 to 0.28 second.
    QRS: About 0.05 second.
    Intrp: Sinus rhythm with second-degree AV block (probably Type I [Wenckebach]).

180. Rate: 96 beats/minute.
    Rhythm: Irregular. An incomplete compensatory pause follows the fourth QRS complex.
    P Waves: Present; precede the second, third, fifth, and sixth QRS complexes.
    P-R Int: 0.18 second.
    QRS: 0.10 second.
    Intrp: Normal sinus rhythm with an isolated premature junctional contraction.

181. Rate: 60 beats/minute.
    Rhythm: Regular.
    P Waves: Present; precede each QRS complex.
    P-R Int: 0.15 second.
    QRS: 0.09 second.
    Intrp: Normal sinus rhythm.

182. Rate: Unmeasurable.
    Rhythm: Irregular.
    P Waves: None; fine ventricular fibrillation waves are present.
    P-R Int: None.
    QRS: None.
    Intrp: Ventricular fibrillation (fine).

183. Rate: 98 beats/minute.
    Rhythm: Regular.
    P Waves: Present; precede each QRS complex.
    P-R Int: About 0.20 second.
    QRS: About 0.19 second.
    Intrp: Normal sinus rhythm with bundle branch block.

184. Rate: 64 beats/minute.
    Rhythm: Regular.
    P Waves: None.
    P-R Int: None.
    QRS: About 0.16 second.
    Intrp: Accelerated idioventricular rhythm.

185. Rate: 35 beats/minute (atrial rate: 167 beats/minute).
    Rhythm: Undeterminable.
    P Waves: Present, but have no set relation to the QRS complexes.
    P-R Int: None.
    QRS: 0.12 second.
    Intrp: Third-degree AV block with wide QRS complexes.

186. Rate: 79 beats/minute.
    Rhythm: Regular.
    P Waves: Present; precede each QRS complex.
    P-R Int: 0.15 second.
    QRS: 0.08 second.
    Intrp: Normal sinus rhythm.

187. Rate: 87 beats/minute.
    Rhythm: Irregular.
    P Waves: None; atrial flutter waves are present. The AV conduction ratios vary.
    P-R Int: None.
    QRS: 0.10 second.
    Intrp: Atrial flutter.

188. Rate: 181 beats/minute.
    Rhythm: Regular.
    P Waves: None.
    P-R Int: None.
    QRS: About 0.22 second.
    Intrp: Supraventricular tachycardia with wide QRS complexes or ventricular tachycardia.

189. Rate: 103 beats/minute.
    Rhythm: Regular.
    P Waves: None; atrial flutter waves are present.
    P-R Int: None.
    QRS: 0.06 second.
    Intrp: Atrial flutter.

190. Rate: 161 beats/minute.
    Rhythm: Regular.
    P Waves: Present; precede each QRS complex.
    P-R Int: 0.12 second.
    QRS: 0.09 second.
    Intrp: Atrial tachycardia.

191. Rate: 130 beats/minute.
    Rhythm: Regular.
    P Waves: None.
    P-R Int: None.
    QRS: About 0.10 second.
    Intrp: Supraventricular tachycardia.

192. Rate: Ventricular rate: none (atrial rate: 70 beats/minute).
Rhythm: Regular.
P Waves: Present.
P-R Int: None.
QRS: None.
Intrp: Ventricular asystole.

193. Rate: 31 beats/minute (atrial rate 106 beats/minute).
Rhythm: Undeterminable.
P Waves: Present, but have no set relation to the QRS complexes.
P-R Int: None.
QRS: About 0.14 second.
Intrp: Third-degree AV block with wide QRS complexes.

194. Rate: 36 beats/minute.
Rhythm: Undeterminable.
P Waves: None.
P-R Int: None.
QRS: 0.16 second.
Intrp: Junctional escape rhythm with wide QRS complexes or ventricular escape rhythm.

195. Rate: 59 beats/minute.
Rhythm: Regular.
P Waves: Present; negative P waves precede each QRS complex.
P-R Int: 0.05 to 0.06 second.
QRS: About 0.14 second.
Intrp: Junctional escape rhythm with bundle branch block.

196. Rate: 71 beats/minute.
Rhythm: Irregular. A complete compensatory pause follows the third QRS complex.
P Waves: Present; precede each QRS complex.
P-R Int: 0.16 second.
QRS: 0.08 second.
Intrp: Normal sinus rhythm with an isolated premature atrial contraction.

197. Rate: 122 beats/minute.
Rhythm: Regular.
P Waves: None.
P-R Int: None.
QRS: 0.12 second.
Intrp: Junctional tachycardia with wide QRS complexes.

198. Rate: None.
Rhythm: None.
P Waves: None.
P-R Int: None.
QRS: 0.16 second.
Intrp: A single wide QRS complex followed by ventricular asystole.

199. Rate: 169 beats/minute.
Rhythm: Irregular.
P Waves: None; atrial flutter waves are present. The AV conduction ratios vary.
P-R Int: None.
QRS: 0.08 second.
Intrp: Atrial flutter.

200. Rate: 128 beats/minute.
Rhythm: Regular.
P Waves: Present; precede each QRS complex. The P waves are abnormally tall (P pulmonale).
P-R Int: 0.20 second.
QRS: About 0.11 second.
Intrp: Sinus tachycardia with incomplete bundle branch block.

201. Rate: 63 beats/minute.
Rhythm: Regular.
P Waves: None.
P-R Int: None.
QRS: About 0.12 second.
Intrp: Accelerated junctional rhythm with wide QRS complexes or accelerated idioventricular rhythm.

202. Rate: 60 beats/minute.
Rhythm: Regular.
P Waves: Present; precede each QRS complex.
P-R Int: 0.16 second.
QRS: 0.07 second.
Intrp: Normal sinus rhythm.

203. Rate: Unmeasurable.
Rhythm: None.
P Waves: None; fine ventricular fibrillation waves are present.
P-R Int: None.
QRS: None.
Intrp: Ventricular fibrillation (fine).

204. Rate: 238 beats/minute.
Rhythm: Regular.
P Waves: Present; precede each QRS complex.
P-R Int: Unmeasurable.
QRS: 0.04 second.
Intrp: Atrial tachycardia.

205. Rate: 165 beats/minute.
Rhythm: Regular.
P Waves: None.
P-R Int: None.
QRS: About 0.24 second.
Intrp: Ventricular tachycardia.

206. Rate: 72 beats/minute.
Rhythm: Regular.
P Waves: None; atrial flutter waves are present.
P-R Int: None.
QRS: 0.08 second.
Intrp: Atrial flutter.

207. Rate: 33 beats/minute.
Rhythm: Undeterminable.
P Waves: None.
P-R Int: None.
QRS: Unmeasurable; greater than 0.12 second.
Intrp: Ventricular escape rhythm.

208. Rate: 126 beats/minute.
Rhythm: Regular.
P Waves: None.
P-R Int: None.
QRS: 0.11 second.
Intrp: Junctional tachycardia with incomplete bundle branch block.

209. Rate: 81 beats/minute.
Rhythm: Irregular.
P Waves: Present; precede each QRS complex. The shape and direction of the fourth P wave differs from the others.
P-R Int: 0.13 second (first, second, third, and fifth P-R intervals); 0.18 second (fourth P-R interval).
QRS: 0.09 second (first, second, third, and fifth QRS complexes); 0.10 second (fourth QRS complex).
Intrp: Normal sinus rhythm with an isolated premature atrial contraction.

210. Rate: 31 beats/minute (atrial rate: 83 beats/minute).
   Rhythm: Undeterminable.
   P Waves: Present, but have no set relation to the QRS complexes.
   P-R Int: None.
   QRS: 0.12 second.
   Intrp: Third-degree AV block with wide QRS complexes.

211. Rate: 180 beats/minute.
   Rhythm: Regular.
   P Waves: Present; precede each QRS complex.
   P-R Int: 0.08 second.
   QRS: 0.08 second.
   Intrp: Atrial tachycardia.

212. Rate: 45 beats/minute (atrial rate 111 beats/minute).
   Rhythm: Regular.
   P Waves: Present, but have no set relation to the QRS complexes.
   P-R Int: None.
   QRS: 0.10 second.
   Intrp: Third-degree AV block.

213. Rate: 52 beats/minute.
   Rhythm: Regular.
   P Waves: Present; the first, third, and fifth P waves are followed by QRS complexes. The AV conduction ratio is 2:1.
   P-R Int: 0.20 second.
   QRS: 0.14 second.
   Intrp: Sinus rhythm with second-degree, 2:1 AV block and bundle branch block.

214. Rate: 44 beats/minute.
   Rhythm: Irregular.
   P Waves: None; atrial flutter waves are present. The AV conduction ratios vary.
   P-R Int: None.
   QRS: 0.10 second.
   Intrp: Atrial flutter.

215. Rate: 71 beats/minute.
   Rhythm: Regular.
   P Waves: Present; precede each QRS complex.
   P-R Int: 0.26 second.
   QRS: 0.08 second.
   Intrp: Sinus rhythm with first-degree AV block.

216. Rate: 103 beats/minute.
   Rhythm: Regular.
   P Waves: Present; precede each QRS complex.
   P-R Int: 0.12 second.
   QRS: 0.14 second.
   Intrp: Sinus tachycardia with bundle branch block.

217. Rate: 104 beats/minute.
   Rhythm: Regular.
   P Waves: None.
   P-R Int: None.
   QRS: 0.12 second.
   Intrp: Junctional tachycardia with wide QRS complexes or ventricular tachycardia.

218. Rate: 109 beats/minute.
   Rhythm: Irregular.
   P Waves: Present, precede the first, second, third, fourth, and fifth QRS complexes.
   P-R Int: 0.14 second.
   QRS: 0.09 second (first, second, third, fourth, and fifth QRS complexes); 0.11 second (sixth QRS complex).
   Intrp: Normal sinus rhythm with premature ventricular contractions and a fusion beat (third QRS complex).

219. Rate: None.
   Rhythm: None.
   P Waves: None.
   P-R Int: None.
   QRS: None.
   Intrp: Ventricular asystole.

220. Rate: 81 beats/minute.
   Rhythm: Regular.
   P Waves: None.
   P-R Int: None.
   QRS: 0.10 second.
   Intrp: Accelerated junctional rhythm.

221. Rate: 109 beats/minute.
   Rhythm: Irregular.
   P Waves: Present; precede the first, second, fourth, and fifth QRS complexes.
   P-R Int: About 0.12 second.
   QRS: 0.08 second (first, second, fourth, and fifth QRS complexes); 0.12 second (third and sixth QRS complexes).
   Intrp: Normal sinus rhythm with unifocal premature ventricular contractions (trigeminy).

222. Rate: 37 beats/minute.
   Rhythm: Undeterminable.
   P Waves: Present; the second and fifth P waves are followed by QRS complexes. The third and sixth P waves are buried in the preceding T waves. The AV conduction ratio is 3:1.
   P-R Int: 0.14 second.
   QRS: 0.13 second.
   Intrp: Sinus rhythm with second-degree, high-degree AV block and bundle branch block.

223. Rate: 128 beats/minute.
   Rhythm: Irregular.
   P Waves: None; fine atrial fibrillation waves are present.
   P-R Int: None.
   QRS: 0.12 to 0.16 second.
   Intrp: Atrial fibrillation (fine) with bundle branch block.

224. Rate: 108 beats/minute.
   Rhythm: Regular.
   P Waves: None.
   P-R Int: None.
   QRS: 0.16 second.
   Intrp: Ventricular tachycardia.

Glossary

Aberrant ventricular conduction (aberrancy). An electrical impulse originating in the SA node, atria, or AV junction that is temporarily conducted abnormally through the bundle branches resulting in a bundle branch block. This is usually caused by the appearance of the electrical impulse at the bundle branches prematurely, before the bundle branches have been sufficiently repolarized. Aberrancy may occur with atrial fibrillation, atrial flutter, premature atrial and junctional contractions, and sinus, atrial and junctional tachycardias.

Absolute refractory period (ARP) of the ventricles. The period of ventricular depolarization and most of ventricular repolarization during which the ventricles cannot be stimulated to depolarize. It begins with the onset of the QRS complex and ends at about the peak of the T wave.

Accelerated rhythm. Three or more consecutive beats originating in an ectopic pacemaker with a rate faster than the inherent rate of the ectopic pacemaker but less than 100 beats per minute. Examples are accelerated junctional rhythm and accelerated idioventricular rhythm (AIVR).

Accelerated idioventricular rhythm (AIVR). An arrhythmia originating in an ectopic pacemaker in the ventricles with a rate between 40 and 100 beats per minute.

Accelerated junctional rhythm. An arrhythmia originating in an ectopic pacemaker in the AV junction with a rate between 60 and 100 beats per minute.

Action potential. See Cardiac action potential.

Acute myocardial infarction. A condition that is present when gross necrosis of the myocardium occurs because of interruption of blood flow to the area.

Adams-Stokes syndrome. Sudden attacks of unconsciousness, with or without convulsions, caused by a sudden slowing or stopping of the heart beat.

Adrenergic. Having the characteristics of the sympathetic nervous system; sympathomimetic.

Advanced life support. Emergency medical care beyond basic life support including one or more of the following: starting an IV, administering IV fluids, administering drugs, defibrillating, inserting an esophageal obturator airway or endotracheal tube, and monitoring and interpreting the ECG.

Afterdepolarization. Spontaneous depolarization of cardiac cells resulting from a spontaneous and rhythmic increase in the level of phase 4 membrane action potential following a normal depolarization; triggered activity.

Agonal. Occurring at the moment of or just before death.

Agonal rhythm. Cardiac arrhythmia present in a dying heart. Ventricular escape rhythm.

Amplitude (voltage). With respect to ECGs, the height or depth of a wave or complex measured in millimeters (mm).

Anoxia. Absence or lack of oxygen.

Antegrade (or anterograde) conduction. Conduction of the electrical impulse in a forward direction, that is, from the SA node or atria to the ventricles or from the AV junction to the ventricles.

Antishock garment (MAST). An airtight, inflatable device that encloses the legs and lower part of the trunk, used to control hemorrhage in the lower body, to immobilize certain fractures of the pelvis and legs, to prevent or control hypotension and shock, and to manage life-threatening arrhythmias, such as electromechanical dissociation (EMD) and hypotension and shock following defibrillation in ventricular fibrillation.

Apex of the heart. The pointed lower end of the heart formed by the right and left ventricles.

Arrhythmia. A rhythm other than a normal sinus rhythm when the heart rate is less than 60 or greater than 100 beats per minute, when the rhythm is irregular, when premature contractions occur, or when the normal progression of the electrical impulse through the electrical conduction system is blocked. Also known as dysrhythmia, a more appropriate term but one not used as frequently.

Artifacts. Mechanically or electrically produced extraneous spikes and waves recorded on an ECG tracing. Noise.

Artificial pacemaker. An electronic device used to stimulate the heart to beat when the electrical conduction system of the heart malfunctions causing bradycardia or ventricular asystole. An artificial pacemaker consists of an electronic pulse generator, a battery, and a wire lead that senses the electrical activity of the heart and delivers electrical impulses to the atria or ventricles or both when the pacemaker senses an absence of electrical activity.

Asystole. Absence of contractions of the ventricles or the entire heart.

Atrial and ventricular demand pacemaker. An artificial pacemaker that paces either the atria or ventricles when there is no appropriate spontaneous underlying atrial or ventricular rhythm.

Atrial arrhythmias. Arrhythmias originating in the atria, such as atrial tachycardia (nonparoxysmal atrial tachycardia, paroxysmal atrial tachycardia [PAT]), atrial fibrillation, atrial flutter, premature atrial contractions (PACs), and wandering atrial pacemaker (WAP).

Atrial depolarization. The electrical process of discharging the resting (polarized) myocardial cells producing the P, F, and f waves and causing the atria to contract.

Atrial fibrillation. An arrhythmia arising in numerous ectopic pacemakers in the atria characterized by very rapid atrial fibrillation (f) waves and an irregular, often rapid ventricular response.

Atrial fibrillation (f) waves. Irregularly shaped, rounded (or pointed), and dissimilar atrial waves originating in multiple ectopic pacemakers in the atria at a rate between 350 and 600 (average, 400) beats per minute.

Atrial flutter. An arrhythmia arising in an ectopic pacemaker in the atria characterized by abnormal atrial flutter waves with a sawtooth appearance and usually a regular ventricular response.

Atrial flutter (F) waves. Regularly shaped, usually pointed atrial waves with a sawtooth appearance originating in an ectopic pacemaker in the atria at a rate between 240 and 360 (average, 300) beats per minute.

"Atrial kick." Refers to the complete filling of the ventricles brought on by the contraction of the atria during the last part of ventricular diastole just before the ventricles contract.

Atrial repolarization. The electrical process by which the depolarized atria return to their polarized, resting state. Atrial repolarization produces the atrial T (Ta) wave.

Atrial standstill. Absence of electrical activity of the atria.

Atrial synchronous ventricular pacemaker. An artificial pacemaker that is synchronized with the patient's atrial rhythm and paces the ventricles when an AV block occurs.

Atrial tachycardia. An arrhythmia originating in an ectopic pacemaker in the atria with a rate between 160 and 240 beats per minute. Includes nonparoxysmal atrial tachycardia and paroxysmal atrial tachycardia (PAT).

Atrial tachycardia with aberrancy. Atrial tachycardia with abnormal QRS complexes that occur only during the tachycardia.

Atrial T wave (Ta). Represents atrial repolarization; often buried in the following QRS complex.

Atrioventricular (AV) block. See AV block and specific AV blocks.

Atrioventricular (AV) dissociation. Occurs when the atria and ventricles beat independently.

Atrioventricular (AV) junction. The part of the electrical conduction system that normally conducts the electrical impulse from the atria to the ventricles. It consists of the AV node and bundle of His.

Atrioventricular (AV) node. The part of the electrical conduction system, located in the posterior floor of the right atrium near the interatrial septum, through which the electrical impulses are normally conducted from the atria to the bundle of His.

Atropine. A drug that counteracts parasympathetic activity in the heart thereby increasing the heart rate and enhancing the conduction of the electrical impulses through the AV node; used to treat bradycardias, electromechanical dissociation (EMD), second- and third-degree AV blocks, and ventricular asystole.

Automaticity. The property of a cell to reach a threshold potential and generate electrical impulses spontaneously.

Autonomic nervous system. Part of the nervous system that is involved in the control of involuntary bodily functions, including the control of cardiac and blood vessel activity. It includes the sympathetic and parasympathetic nervous systems.

AV. Abbreviation for atrioventricular.

AV block. Delay or failure of conduction of electrical impulses through the AV junction.

AV block, first-degree. An arrhythmia in which there is a constant delay in the conduction of electrical impulses through the AV node. It is characterized by abnormally prolonged P-R intervals (greater than 0.20 second).

AV block, second-degree, type I (Wenckebach). An arrhythmia in which progressive prolongation of the conduction of electrical impulses through the AV node occurs until conduction is completely blocked. It is characterized by progressive lengthening of the P-R interval until a QRS complex fails to appear after a P wave. This phenomenon is cyclical.

AV block, second-degree, type II. An arrhythmia in which a complete block of conduction of the electrical impulses occurs in one bundle branch and an intermittent block in the other. It is characterized by regularly or irregularly absent QRS complexes (producing, commonly, an AV conduction ratio of 4:3 or 3:2) and a bundle branch block.

AV block, second-degree, 2:1 and high-degree (advanced). An arrhythmia caused by defective conduction of electrical impulses through the AV node or bundle branches or both. It is characterized by regularly or irregularly absent QRS complexes (producing, commonly, an AV conduction ratio of 2:1 or greater) with or without a bundle branch block.

AV block, third-degree. An arrhythmia in which there is a complete block of the conduction of electrical impulses through the AV node, bundle of His, or bundle branches. It is characterized by independent beating of the atria and ventricles.

AV conduction ratio. The ratio of P waves to QRS complexes. For example, an AV conduction ratio of 4:3 indicates that for every four P waves, three are followed by QRS complexes.

AV dissociation. Occurs when the atria and ventricles beat independently.

AV node. See Atrioventricular (AV) node.

AV sequential pacemaker. An artificial pacemaker that paces either the atria or ventricles or both sequentially when spontaneous ventricular activity is absent.

Bachmann's bundle. A branch of the internodal atrial conduction tracts that extends across the atria, conducting the electrical impulses from the SA node to the left atrium.

Baseline. The part of the ECG during which electrical activity of the heart is absent. Commonly the interval between the end of the T wave and the onset of the P wave (the T-P interval) is considered the baseline and is used as the reference for the measurement of the amplitude of the ECG waves and complexes.

Bidirectional tachycardia. Ventricular tachycardia characterized by two distinctly different forms of QRS complexes alternating with each other, indicating the presence of two ventricular ectopic pacemakers.

Bigeminy. An arrhythmia in which every other beat is a premature contraction.

Biological death. Present when irreversible brain damage has occurred, usually within five to ten minutes after cardiac arrest, if untreated.

Bipolar limb leads. Leads I, II, and III.

Block. Delay or failure of conduction of an electrical impulse through the electrical conduction system because of tissue damage or increased parasympathetic (vagal) tone.

Blocked PAC. A P′ wave not followed by a QRS complex.

Bolus. A single large dose of a drug that provides an initial high therapeutic blood level of the drug.

Bradycardia. An arrhythmia with a rate of less than 60 per minute.

Bradycardias. Arrhythmias with rates of less than 60 per minute, e.g., junctional escape rhythm; second-degree, type I AV block (Wenckebach); second-degree, type II AV block; second-degree, 2:1 and high-degree (advanced) AV block; sinus arrest and sinoatrial (SA) exit block; sinus bradycardia; third-degree AV block; and ventricular escape rhythm.

Bretylium tosylate. An antiarrhythmic used in the treatment of premature ventricular contractions (PVCs), ventricular fibrillation, and ventricular tachycardia.

Bundle branch block (BBB). Defective conduction of electrical impulses through the right or left bundle branch from the bundle of His to the Purkinje network causing a right or left bundle branch block. It may be complete or incomplete or permanent or intermittent.

Bundle branches. The part of the electrical conduction system in the ventricles consisting of the right and left bundle branches that conducts the electrical impulses from the bundle of His to the Purkinje network of the myocardium.

Bundle of His. The part of the electrical conduction system located in the upper part of the interventricular septum that conducts the electrical impulses from the AV node to the right and left bundle branches. The bundle of His and the AV node form the AV junction.

Bursts. Refers to the occurrence of two or more consecutive premature contractions.

Capture. Refers to the ability of a pacemaker's electrical impulse to depolarize the atria or ventricles or both.

Capture beat. A normally conducted QRS complex of the underlying rhythm occurring within a ventricular tachycardia.

Cardiac action potential. Refers to the membrane potential of a myocardial cell and the changes it undergoes during depolarization and repolarization.
    phase 0—the rapid depolarization phase of the action potential.
    phase 1—the early rapid repolarization phase of the action potential.
    phase 2—the plateau phase of repolarization of the action potential.
    phase 3—the terminal phase of rapid repolarization of the action potential.
    phase 4—the period between action potentials.

Cardiac arrest. The sudden and unexpected cessation of an adequate circulation to maintain life in a patient who was not expected to die.

Cardiac cycle. The interval from the beginning of one heart beat to the beginning of the next one. The cardiac cycle normally consists of a P wave, a QRS complex, and a T wave, representing a sequence of atrial contraction and relaxation and ventricular contraction and relaxation, in that order.

Cardiac standstill. Absence of atrial and ventricular contractions. This term is used interchangeably with ventricular asystole.

Cardiogenic. Originating in the heart.

Cardiogenic shock. A life-threatening complication of acute myocardial infarction caused by the inability of the damaged ventricles to maintain an adequate systemic circulation.

Cardioversion. Application of a direct-current (DC) countershock to convert certain arrhythmias—atrial fibrillation, atrial flutter, nonparoxysmal atrial tachycardia without block, paroxysmal atrial tachycardia (PAT), paroxysmal junctional tachycardia (PJT), ventricular tachycardia (pulseless), and ventricular tachycardia (with pulse) in a patient hemodynamically unstable—to an organized supraventricular rhythm.

Carotid sinus. A slightly dilated section of the common carotid artery at the point where it bifurcates, containing sensory nerve endings necessary in the regulation of blood pressure and heart rate.

Carotid sinus massage. Application of pressure to the carotid sinus with the fingertips to convert paroxysmal atrial tachycardia (PAT) and paroxysmal junctional tachycardia (PJT) to an organized supraventricular rhythm.

Catecholamines. Hormonelike substances such as epinephrine and norepinephrine that have a strong sympathetic action on the heart and peripheral blood vessels, increasing the cardiac output and blood pressure.

cc. Abbreviation for cubic centimeter. It is often substituted for ml.

Cell membrane potential. The difference between the electrical potential within the cell and a reference potential in the extracellular fluid surrounding the cell.

Clinical death. Present the moment the patient's pulse and blood pressure are absent; occurs immediately after the onset of cardiac arrest.

Coarse atrial fibrillation. Atrial fibrillation with large fibrillatory waves—greater than 1 mm in height.

Coarse ventricular fibrillation. Ventricular fibrillation with large fibrillatory waves—greater than 3 mm in height.

Compensatory pause. The R-R interval following a premature contraction. It may be full or incomplete depending on whether or not the SA node, for example, is depolarized by the premature contraction. If the SA node is not depolarized by the premature contraction, the compensatory pause is called "full"; the sum of a "full" compensatory pause and the preceding R-R interval is equal to the sum of two R-R intervals of the underlying rhythm. If the SA node is depolarized by the premature contraction, resetting the timing of the SA node, the compensatory pause is called "incomplete"; the sum of an "incomplete" compensatory pause and the preceding R-R interval is less than the sum of two R-R intervals of the underlying rhythm.

Complete bundle branch block. Complete disruption of the conduction of electrical impulses through the right or left bundle branch.

Components of the electrocardiogram. Includes the P wave, P-R interval, P-R segment, QRS complex, S-T segment, T wave, U wave, T-P segment, and R-R interval.

Conducted PAC. A positive P′ wave (in Lead II) followed by a QRS complex.

Conducted PJC. A negative P′ wave (in Lead II) followed by a QRS complex.

Conductivity. The property of cardiac cells to conduct electrical impulses.

Congestive heart failure. Excessive blood or tissue fluid in the lungs or body or both caused by the inefficient pumping of the ventricles.

Contractile filament. See Myofibril.

Contractility. The property of cardiac cells to contract when they are depolarized by an electrical impulse.

Controlled atrial flutter. A "treated" atrial flutter with a slow ventricular rate of about 60 to 75 beats per minute.

Coronary artery disease. Progressive narrowing and eventual obstruction of the coronary arteries by atherosclerosis.

Coronary sinus. The outlet in the right atrium draining the coronary venous system.

Couplet. Two consecutive premature contractions.

Coupling. Ventricular bigeminy with the premature ventricular contractions following the QRS complexes of the underlying rhythm at the same intervals.

Coupling interval. The R-R interval between a premature contraction and the preceding QRS complex of the underlying rhythm.

Cyanosis. Slightly bluish, greyish, slatelike or purplish discoloration of the skin caused by the presence of unoxygenated blood.

Delta wave. The initial slurring of the QRS complex found in anomalous AV conduction or preexcitation syndrome.

Demand pacing. Refers to a mode of artificial pacing in which the pacemaker is turned on when an appropriate underlying spontaneous atrial or ventricular rhythm is absent.

Depolarization. The electrical process by which the resting potential of a polarized, resting cell is reduced to a less negative value.

Depolarization waves. The parts of the ECG representing the depolarization of the atria and ventricles—the P wave (atrial depolarization) and the QRS complex (ventricular depolarization).

Depolarized state. The condition of the cell when it has been completely depolarized.

Diastole (electrical). Phase 4 of the action potential.

Diastole (mechanical). The period of atrial or ventricular relaxation.

Diazepam. An antianxiety agent used to produce amnesia in conscious patients before cardioverting atrial fibrillation, atrial flutter, nonparoxysmal atrial tachycardia without block, paroxysmal atrial tachycardia (PAT), paroxysmal junctional tachycardia (PJT), ventricular tachycardia (pulseless), and ventricular tachycardia (with pulse) in a patient hemodynamically unstable.

Digitalis. A drug used to decrease rapid ventricular rate in atrial fibrillation, atrial flutter, nonparoxysmal atrial tachycardia without block, paroxysmal atrial tachycardia (PAT), and paroxysmal junctional tachycardia (PAT) and to improve ventricular contraction in congestive heart failure.

Digitalis overdose. Excessive administration of digitalis, often accompanied by signs and symptoms of digitalis toxicity which includes the appearance of arrhythmias, such as accelerated idioventricular rhythm (AIVR), AV blocks, junctional tachycardia, nonparoxysmal atrial tachycardia with or without block, premature atrial contractions (PACs), premature junctional contractions (PJCs), ventricular fibrillation, and ventricular tachycardia. In fact, almost any arrhythmia may be caused by excess digitalis.

Digitalis toxicity. Digitalis overdose.

Digitalization. The process of administering an adequate amount of digitalis over a period of time in the treatment of certain arrhythmias. See Digoxin.

Digoxin. A drug used in the treatment of atrial fibrillation, atrial flutter, nonparoxysmal atrial tachycardia without block, paroxysmal atrial tachycardia (PAT), and paroxysmal junctional tachycardia (PAT).

Direct-current (DC) countershock. Used in the treatment of atrial fibrillation, atrial flutter, nonparoxysmal atrial tachycardia without block, paroxysmal atrial tachycardia (PAT), paroxysmal junctional tachycardia (PJT), ventricular tachycardia (pulseless), and ventricular tachycardia (with pulse) in a patient hemodynamically unstable.

Direct-current (DC) shock. Used in the treatment of ventricular fibrillation.

Diuretic. A drug to used in congestive heart failure to decrease excess body fluid by increasing the secretion of urine by the kidney.

Dominant pacemaker of the heart. The SA node.

Dopamine hydrochloride. A sympathomimetic that increases blood pressure; used in the treatment of hypotension and shock.

Dropped beats. Nonconducted P waves in AV blocks.

Dropped P waves. Absent P waves in sinus arrest and sinoatrial (SA) exit block.

Dying heart. A heart with feeble ineffectual ventricular contractions and an ECG showing markedly abnormal QRS complexes, usually a ventricular escape rhythm.

Dysrhythmia. A rhythm other than a normal sinus rhythm. A term more correct than "arrhythmia" but less frequently used.

ECG. Abbreviation for electrocardiogram.

ECG artifacts. See Artifacts.

ECG grid. The grid on ECG paper formed by the dark and light horizontal and vertical lines.

Ectopic beats. Premature beats originating in ectopic pacemakers in the atria, AV junction, and ventricles, e.g., premature atrial contractions (PACs), premature junctional contractions (PJCs), and premature ventricular contractions (PVCs).

Ectopic focus. A pacemaker other than the SA node.

Ectopic pacemakers. Abnormal pacemakers in the atria, AV junction, bundle branches, Purkinje network, and ventricular myocardium.

Ectopic rhythms. Arrhythmias originating in ectopic pacemakers in the atria, AV junction, and ventricles, e.g., accelerated idioventricular rhythm (AIVR), atrial fibrillation, atrial flutter, atrial tachycardia (nonparoxysmal atrial tachycardia, paroxysmal atrial tachycardia [PAT]), nonparoxysmal junctional tachycardia (accelerated junctional rhythm, junctional tachycardia), paroxysmal junctional tachycardia (PJT), premature atrial contractions (PACs), premature junctional contractions (PJCs), premature ventricular contractions (PVCs), ventricular fibrillation (VF), ventricular tachycardia (VT), and wandering atrial pacemaker (WAP).

Ectopic tachycardias. Abnormal rhythms originating in ectopic pacemakers having a rate of over 100 beats per minute, e.g., atrial fibrillation, atrial flutter, atrial tachycardia, (nonparoxysmal atrial tachycardia, paroxysmal atrial tachycardia [PAT]), junctional tachycardia, paroxysmal junctional tachycardia (PJT), and ventricular tachycardia (VT).

Ectopic ventricular arrhythmias. Abnormal rhythms originating in ectopic pacemakers in the ventricles, e.g., accelerated idioventricular rhythm (AIVR), premature ventricular contractions (PVCs), ventricular fibrillation, and ventricular tachycardia.

Edema. A condition in which the body tissues have accumulated excessive tissue fluid or exudate (as in congestive heart failure).

Electrical activity of the heart. The electric current generated by the depolarization and repolarization of the atria and ventricles, which can be graphically displayed on the ECG.

Electrical conduction system of the heart. Includes the sinoatrial (SA) node, internodal atrial conduction tracts, interatrial conduction tract (Bachmann's bundle), atrioventricular (AV) node, bundle of His, right and left bundle branches, and Purkinje network.

Electrical conduction system of the ventricles. The His-Purkinje system which includes the bundle of His, the right and left bundle branches, and the Purkinje network.

Electrical impulse. The tiny electrical current that normally originates in the SA node automatically and is conducted through the electrical conduction system to the atria and ventricles, causing them to depolarize and contract.

Electrocardiogram (ECG). The graphic display of the electrical activity of the heart generated by the depolarization and repolarization of the atria and ventricles. The ECG includes the QRS complex; the P, T, and U waves; the P-R, S-T, and T-P segments; and the P-R, Q-T, and R-R intervals.

Electrode. A sensing device that detects electrical activity such as that of the heart.

Electrolyte. A substance that when in solution dissociates into cations and anions, thus becoming capable of conducting electricity.

Electrolyte imbalance. Abnormal concentrations of serum electrolytes caused by excessive intake or loss of such electrolytes as calcium, carbonate, chloride, potassium and sodium.

Electromechanical dissociation (EMD). A condition of the heart in which the electrical activity of the heart is present and can be recorded on the ECG, but effective ventricular contractions and pulses are absent.

Embolism. Obstruction of a blood vessel by an embolus that reduces or stops blood flow, resulting in ischemia or necrosis of the tissue supplied by the blood vessel.

Embolus. A mass of solid, liquid or gaseous material carried from one part of the circulatory system to another.

End-diastolic PVC. A PVC occurring at about the same time that a QRS complex of the underlying rhythm is expected to occur.

Endocardium. The thin membrane lining the inside of the heart.

Enhanced automaticity. An abnormal condition of latent pacemaker cells in which their firing rate is increased beyond their inherent rate because of an increase in the phase 4 slope of spontaneous depolarization.

Epicardial surface. The outside surface of the heart.

Epicardium. The thin membrane lining the outside of the heart.

Epinephrine. Hormone and drug used in the treatment of electromechanical dissociation (EMD), ventricular asystole, ventricular fibrillation, and ventricular tachycardia (pulseless).

Escape beat or complex. A QRS complex arising in an escape or secondary pacemaker when the underlying rhythm slows to less than the escape or secondary pacemaker's inherent firing rate.

Escape or secondary pacemaker. A latent pacemaker that takes over pacing the heart when the pacemaker of the underlying rhythm slows to less than the latent pacemaker's inherent firing rate.

Escape rhythm. Three or more consecutive QRS complexes that result when the underlying rhythm slows to less than the escape or secondary pacemaker's inherent firing rate and the escape pacemaker takes over. Examples of escape rhythms are junctional escape rhythm and ventricular escape rhythm.

Essentially regular rhythm. A rhythm in which the shortest and longest R-R intervals vary by less than 0.16 seconds (four small squares) in an ECG tracing.

Excitability. The ability of a cell to respond to stimulation.

External cardiac pacing. A technique to treat bradycardias, electromechanical dissociation (EMD), and ventricular asystole using an external artificial pacemaker.

Extrasystole. A premature beat or contraction independent of the underlying rhythm caused by an electrical impulse originating in an ectopic focus in the atria, AV junction, or ventricles. Examples of extrasystoles are premature atrial contractions (PACs), premature junctional contractions (PJCs), and premature ventricular contractions (PVCs).

Fascicular premature ventricular contraction. A PVC with an almost normal QRS complex originating in the ventricles near the bifurcation of the bundle of His.

Fast sodium channels. Structures in the cell membrane called "pores" which facilitate the rapid flow of sodium ions into the cell during depolarization, rapidly changing the electrical potential within the cell from negative to positive.

Fibrillation. Chaotic, disorganized beating of the myocardium in which each myofibril contracts and relaxes independently, producing rapid, tremulous and ineffectual contractions. Fibrillation may occur in both the atria and ventricles.

Fibrillation waves. On the ECG, these waves appear as numerous irregularly shaped, rounded (or pointed) and dissimilar waves originating in multiple ectopic foci in the atria or ventricles.

Fine atrial fibrillation. Atrial fibrillation with fine fibrillatory waves—less than 1 mm in height.

Fine ventricular fibrillation. Ventricular fibrillation with small fibrillatory waves—less than 3 mm in height.

Firing rate. The rate at which electrical impulses are generated in a pacemaker, whether it is the SA node or an ectopic or escape pacemaker.

First-degree AV block. An arrhythmia in which there is a constant delay in the conduction of electrical impulses through the AV node. It is characterized by abnormally prolonged P-R intervals (greater than 0.20 second).

Flutter. Rapid, regular, repetitive beating of the atria or ventricles.

Flutter-fibrillation. Refers to the simultaneous occurrence of flutter and fibrillation as in atrial flutter-fibrillation.

Flutter waves. On the ECG, these waves appear as numerous repetitive similar, usually pointed waves originating in an ectopic pacemaker in the atria or ventricles.

Frequent PVCs. Five or more PVCs per minute.

Fusion beat, ventricular. A ventricular complex unlike the QRS complexes of the underlying rhythm and those of the ventricular arrhythmia in a given ECG lead, having features of both. This results from the stimulation of the ventricles by two electrical impulses, one originating in the SA node or an ectopic focus in the atria or AV junction and the other in an ectopic focus in the ventricles. A fusion beat can occur in accelerated idioventricular rhythm (AIVR), pacemaker rhythm, premature ventricular contractions (PVCs), and ventricular tachycardia.

f waves. See Atrial fibrillation (f) waves.

F waves. See Atrial flutter (F) waves.

Gap junction. A structure within the intercalated disks located at the junctions of the branches of myocardial cells, permitting very rapid conduction of electrical impulses from one cell to another.

Gram (gm). Measurement of metric weight equal to about one cubic centimeter (cc) or one milliliter (ml) of water. 1,000 grams is equal to 1 kilogram.

Grid, ECG. See ECG grid.

Ground electrode. The ECG lead other than the positive and negative leads that grounds the input to prevent extraneous noise from entering the amplifier circuit.

Group beating. Repetitive sequence of two or more consecutive beats followed by a dropped beat as seen in AV block.

Group beats. Occurrence of two or more consecutive premature contractions preceded and followed by the underlying rhythm.

His-Purkinje system (of the ventricles). The part of the electrical system consisting of the bundle of His, bundle branches, and Purkinje network.

Horizontal lines. Refer to the horizontal lines forming, with the vertical lines, the grid on ECG paper.

Hypercalcemia. Elevated levels of calcium in the blood.

Hypercapnia. Excessive amount of carbon dioxide in the blood.

Hypercarbia. Hypercapnia.

Hyperkalemia. Excessive amount of potassium in the blood.

Hypertension. Blood pressure over 140/90 mm Hg.

Hyperventilation. Increased ventilation of the alveoli caused by abnormally rapid, deep, and prolonged respirations; the result is a loss of carbon dioxide from the body and eventually alkalosis.

Hypocalcemia. Low amount of calcium in the blood.

Hypocarbia. Low amount of carbon dioxide in the blood.

Hypokalemia. Low amount of potassium in the blood.

Hypotension. Low blood pressure; generally considered to be a systolic blood pressure of 80 to 90 mm Hg or less.

Hypoventilation. Decreased ventilation of the alveoli.

Hypovolemia. Decreased amount of blood in the body's cardiovascular system.

Hypoxemia. Reduced oxygenation of the blood.

Hypoxia. Reduced amount of oxygen. Hypoxia is used interchangeably with the term anoxia.

Idioventricular. Pertaining to the ventricle.

IM. Abbreviation for intramuscular.

Incomplete bundle branch block. Defective conduction of electrical impulses through the right or left bundle branch from the bundle of His to the Purkinje network in the myocardium resulting in a slightly widened QRS complex, i.e., greater than 0.10 second but less than 0.12 second.

Incomplete compensatory pause. The R-R interval following a premature contraction that if added to the R-R interval preceding the premature complex would result in a sum less than the sum of two R-R intervals of the underlying rhythm. See Compensatory pause.

Infarction. Death (necrosis) of tissue caused by interruption of the blood supply to the affected tissue.

Inferior vena cava. One of the two largest veins in the body that empty venous blood into the right atrium.

Infrequent PVCs. Less tan five PVCs per minute.

Inherent firing rate. The rate at which a given pacemaker of the heart normally generates electrical impulses.

Interatrial conduction tracts. See Bachmann's bundle.

Interatrial septum. The membranous wall dividing the right and left atria.

Intercalated disks. Specialized structures located at the junctions of the branches of myocardial cells that permit very rapid conduction of electrical impulses from one cell to another.

Internodal atrial conduction tracts. Part of the electrical conduction system of the heart consisting of three pathways of specialized conducting tissue located in the walls of the right atrium between the SA node and AV node.

Interpolated PVC. A PVC that occurs between two normally conducted QRS complexes without greatly disturbing the underlying rhythm. A full compensatory pause, as is commonly present with PVCs, is absent.

Interventricular septum. The membranous, muscular wall dividing the right and left ventricles.

Interval(s). The sections of the ECG between waves and complexes of the ECG. See P-P interval, P-R interval, Q-T interval, and R-R interval.

Intracardiac. Within the heart.

Intravenous (IV) drip. The administration of fluid into a vein very slowly.

Ion. An atom or group of atoms having a positive charge (cation) or a negative one (anion).

Ischemia. Reduced blood flow to tissue caused by narrowing or occlusion of the artery supplying blood to it. Ischemia results in tissue anoxia.

Isoelectric line. The flat line in an ECG during which electrical activity is absent.

Isolated beat. A premature contraction occurring singly.

Isoproterenol. A potent beta receptor stimulating drug, especially effective in stimulating the beta receptors of the heart; used in the treatment of bradycardias, electromechanical dissociation (EMD), and ventricular asystole.

IV. Abbreviation for intravenous.

Joules. Unit of electrical energy delivered for 1 second by an electrical source, such as a defibrillator. Used interchangeably with Watt-seconds.

J point. The point where the QRS complex becomes the S-T segment or the S-T,T wave.

Junction (AV). See Atrioventricular (AV) junction.

Junctional arrhythmia. An arrhythmia arising in an ectopic or escape pacemaker in the AV junction, e.g., premature junctional contractions, junctional escape rhythm, nonparoxysmal junctional tachycardia (accelerated junctional rhythm, junctional tachycardia), and paroxysmal junctional tachycardia (PJT).

Junctional escape rhythm. An arrhythmia originating in an escape pacemaker in the AV junction with a rate of 40 to 60 beats per minute.

Junctional tachycardia. An arrhythmia originating in an ectopic pacemaker in the AV junction with a rate greater than 100 beats per minute.

Junctional tachycardia with aberrancy. Junctional tachycardia with abnormal QRS complexes that occur only during the tachycardia.

K+. Symbol for potassium.

Kg. Abbreviation for kilogram.

Kilogram. A unit of metric weight measurement. One kilogram (kg) is equal to 1,000 grams, or 2.2 pounds.

KVO Abbreviation for "keep the vein open."

L. Abbreviation for liter.

Lactated Ringer's. Frequently used sterile IV solution containing sodium, potassium, calcium, and chloride ions in about the same concentrations as present in blood in addition to lactate ions.

Large squares. The areas on ECG paper enclosed by the dark horizontal and vertical lines of the grid.

Left bundle branch block (LBBB). Defective conduction of electrical impulses through the left bundle branch. Left bundle branch block may be complete or incomplete.

Lidocaine. An antiarrhythmic used to treat premature ventricular contractions (PVCs), ventricular fibrillation, and ventricular tachycardia.

Life-threatening arrhythmias Include electromechanical dissociation (EMD), ventricular asystole, ventricular fibrillation, and ventricular tachycardia.

Liter (L). A metric measurement of volume. One liter is equal to 1,000 milliliters (ml), or 1.1 quarts.

Loading dose. A single large dose of a drug that produces an initial high therapeutic blood level necessary to treat certain conditions.

Marked sinus bradycardia. A bradycardia with a heart rate between 30 and 45 beats per minute or less, hypotension, and signs and symptoms of decreased perfusion of the brain and other organs.

MAST. Abbreviation for "Military Antishock Trousers" or "Medical Antishock Trouser." Used interchangeably with antishock garment.

MAT. See Multifocal atrial tachycardia.

Membrane potential. The electrical potential measuring the difference between the interior of a cell and the extracellular fluid.

mEq. Abbreviation for milliequivalents.

Meter. A metric unit of linear measurement. One meter is equal to 1,000 millimeters, or 39.37 inches.

mg. Abbreviation for milligrams.

microgram (μg). A metric unit of measurement of weight. One thousand micrograms are equal to one milligram.

μg. Abbreviation for microgram.

Midclavicular line. An imaginary line beginning in the middle of the left clavicle and running parallel to the sternum slightly inside the left nipple.

Military antishock trouser (MAST). See Antishock garment (MAST).

Mild sinus bradycardia. A bradycardia with a heart rate between 50 and 59 beats per minute and absence of hypotension and signs and symptoms of decreased perfusion of the brain or other organs.

Milliequivalents (mEq). The weight of a substance dissolved in one milliliter of solution.

Milligram (mg). A metric unit of weight. One thousand milligrams are equal to 1 kilogram, or 2.2 pounds.

Milliliter (ml). A metric unit of measurement of volume. One thousand milliliters are equal to 1 liter, or 1.1 quarts.

Millimeter (mm). A metric unit of linear measurement. One thousand millimeters are equal to 1 meter, or 39.37 inches.

Millimeter of mercury (mm Hg). A metric unit of weight used in the determination of blood pressure.

Millivolt (mV). A unit of electrical energy. One thousand millivolts are equal to 1 volt.

ml. Abbreviation for milliliter.

mm. Abbreviation for millimeter.

mm Hg. Abbreviation for millimeters of mercury.

Morphine sulfate. A narcotic analgesic used in conscious patients before cardioverting atrial fibrillation, atrial flutter, nonparoxysmal atrial tachycardia without block, paroxysmal atrial tachycardia (PAT), paroxysmal junctional tachycardia (PJT), ventricular tachycardia (pulseless), and ventricular tachycardia (with pulse) in a patient hemodynamically unstable.

Multifocal atrial tachycardia (MAT). Atrial tachycardia originating in three or more different atrial ectopic pacemaker sites, characterized by P′ waves that differ in size, shape, and direction.

Multifocal premature ventricular contractions. Different appearing premature ventricular contractions in the same tracing that originate from different ectopic pacemaker sites in the ventricles.

Multiform premature ventricular contractions. Different appearing premature ventricular contractions in the same tracing that originate in the same ectopic pacemaker site in the ventricles.

Multiform ventricular tachycardia. Ventricular tachycardia with QRS complexes that differ markedly from beat to beat.

Muscle tremor. The cause of extraneous spikes and waves in the ECG brought on by voluntary or involuntary muscle movement or shivering; often seen in elderly persons or in a cold environment.

mV. Abbreviation for millivolt.

Myocardial. Pertaining to the muscular part of the heart.

Myocardial infarction. See Acute myocardial infarction.

Myocardium. Cardiac muscle.

Myofibril. Tiny structure within a muscle cell that contracts when stimulated.

Na+. Symbol for sodium ion.

Necrosis. Death of tissue.

Noise. Extraneous spikes, waves, and complexes in the ECG signal caused by muscle tremor, 60-cycle AC interference, improperly attached electrodes, and biomedical telemetry-related events, such as out-of-range ECG transmission and weak transmitter batteries.

Nonconducted PAC. A positive P′ wave (in Lead II) not followed by a QRS complex.

Nonconducted PJC. A negative P' wave (in Lead II) not followed by a QRS complex.

Nonparoxysmal junctional tachycardia. See Accelerated junctional rhythm and junctional tachycardia.

Nonsustained ventricular tachycardia. Paroxysms of three or more PVCs separated by the underlying rhythm. Paroxysmal ventricular tachycardia.

Norepinephrine base (Levophed, levarterenol). A sympathomimetic used in the treatment of hypotension and shock.

Normal saline. Incorrect term for the intravenous saline solution containing 0.9 percent sodium chloride.

Normal sinus rhythm (NSR). Normal rhythm of the heart, originating in the SA node with a rate of 60 to 100 beats per minute.

Notch. A sharply pointed upright or downward wave in the QRS complex or T wave that does not go below or above the baseline, respectively.

Optimal sequential pacemaker. An artificial pacemaker that paces the atria or ventricles or both when spontaneous atrial or ventricular activity is absent.

Overdrive suppression. A delay in the generation of an electrical impulse in the SA node, for example, caused by a premature atrial or ventricular contraction; the result is a slight delay in the appearance of the next expected P wave.

Pacemaker cell. A cell with the property of automaticity.

Pacemaker, artificial. An electronic device used to stimulate the heart to beat when the electrical conduction system of the heart malfunctions causing bradycardia or ventricular asystole. An artificial pacemaker consists of an electronic pulse generator, a battery, and a wire lead that senses the electrical activity of the heart and delivers electrical impulses to the atria or ventricles or both when the pacemaker senses an absence of electrical activity.

Pacemaker of the heart. The SA node or an escape or ectopic pacemaker in the electrical system of the heart or in the myocardium.

Pacemaker rhythm. An arrhythmia produced by an artificial pacemaker.

Pacemaker site. The site of the origin of an electrical impulse. It can be the SA node or an escape or ectopic pacemaker in any part of the electrical system of the heart or in the myocardium.

Pacemaker spike. The narrow sharp wave in the ECG caused by the electrical impulse generated by an artificial pacemaker.

PAC. Abbreviation for premature atrial contraction.

Paired PVCs. Two consecutive PVCs.

Parasympathetic nervous system. Part of the autonomic nervous system involved in the control of involuntary bodily functions, including the control of cardiac and blood vessel activity. Activation of this system depresses cardiac activity and produces effects opposite to those of the sympathetic nervous system. Some effects of parasympathetic stimulation are slowing of the heart rate, decreased cardiac output, drop in blood pressure, nausea, vomiting, bronchial spasm, sweating, faintness, and hypersalivation.

Parasympathetic (vagal) tone. Pertains to the degree of parasympathetic activity.

Paroxysm. Sudden occurrence; spasm or seizure.

Paroxysmal atrial tachycardia (PAT). An arrhythmia originating in an ectopic pacemaker in the atria with a rate between 160 and 240 beats per minute. It typically starts and ends abruptly, occurring in paroxysms which may last from a few seconds to many hours and recur for many years.

Paroxysmal junctional tachycardia (PJT). An arrhythmia originating in an ectopic pacemaker in the AV junction with a rate between 160 and 240 beats per minute. It typically starts and ends abruptly, occurring in paroxysms which may last from a few seconds to many hours and recur for many years.

Paroxysmal supraventricular tachycardia (PSVT). A commonly used term to indicate a paroxysmal tachycardia with a rate between 160 and 240 beats per minute originating in the atria or AV junction when the origin of the tachycardia is not clearly evident.

Perfusion. Passage of a fluid such as blood through the vessels of a tissue or organ.

Pericardium. The tough fibrous sac containing the heart and origins of the superior vena cava, inferior vena cava, aorta, and pulmonary artery. The pericardium consists of an inner serous layer (visceral pericardium or epicardium) and an outer fibrous layer (parietal pericardium).

Peripheral vascular resistance. The resistance to blood flow in the systemic circulation that depends on the degree of constriction or dilation of the small arteries, arterioles, venules, and small veins making up the peripheral vascular system.

Peripheral vasoconstriction. Constriction of blood vessels, especially the small arteries, arterioles, venules, and small veins, causing an increase in blood pressure and a decrease in the circulation of blood beyond the point of vasoconstriction.

Peripheral vasodilatation. Dilation of blood vessels, especially the small arteries, arterioles, venules, and small veins, causing a decrease in blood pressure.

pH. Symbol for the concentration of hydrogen ions (H+) in a solution.

Physiological AV block. An AV block that occurs only when an atrial arrhythmia, such as atrial fibrillation, atrial flutter, and atrial tachycardia, is present.

PJC. Abbreviation for premature junctional contraction.

P mitrale. A wide notched P wave occurring in the presence of left atrial dilatation and hypertrophied. Typically associated with severe mitral stenosis.

Polarized (or resting) state of the cell. The condition of the cell following repolarization when the interior of the cell is negative and the outside positive.

Potential (electrical). The difference in the concentration of ions across a cell membrane, for instance, measured in millivolts.

P prime (P'). An abnormal P wave originating in an ectopic pacemaker in the atria or AV junction.

P pulmonale. A wide, tall P wave (greater than 2.5 mm in height) occurring in the presence of right atrial dilatation and hypertrophy. Typically associated with pulmonary disease such as COPD and increased pulmonary artery pressure.

Precordial. Pertaining to the precordium.

Precordial thump. A sharp brisk blow delivered to the midportion of the sternum for the purpose of terminating ventricular fibrillation and ventricular tachycardia or initiating an electrical impulse in bradycardias, electromechanical dissociation (EMD), and ventricular asystole.

Precordium. The region of the thorax over the heart, the midportion of the sternum.

Preexcitation syndrome. An abnormal condition in which the electrical impulses enter the ventricles from the atria through an accessory pathway that bypasses the AV junction resulting in a short P-R interval, a wide QRS complex with an initial slurring (delta wave) of the upward slope, and a tendency to atrial flutter and fibrillation with rapid ventricular rates and paroxysmal supraventricular tachycardia. A common type of preexcitation syndrome is the Wolff-Parkinson-White (WPW) syndrome.

Premature atrial contraction (PAC). An extra beat consisting of an abnormal P wave originating in an ectopic pacemaker in the atria followed by a normal or abnormal QRS complex.

Premature ectopic beats (contractions). Extra beats or contractions originating in the atria, AV junction or ventricles, e.g., premature atrial contractions (PACs), premature junctional contractions (PJCs), and premature ventricular contractions (PVCs).

Premature junctional contractions (PJC). An extra beat originating in an ectopic pacemaker in the AV junction and consisting of a normal or abnormal QRS complex with or without an abnormal P wave. If a P wave is present, the P-R interval is shorter than normal.

Premature junctional contractions with aberrancy. PJCs with abnormal QRS complexes that occur only with the PJCs.

Premature ventricular contraction (PVC). An extra beat consisting of an abnormally wide and bizarre QRS complex originating in an ectopic pacemaker in the ventricles.

P-R interval. The section of the ECG between the onset of the P wave and the onset of the QRS complex.

Procainamide. An antiarrhythmic used to treat premature ventricular contractions and ventricular tachycardia.

Prophylaxis. Preventive treatment.

Propranolol (Inderal). An antiarrhythmic used to treat atrial fibrillation, atrial flutter, nonparoxysmal atrial tachycardia without block, paroxysmal atrial tachycardia (PAT), and paroxysmal junctional tachycardia (PJT). Propranolol is one of several agents called beta blockers.

P-R segment. The section of the ECG between the end of the P wave and the onset of the QRS complex.

Purkinje network of the ventricles. The part of the electrical conduction system between the bundle branches and the ventricular myocardium consisting of the Purkinje fibers and their terminal branches.

PVC. Abbreviation for premature ventricular contraction.

P wave. Normally, the first wave of the P-QRS-T complex representing the depolarization of the atria.

QRS complex. Normally, the wave following the P wave, consisting of the Q, R, and S waves and representing ventricular depolarization.

QS wave. A QRS complex that consists entirely of a single, large negative deflection.

Q-T interval. The section of the ECG between the onset of the QRS complex and the end of the T wave, representing ventricular depolarization and repolarization.

Quadrigeminy. A series of groups of four beats, usually consisting of three normally conducted QRS complexes followed by a premature contraction.

Quinidine sulfate. An antiarrhythmic used to treat premature atrial and junctional contractions.

Q wave. The first negative deflection of the QRS complex not preceded by an R wave.

Rate conversion table. A table converting the number of small squares between two adjacent R waves into the heart rate per minute.

R double prime (R″). The third R wave in a QRS complex.

Reentry mechanism. A mechanism by which an electrical impulse repeatedly exits and reenters an area of the heart causing one or more ectopic contractions.

Refractory. Inability to respond to a stimulus.

Refractory period. The time during which a cell or fiber may or may not be depolarized by an electrical stimulus depending on the strength of the electrical impulse. It extends from phase 0 to the end of phase 3 and is divided into the absolute refractory period (ARP) and relative refractory period (RRP). The absolute refractory period extends from phase 0 to about midway through phase 3. The relative refractory period extends from about midway through phase 3 to the end of phase 3.

Relative refractory period (RRP) of the ventricles. The period of ventricular repolarization during which the ventricles can be stimulated to depolarize by an electrical impulse stronger than usual. It begins at about the peak of the T wave and ends with the end of the T wave.

Repolarization. The electrical process by which a depolarized cell returns to its polarized, resting state.

Repolarization wave. The progression of the repolarization process through the atria and ventricles that appears on the ECG as the atrial and ventricular T waves.

Repolarized state. The condition of the cell when it has been completely repolarized.

Resting membrane potential. Electrical measurement of the difference between the electrical potential of the interior of a fully repolarized, resting cell and that of the extracellular fluid surrounding it.

Resuscitation. The restoration of life by artificial respiration and external chest compression.

Retrograde atrial depolarization. Abnormal depolarization of the atria that begins near the AV junction, producing a negative P′ wave in Lead II. Typically associated with junctional arrhythmias.

Retrograde AV block. Delay or failure of backward conduction through the AV junction into the atria of electrical impulses originating in the bundle of His or the ventricles.

Retrograde conduction. Conduction of an electrical impulse in a direction opposite from normal, that is, from the AV junction or ventricles to the atria or SA node.

Right bundle branch block (RBBB). Defective conduction of electrical impulses through the right bundle branch. It may be complete or incomplete.

Ringer's solution. See Lactated Ringer's solution.

R-on-T phenomenon. An ominous type of premature ventricular contraction that falls on the T wave of the preceding QRS-T complex. This can cause ventricular tachycardia or ventricular fibrillation.

R prime (R′). The second R wave in a QRS complex.

R-P′ interval. The section of the ECG between the onset of the QRS complex and the onset of the P′ wave following it. This is present in junctional arrhythmias and occasionally in ventricular arrhythmias.

R-R interval. The section of the ECG between the onset of one QRS complex and the onset of an adjacent QRS complex or between two adjacent R waves.

R wave. The positive wave or deflection in the QRS complex.

Salvos. Refers to two or more consecutive premature contractions. Bursts.

Saw-toothed appearance. Description given atrial flutter waves.

SA node. The dominant pacemaker of the heart located in the wall of the right atrium near the inlet of the superior vena cava.

S double prime (S″). The third S wave in the QRS complex.

Secondary pacemaker of the heart. A pacemaker in the electrical system of the heart other than the SA node; an escape or ectopic pacemaker.

Second-degree AV block. An arrhythmia in which one or more P waves are not conducted to the ventricles. See AV block, second-degree, type I (Wenckebach); AV block, second-degree, type II; and AV block, second-degree, 2:1 and high-degree (advanced).

Second-degree, type I AV block (Wenckebach). An arrhythmia in which progressive prolongation of the conduction of electrical impulses through the AV node occurs until conduction is completely blocked. It is characterized by progressive lengthening of the P-R interval until a QRS complex fails to appear after a P wave. This phenomenon is cyclical.

Second-degree, type II AV block. An arrhythmia in which a complete block of conduction of the electrical impulses occurs in one bundle branch and an intermittent block in the other. It is characterized by regularly or irregularly absent QRS complexes (producing, commonly, an AV conduction ratio of 4:3 or 3:2) and a bundle branch block.

Second-degree, 2:1 and high-degree (advanced) AV block. An arrhythmia caused by defective conduction of the electrical impulses through the AV node or the bundle branches or both. It is characterized by regularly or irregularly absent QRS complexes (producing, commonly, an AV conduction ratio of 2:1 or greater) with or without a bundle branch block.

Segment. A section of the ECG between two waves, e.g., P-R segment and S-T segment.

Septum. A wall separating two cavities.

Shock. A state of cardiovascular collapse caused by numerous factors such as severe AMI, hemorrhage, anaphylactic reaction, severe trauma, pain, strong emotions, drug toxicity, or other causes. A patient in decompensated shock typically has dulled senses and staring eyes, a pale and cyanotic color, cold and clammy skin, systolic blood pressure of 80 to 90 mm Hg or less, a feeble rapid pulse (over 110 beats per minute), and a urinary output of less than 20 milliliters per hour.

Short vertical lines. The vertical lines inscribed at every three-second interval along the top of the ECG paper.

Sinoatrial (SA) node. See SA node.

Sinoatrial (SA) exit block. An arrhythmia caused by a block in the conduction of the electrical impulse from the SA node to the atria, resulting in bradycardia, episodes of asystole, or both.

Sinus arrest. An arrhythmia caused by a decrease in the automaticity of the SA node resulting in bradycardia, episodes of asystole, or both.

Sinus arrhythmia. Irregularity of the heart rate caused by fluctuations of parasympathetic activity on the SA node during breathing.

Sinus bradycardia. An arrhythmia originating in the SA node with a rate of less than 60 beats per minute.

Sinus tachycardia. An arrhythmia originating in the SA node with a rate of over 100 beats per minute.

Six-second count method. A method of determining the heart rate by counting the number of QRS complexes within a six-second interval and multiplying this number by 10 to get the heart rate per minute.

Six-second intervals. The period of time between every third three-second interval mark.

Slow calcium channels. A mechanism in the membrane of certain cardiac cells, predominantly those of the SA and AV nodes, by which calcium ions enter the cells slowly during depolarization, changing the potential within these cells from negative to positive.

Slurring of the QRS complex. The delta wave.

Small squares. The areas on ECG paper enclosed by the light horizontal and vertical lines of the grid.

Sodium bicarbonate. Chemical substance with alkaline properties used to increase the pH or alkalinity of the body when acidosis is present; considered in the treatment of electromechanical dissociation (EMD), ventricular asystole, ventricular fibrillation, and ventricular tachycardia.

Spikes. Artifacts in the ECG. If numerous and occurring randomly, they are most likely caused by muscle tremor, AC interference, loose electrodes, or biotelemetry-related interference. If they are regular, occurring at a rate of about 60 to 80, they are most likely caused by an artificial pacemaker.

Spontaneous depolarization. Property possessed by pacemaker cells allowing them to achieve threshold potential and depolarize without external stimulation.

S prime (S′). The second S wave in the QRS complex.

Standardization of the ECG tracing. A means of standardizing the amplitude of the waves and complexes of the ECG using a one millivolt/10 mm standardization impulse.

Standard limb leads. Leads I, II, and III.

Standard paper speed. A rate of 25 mm per second.

S-T segment. The section of the ECG between the end of the QRS complex and onset of the T wave.

S-T,T wave. The section of the ECG between the end of the QRS complex and the end of the T wave that includes the S-T segment and T wave.

Substernal. Under the sternum (retrosternal).

Sudden death. Sudden and unexpected death usually from coronary artery disease in patients with relatively minor or vague premonitory symptoms, who appear well and are not expected to die.

Superior vena cava. One of the largest veins in the body that empty venous blood into the right atrium.

Supernormal period of ventricular repolarization. The last phase of repolarization during which the cell can be stimulated to depolarize by an electrical stimulus smaller than usual, i.e., a subthreshold stimulus.

Supraventricular. Refers to the part of the heart above the bundle branches; includes the SA node, atria and AV junction.

Supraventricular arrhythmia. An arrhythmia originating above the bifurcation of the bundle of His.

Supraventricular tachycardia. An arrhythmia originating above the bifurcation of the bundle of His with a rate of over 100 beats per minute.

Sustained ventricular tachycardia. Prolonged ventricular tachycardia.

S wave. The first negative or downward wave of deflection of the QRS complex that is preceded by an R wave.

Sympathetic nervous system. Part of the autonomic nervous system involved in the control of involuntary bodily functions, including the control of cardiac and blood vessel activity. This system stimulates cardiac activity and produces effects opposite to those of the parasympathetic nervous system, which depresses cardiac activity. Some effects of sympathetic stimulation are an increase in heart rate, cardiac output and blood pressure.

Sympathetic tone. Pertains to the degree of sympathetic activity.

Sympathomimetic drugs. Drugs that mimic the effects of stimulation of the sympathetic nervous system, e.g., epinephrine, isoproterenol and norepinephrine.

Synchronized direct-current (DC) countershock. DC countershock synchronized with a QRS complex used in the treatment of atrial fibrillation, atrial flutter, nonparoxysmal atrial tachycardia without block, paroxysmal atrial tachycardia (PAT), paroxysmal junctional tachycardia (PJT), and ventricular tachycardia (with pulse).

Systole (electrical). The period of time from phase 0 to the end of phase 3 of the cardiac action potential.

Systole (mechanical). Period of contraction.

Tachycardia. Considered to be three or more beats occurring at a rate exceeding 100 beats per minute.

Ta wave. Atrial T wave; usually buried in the following QRS complex.

Third-degree AV block. Complete absence of conduction of the electrical impulse from the atria to the ventricles through the AV junction. See AV block, third-degree.

Three-second intervals. The time period between two adjacent three-second interval lines.

Threshold potential. The value of intracellular negativity at which point a cardiac cell can be depolarized after being electrically stimulated.

Torsades de pointes. A form of ventricular tachycardia characterized by QRS complexes that gradually change back and forth from one shape and direction to another over a series of beats.

T-P segment. The section of the ECG between the end of the T wave and the onset of the P wave. Used as the baseline reference for the measurement of the amplitude of the ECG waves and complexes.

Trigeminy. A series of groups of three beats, usually consisting of two normally conducted QRS complexes followed by a premature contraction.

Triggered activity. Spontaneous depolarization of cardiac cells resulting from a spontaneous and rhythmic increase in the level of phase 4 membrane action potential following a normal depolarization; afterdepolarization.

Triplicate method. A method used to determine the heart rate.

T wave. The part of the ECG representing repolarization of the ventricles.

12-lead electrocardiogram. The routine ECG.

Underlying rhythm. The basic rhythm upon which certain arrhythmias are superimposed, e.g., sinus arrest and sinoatrial (SA) exit block, AV blocks, pacemaker rhythm, and premature atrial, junctional, and ventricular contractions.

Unifocal. Pertains to a single ectopic pacemaker site.

Unifocal PVCs. PVCs originating in the same ventricular ectopic pacemaker site.

Unipolar chest leads. ECG Leads V1 to V6.

Unipolar limb leads. ECG Leads AVR, AVL, and AVF.

Unsynchronized, DC countershock. DC countershock not synchronized with the QRS complex used to treat ventricular tachycardia (pulseless), and ventricular tachycardia (with pulse) in a patient hemodynamically unstable.

U wave. The wave superimposed on or following the T wave. Possibly represents the final phase of repolarization of the ventricles.

Vagal maneuvers. Methods to increase the vagal (parasympathetic) tone to convert paroxysmal atrial and junctional tachycardias. See Valsalva maneuver.

Vagal (parasympathetic) tone. See Parasympathetic (vagal) tone.

Vagus. The parasympathetic nerve.

Valsalva maneuver. Forceful act of expiration with the mouth and nose closed producing a bearing down on the abdomen. Used to increase the parasympathetic tone to convert paroxysmal atrial and junctional tachycardias.

Vasoconstriction. Narrowing the diameter of blood vessels.

Vasoconstrictor. A drug, hormone, or substance that constricts the diameter of blood vessels.

Vasodilatation. Widening the diameter of blood vessels.

Vasodilator. A drug, hormone, or substance that dilates or widens the diameter of blood vessels.

Vasopressor. A drug that causes vasoconstriction.

Vasovagal. Pertaining to a vascular and neurogenic cause.

Ventricular arrhythmia. An arrhythmia originating in an ectopic pacemaker in the ventricles.

Ventricular asystole (cardiac standstill). Cessation of ventricular contractions.

Ventricular escape rhythm. An arrhythmia arising in an escape or ectopic pacemaker in the ventricles with a rate of less than 40 beats per minute.

Ventricular fibrillation. An arrhythmia originating in multiple ectopic pacemakers in the ventricles characterized by numerous ventricular fibrillatory waves and no QRS complexes.

Ventricular fibrillation (VF) waves. Bizarre, irregularly shaped, rounded or pointed, and markedly dissimilar waves originating in multiple ectopic pacemakers in the ventricles.

Ventricular fusion beat. See Fusion beat, ventricular.

Ventricular repolarization. The electrical process by which the depolarized ventricles return to their polarized, resting state. Ventricular depolarization is represented by the T wave on the ECG.

Ventricular tachycardia. An arrhythmia originating in an ectopic pacemaker in the ventricles with a rate between 110 and 250 beats per minute.

Ventricular T wave. Represents ventricular repolarization.

Verapamil. An antiarrhythmic used to treat paroxysmal atrial and junctional tachycardias.

Voltage (amplitude). See Amplitude (voltage).

Vulnerable period of ventricular repolarization. The part of the last phase of repolarization during which the ventricles can be stimulated to depolarize prematurely by a greater than normal electrical stimulus. This corresponds to the downslope of the T wave.

Wandering atrial pacemaker (WAP). An arrhythmia originating in pacemakers that shift back and forth between the SA node and an ectopic pacemaker in the atria or AV junction. It is characterized by P waves varying in size, shape, and direction in any given lead.

Watt/seconds. A unit of electrical energy delivered by a source of energy, such as a defibrillator. Joules.

Wenckebach phenomenon. A progressive prolongation of the conduction of electrical impulses through the AV junction until conduction is completely blocked, occurring in cycles.

Wolff-Parkinson-White (WPW) syndrome. See Preexcitation syndrome.

Index